Praise for Co-Occuring Disorders, Second Edition

"I adopted the first edition of this book as soon as it became available six years ago. I use it in more than one of my courses in the three-year co-occurring disorders cohort MSW program. Students find it to be a truly valuable resource."

– Jaak Rakfeldt, PhD, Professor and Coordinator of the Co-Occurring Disorders MSW Cohort Program at Southern Connecticut State University

"I found this book very helpful and clear for my students, who are approaching the material from all different backgrounds. I appreciate the material, which includes common presenting problems, risk issues, treatment planning, and interventions."

– Josh Kirsch, LCSW, Instructor at UC Berkeley Extension and Therapist at Kaiser Permanente

"So much valuable information in a user-friendly manner…"

– Colette Anderson, LCSW, CEO of The Connecticut Women's Consortium

"A clinical road map beginning with an outline of key issues and ending with treatment planning…"

–Eileen M. Russo, MA, LADC

"As a person that has lived with bipolar disorder for many years and has proudly disclosed my personal journey of recovery, I know there are many people who would greatly benefit from the treatments suggested in this powerful book. Co-occurring services are rarely done in such a comprehensive way."

–Karen A. Kangas, EdD

"Dr. Atkins provides a thorough analysis in which he presents the information in a clear and well-organized manner. Throughout the entire book, his tone is compassionate, respectful, and gives an inspiring message of hope. This book is a sound guide for both experienced clinicians, as well as students."

– **Gabriela Krainer, LCSW, LADC**, Substance Abuse Program Director and Team Lead at Family & Children's Aid

"Dr. Atkins has provided the treatment community with an invaluable resource for understanding the nuances of co-occurring disorders. This clear and concise book makes the theoretical underpinnings of the evidence-based treatment of complex disorders accessible to non-medical providers and gives students a strong foundation. Weaving case examples throughout the text, Dr. Atkins provides relatable scenarios that will help the reader see how to move from theory to practice. Above all, Dr. Atkins instills in the reader an appreciation for the humanity of clients struggling with co-occurring disorders and the hope that recovery is possible."

– **Lauren Doninger, EdD, LADC, LPC**

CO-OCCURRING
DISORDERS

Second Edition

A Whole-Person Approach to
the Assessment & Treatment of
Substance Use and Mental Disorders

Charles Atkins, MD

Published by
PESI Publishing
3839 White Ave
Eau Claire, WI 54703

Cover: Amy Rubenzer
Editing: Jenessa Jackson, PhD
Layout: Bookmasters & Amy Rubenzer

ISBN: 9781683733829

Printed in the United States of America.

Neither the publisher or the author is engaged in rendering professional advice or services to the individual reader. The ideas, procedures, and suggestions contained in this book are not intended as a substitute for consulting with your physician. All matters regarding your health require medical supervision. Neither the author nor the publisher shall be liable or responsible for any loss or damage allegedly arising from any information or suggestion in this book.

Library of Congress Cataloging-in-Publication Data

Names: Atkins, Charles, author.
Title: Co-occurring disorders : a whole-person approach to the assessment and treatment of substance use and mental disorders / Charles Atkins.
Description: 2nd edition. | Eau Claire : PESI Publishing, 2021. | Includes bibliographical references and index.
Identifiers: LCCN 2021015585 (print) | LCCN 2021015586 (ebook) | ISBN 9781683733829 (paperback) | ISBN 9781683733843 (epub)
Subjects: LCSH: Substance abuse--Patients--Rehabilitation. | Mentally ill--Rehabilitation. | Dual diagnosis.
Classification: LCC RC564 .A88 2021 (print) | LCC RC564 (ebook) | DDC 362.29--dc23
LC record available at https://lccn.loc.gov/2021015585
LC ebook record available at https://lccn.loc.gov/2021015586

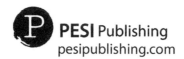

PESI Publishing
pesipublishing.com

Books by Charles Atkins

Nonfiction:

Co-Occurring Disorders:
Integrated Assessment and Treatment of Substance Use and Mental Disorders
Opioid Use Disorder: A Holistic Guide to Assessment, Treatment & Recovery
The Bipolar Disorder Answer Book
The Alzheimer's Answer Book

Fiction:

Best Place to Die
Elixir
Vultures at Twilight
Mother's Milk
Ashes Ashes
The Prodigy
Go to Hell
Cadaver's Ball
Risk Factor
The Portrait

Fiction as Caleb James:
Dark Blood
Hound
Exile
Haffling

About the Author

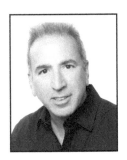

Charles Atkins, MD, is a board-certified psychiatrist, national speaker, and author of fiction and nonfiction books. His short stories and articles have appeared in publications from the *Journal of the American Medical Association* (JAMA) to *Writer's Digest Magazine*. His books on co-occurring substance use and mental disorders, and opioid use disorders, are used in schools and practices nationwide. He has written two plain-speak books on Alzheimer's disease and bipolar disorder, and a special-edition magazine on the science of sleep for PARADE. He writes thrillers, mysteries, and urban fantasy both under his own name and as Caleb James. Dr. Atkins has served as a regional medical director for the Connecticut Department of Mental Health and Addiction Services, and as the chief medical officer for Waterbury Hospital and Community Mental Health Affiliates. He is on the volunteer faculty at Yale School of Medicine and is a member of the Connecticut Commissioners' Alcohol and Drug Policy Council.

To Harvey and Cynthia Atkins

Table of Contents

Acknowledgments

I am grateful to all of those who helped me develop this book. It's a long list and includes my family, friends, colleagues at PESI, the Connecticut Women's Consortium, Community Mental Health Affiliates, Community Health and Wellness Center, West Main Behavioral Health of Waterbury Hospital, and all those who found their way to the first edition and have been so generous with their time and input with this second.

Introduction to the Second Edition

Much has changed in the six years since the first edition of this book. We have seen significant changes in the national dialogue on substance use and, to a lesser extent, mental health. Research into important wellness strategies, such as restorative sleep, mindfulness, and meaningful pursuit, have helped shift the dialogue about what moves us forward in recovery. The opioid epidemic, with its wake of death, has worsened, and the connections between childhood trauma, disease, and early death from all causes have moved into mainstream awareness. New medications and therapies have entered the treatment arena, while others have been deemphasized or proven less effective. There is a greater shift toward health care integration, and our shared experiences with the coronavirus pandemic have underscored the need to rethink, rework, and do what is required. For all the above reasons and many more, it was time to sit down and do a thorough and updated revision.

To begin, more than eight million Americans meet DSM criteria for at least one co-occurring substance use and mental health disorder. It's the CEO of a Fortune 500 company who drinks to dampen her crippling obsessive-compulsive disorder (OCD) and the homeless man with a diagnosis of schizophrenia who drinks, smokes cannabis, and snorts or injects fentanyl-laced heroin and has been in and out of psychiatric hospitals. The spectrum of co-occurring disorders presents us with an almost infinite number of diagnostic combinations. Assessment and treatment must fit the person and their real-life circumstances, priorities, and goals. Strategies to help that man with schizophrenia who has overdosed twice in the past year will miss the mark with the germ-phobic executive who drinks to mute intrusive obsessive thoughts and vice versa.

This co-occurring matrix, because of its complexity and multiple variables, almost defies careful study. On balance, the research shows that integrated treatment (i.e., approaches that address both mental disorders and substance use) leads to better outcomes. But a problem must first be correctly identified before it can be solved. Programs, practitioners, clinics, and others who identify as either substance use or mental health providers, but not both, must expand their ability to screen and refer out for what they don't treat. Better still, and what I encourage throughout this book, they must work with the entire person. Your outcomes, and theirs, will improve.

There is nothing magical about how and why someone develops coexistent substance use and mental health challenges. We are the sum of our experiences, upbringing, genetics, epigenetics, family history, lifestyle, habits, trauma, and temperament. Perhaps they got into trouble with drugs to medicate crippling anxiety and depression. Perhaps they struggled with attention-deficit/hyperactivity disorder (ADHD) and began to misuse their prescribed stimulants (e.g., Ritalin, Adderall, etc.) or discovered cocaine helped them focus. Opioids, with their potent psychological effects, can provide a welcome balm to trauma survivors with that first pill or snort. And the rapid euphoria of alcohol is used by hundreds of millions each day to get high, happy, and numb or to pass out when the racing voices of a bipolar high or intractable anxiety make sleep impossible.

In some instances, drugs and/or alcohol come first, and serious psychiatric symptoms follow. Studies show that, for certain people, drugs are like pressing the "on" button to serious mental illnesses like schizophrenia. We also know that the earlier someone uses mood-altering substances—including alcohol, tobacco, and marijuana—the more likely they are to have a substance use disorder later in life, which in turn increases the risk for one or more psychiatric disorders.

In other cases, a person with no history of mental illness can change dramatically following a trauma—the experience or witnessing of life-threatening circumstances like war, sexual assault, prison, or natural or human-made disasters, such as 9/11. There is no more frightening experience than to have your mind, which you thought was under your control, play horrible and frightening tricks that can include vivid flashbacks, recurrent nightmares, paralyzing fear and anxiety, and the reexperiencing of horrific events.

When we are in physical or emotional pain, we want relief, even if temporary. But for someone with disabling anxiety and panic attacks, the calming effects of alcohol can quickly turn into a daily habit. Likewise, the euphoria of opioids—from pain pills to heroin and now over twenty fentanyl analogs—can quickly change from occasional indulgence to enslaving addiction, where even a few hours without a pill or a hit of dope leads to unbearable symptoms of withdrawal.

I use the metaphor that treatment of and recovery from co-occurring disorders is like firing on all burners to prepare a Thanksgiving meal. Some dishes must be carefully watched or they'll boil over, while others can simmer for hours. And the special needs, dietary restrictions, and religious beliefs of every guest require attention. In this analogy, the front-burner items that must be immediately tended to include active withdrawal syndromes, suicidality, homelessness, serious legal issues, child safety concerns, and dangerous behaviors. Once those are managed, or at least not about to boil over, the focus shifts to less pressing but still serious concerns, such as untreated depression or anxiety.

My goal with this book is to give you both the framework for understanding treatment and recovery and the tools with which to create positive change. It is written for clinicians and educators, as well as for people in recovery and their families and loved ones.

- The first part explores major topics in co-occurring mental illness and substance use. This includes how to conduct a comprehensive and ongoing assessment, clarify diagnoses, and establish and understand the person's goals and level of motivation (both to change the substance use behavior and to work on mental health problems). More importantly, what do they want out of life? These first chapters lay down a step-by-step process to construct problem/need lists, establish goals and priorities, and map out treatment. The wellness chapter sets out important factors that provide the critical foundations of health and wellness, such as sleep, exercise, attention to physical conditions, nutrition, relationships, and a sense of purpose.

- The second portion of this book goes through the major classes of mental disorders. Each of these chapters utilizes case studies to demonstrate the tight connections between mental disorders and substance use, and each includes specific therapeutic approaches, wellness regimens, and medications when indicated.

- The final section covers topics related to specific substances, such as alcohol, opioids, over-the-counter medications, substances obtained through the internet, and so forth. I will review therapies approved by the Food and Drug Administration (FDA) for particular drugs, along with other "off-label" and alternative treatments and the evidence—or lack thereof—to support their efficacy.

- References and resources specific to each chapter are included at the back of the book.

Since the release of the first edition, I've become aware that this book has found its way into many schools of social work, substance abuse counseling, and related fields from coast to coast. As part of my process in this update, I've reached out to several educators to make the material even more classroom friendly. To this end, most of the comprehensive case studies (which are fictional) and related discussions are new, but those from the first edition will be made available to educators via a password and username and can be easily incorporated into homework assignments, quizzes, and class exercises.

This work is challenging and gratifying. People can and do transform their lives. It's wonderful to be a part of that.

GETTING
STARTED

CHAPTER 1

·····················

Co-Occurring Basics:
Overview, Terms, Key Concepts, and a Bit of History

OVERVIEW

It's easy to drown in data. Numbers are important, but they can obscure the faces of people in need. As we discuss coexisting mental health and substance use disorders, I'd like to start with a couple of facts. Most people with mental health problems never come to the attention of mental health professionals. The same is truer for people who meet criteria for a substance use disorder. Those two statements are bolstered by statistics, such as the fact that only one in five people who die by suicide sought professional help beforehand or that deaths from substance-related causes (overdoses and alcohol- and tobacco-related deaths) rank among the top ten causes of death in this country.

How and when do people seek clinical help—and from whom? Usually it's when the issue has exceeded their ability to manage and they recognize that they can't do it alone or with their existing resources of family, friends, or clergy. This may be a self-realization, or it may be brought on by an outside entity, such as a family member, spouse, friend, the court system (mandated treatment), or other motivator, such as an employer or child protective services.

Though it is often not apparent and requires up-front and ongoing assessment, the majority of those who walk through our collective mental health and substance use treatment doors have issues with both mental health and substance-related problems.

Data might be impersonal, but it matters. Why bother fixing a problem if there's no evidence it exists? In the case of co-occurring disorders, we'll start with results of the 2018 National Survey on Drug Use and Health (NSDUH).

What is the National Survey on Drug Use and Health (NSDUH)? Founded in 1971, the NSDUH is the Substance Abuse and Mental Health Services Administration's (SAMHSA) annual survey of noninstitutionalized Americans and covers a broad range of mental health and substance use indicators in fifty states and the District of Columbia for people twelve and older. In 2018, there were 67,791 completed surveys.

Here are some key findings from the 2018 report:

- 47.6 million American adults (eighteen and older) had at least one mental illness in the past year (19.1 percent of the population).
- A major depressive disorder was estimated in one out of seven adolescents (14.4 percent) and 13.8 percent of young adults (ages eighteen to twenty-five).
- Suicidal thoughts and behaviors were estimated in 10.7 million adults (4.3 percent). And 1.4 million made a nonfatal attempt.
- 11.4 million had a serious mental illness (4.6 percent of the population).
- 20.8 million people twelve and older had a substance use disorder.
  - 14.8 million had an alcohol use disorder.
  - 8.1 million had an illicit-drug use disorder.
- **Co-occurring mental health and substance use disorders were estimated in 358,000 adolescents (1.5 percent) and 9.2 million adults (3.7 percent).**
  - Substance use and related disorders are far more common among individuals (both adults and adolescents) with mental health issues.
- 164.8 million people twelve and older were past-month substance users (e.g., tobacco, alcohol, illicit drugs).

- 139.8 million Americans had consumed some alcohol in the past month, while 67.7 million had binged.
- 16.6 million (6.1 percent) people were heavy drinkers.
- 2.3 million adolescents (ages twelve to seventeen) drank in the past month, while 1.2 million binged.
- Illicit drug use was reported by 19.4 percent of those twelve and older.
  - The largest percentage was marijuana use (by 43.5 million people).
  - Prescription pain medication misuse was second highest (at 3.6 percent).
  - Opioid misuse (e.g., heroin, prescription pain pills, fentanyl) was estimated in 10.3 million people—9.9 million with prescription pills and 808,000 with heroin (including illicit fentanyl).
- Tobacco use was estimated in 47 million people twelve and older, with 27.3 million daily smokers. Of note, vaping was not yet incorporated into this survey.
- Substance use initiation (first-time users in 2018):
  - Alcohol—4.9 million
  - Marijuana—3.1 million
  - Prescription pain medications—1.9 million

Notable trends in NSDUH data from recent years include a relative consistency in the numbers for substance use and mental health disorders, with some exceptions:

- A decline in cigarette smoking in all age groups, though vaping and e-cigarettes are not adequately captured in the new data
- An increase in younger adults who meet criteria for serious mental illness
- An upward trend in suicidal thoughts and behaviors in adults and adolescents
- An increase in marijuana use among younger Americans
- An uptick in first-time cocaine use (initiation), especially among those aged eighteen to twenty-five
- A decline in first-time heroin use, combined with an increase in those who meet criteria for an opioid use disorder
- A decline in alcohol use disorders among those eighteen to twenty-five

For clinicians, the question becomes not "Did you use drugs?" but "What drugs did you use and why? Did you use drugs to get high? To be social? Or was it to medicate away painful memories, depression, anxiety, or other symptoms of mental health problems?"

- The scope and magnitude of co-occurring disorders include the following:
- More than nine million Americans have co-occurring disorders.

- Mental illness rates in people seeking substance abuse treatment range from 50 to 75 percent.
- Substance use disorders are present in 50 percent of people seeking mental health services.

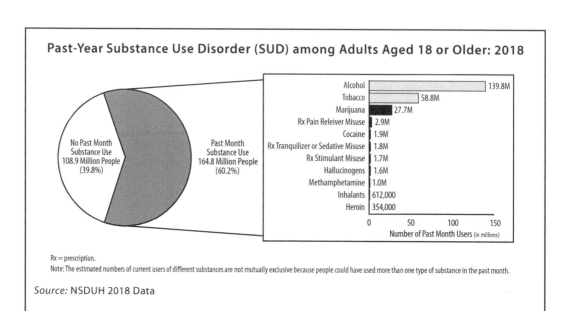

Past-Year Substance Use Disorder (SUD) among Adults Aged 18 or Older: 2018

No Past Month Substance Use 108.9 Million People (39.8%)

Past Month Substance Use 164.8 Million People (60.2%)

Substance	Number of Past Month Users (in millions)
Alcohol	139.8M
Tobacco	58.8M
Marijuana	27.7M
Rx Pain Reliever Misuse	2.9M
Cocaine	1.9M
Rx Tranquilizer or Sedative Misuse	1.8M
Rx Stimulant Misuse	1.7M
Hallucinogens	1.6M
Methamphetamine	1.0M
Inhalants	612,000
Heroin	354,000

Rx = prescription.
Note: The estimated numbers of current users of different substances are not mutually exclusive because people could have used more than one type of substance in the past month.

Source: NSDUH 2018 Data

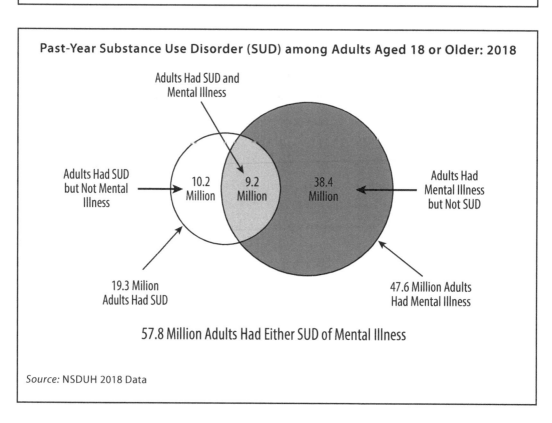

Past-Year Substance Use Disorder (SUD) among Adults Aged 18 or Older: 2018

Adults Had SUD and Mental Illness

Adults Had SUD but Not Mental Illness → 10.2 Million

9.2 Million

38.4 Million ← Adults Had Mental Illness but Not SUD

19.3 Milion Adults Had SUD

47.6 Million Adults Had Mental Illness

57.8 Million Adults Had Either SUD of Mental Illness

Source: NSDUH 2018 Data

- People with co-occurring disorders are far more likely to require hospitalization than people with either just a mental illness or just a substance use disorder.

- Across mental health diagnoses, people who have co-occurring substance use disorders have worse outcomes that include more hospitalizations, lower quality of life, more physical health problems, and more psychiatric diagnoses.

- Higher rates of suicidal thoughts, plans, and attempts are seen in people with co-occurring disorders.

- Rates of illicit substance, tobacco, and alcohol use are higher among people with mental illness.

And when we turn to people with more serious mental health problems, all the above facts and figures pale, and life expectancy is diminished by fifteen to twenty-four years. Those lost years will be echoed when we discuss the impact of severe and persistent trauma and high adverse childhood experiences (ACE) scores.

HISTORICAL PERSPECTIVE

The mid- to late-twentieth century saw a movement away from long-term hospitalization of people with serious mental illnesses, such as schizophrenia, bipolar disorder, and disabling depression. Many of these individuals had spent much of their lives in institutionalized settings. Although efforts at deinstitutionalization were deemed humanitarian and the emphasis was placed on "least restrictive settings," the transition into the community was not smooth.

As large state hospitals emptied and then closed, their prior residents experienced high rates of homelessness, exposure to violence, infections (HIV and hepatitis), legal problems, and substance misuse. At the same time, younger individuals with serious mental illness, for whom these long-term hospitalizations were no longer an option, came to the attention of researchers as they too turned to drugs and alcohol.

In the late 1980s, the terms *dual diagnosis* and *co-occurring* emerged to describe individuals who had both serious mental illness and substance use disorders. It became clear that services for substance use disorders and mental illness were not linked and had separate criteria that created barriers. The norm was for a substance abuse treatment program to exclude people with significant mental illness, and mental health providers were reluctant to work with people who actively used drugs or alcohol. A catch-22 developed where a person who heard voices and drank could not find mental health treatment until they were sober, and clinicians would counsel their clients to conceal their psychiatric symptoms and histories if they wanted to be admitted to a detox or rehab program.

By the 1990s, links between substance use disorders and mental illness became clear, along with associated risks of co-occurring disorders that ranged from increased rates of hospitalization, homelessness, poverty, arrests, violence, traumatization, HIV and hepatitis infection, and functional impairment. The concept of integrated treatment emerged to address this, and early studies and efforts to treat both disorders simultaneously showed improved outcomes with decreased rates of relapse and hospitalization and better quality of life.

In the past three decades, greater attention has surrounded the issues of co-occurring disorders. In 2005, the Center for Substance Abuse Treatment, a part of SAMHSA, released a treatment improvement protocol (TIP 42) that explored the scope of the issue and urged clinicians, programs, and mental health and substance abuse systems to move toward integrated care.

In TIP 42, as well as in other publications since, there is an acknowledgment that any discussion of co-occurring disorders involves a vast matrix of people and diagnoses. What has been carefully studied—mostly among those with more serious mental illnesses and disabilities—is the tip of the iceberg.

For researchers, the task is daunting. Co-occurring disorders, by definition, imply multiple variables. This makes for complex questions, such as whether a medication or therapy works with a certain group of people who have a certain psychiatric diagnosis *and* a particular substance use disorder. Because of this, few careful studies have looked at specific medications and therapies in people with co-occurring disorders. For instance, little is known about the specific benefits of any FDA-approved antipsychotic medication for people who have both schizophrenia and a cocaine or alcohol use disorder or which medication might be the best choice for a person with a panic disorder who also misuses alcohol.

On the plus side, there is more research around psychosocial and psychotherapeutic approaches for people with co-occurring disorders, such as treatments for trauma survivors who also have substance use disorders. So even though research and empirical evidence are important, they often fall short of what clinicians and people with co-occurring disorders need in order to construct effective and realistic recovery and treatment plans.

It all comes down to the individual. What is it they'd like to change? What are their true goals and priorities? What strengths do they bring to the table, and what challenges do they face? What may work for the tax attorney who drinks too much and has a panic disorder may not help the woman who lives in a shelter and has bipolar disorder, hepatitis, and a severe cocaine problem, or the adolescent with ADHD who has just been arrested for bartering his prescribed stimulants to buy fentanyl-laced heroin.

As integrated treatment progresses, the challenge continues to be how to create services and treatments that meet the entire needs of a person. As we look toward best practices and directions for the future, what emerges are models of fully integrated care that move us beyond just mental health and substance use into primary and specialty medical care and wellness.

KEY CONCEPTS AND DEFINITIONS

Recovery

The use of the term *recovery* is rooted in the self-help 12-step movement, such as Alcoholics Anonymous (AA), Narcotics Anonymous (NA), and so on. In the past, recovery was often equated to time abstinent from drugs and/or alcohol: "I've been in recovery for ten years now." In current usage, *recovery* is an overarching term for all behavioral health and substance use goals. Although the following guidelines, which emphasize respect, hope, meaning, and autonomy, seem like common sense, the notion of recovery from mental disorders is relatively new. It replaces prior attitudes that mental disorders, especially serious ones, were chronic conditions for which true recovery was not possible. Embedded in that older belief was a paternalistic approach to the individual: "They're not responsible for their actions, so we need to take care of them." This attitude resulted in a system in which the rights and civil liberties of people with mental disorders were disregarded. Up until the early 1980s, it was standard practice for people with serious mental illness to find themselves involuntarily hospitalized for extended periods of time, with little or no due process. A diagnosis of schizophrenia could result in a person being locked away in a state hospital for months, years, or even decades.

In 2013, SAMHSA published a working definition of recovery, along with four dimensions and ten guiding principles:

- SAMHSA's working definition of recovery: "A process of change through which individuals improve their health and wellness, live a self-directed life, and strive to reach their full potential."
- Four dimensions of recovery:
  1. Health: Attending to physical, mental, and substance use disorders and symptoms
  2. Home: Safe and stable housing
  3. Purpose: A full and meaningful life that includes work, volunteerism, hobbies, family, and the ability to participate fully in society
  4. Community: Nurturing of social connections that provide support, friendship, and love
- Ten guiding principles of recovery:
  1. Recovery emerges from hope.
  2. Recovery is person-driven.
  3. Recovery occurs via many pathways.
  4. Recovery is holistic.
  5. Recovery is supported by peers and allies.
  6. Recovery is supported through relationship and social networks.
  7. Recovery is culturally based and influenced.

8. Recovery is supported by addressing trauma.

9. Recovery involves individual, family, and community strengths and responsibility.

10. Recovery is based on respect.

Co-Occurring Disorders

For the purposes of this book, co-occurring disorders are those that involve one or more non-tobacco/nicotine substance use disorder and one or more mental disorder. Specific disorders are based on criteria in the fifth edition of the *Diagnostic and Statistical Manual of Mental Disorders* (DSM-5), which is the current standard diagnostic system in use in the United States at the time of publication. DSM-5 criteria and diagnoses are closely linked and "harmonized" with those found in the tenth edition of the *International Classification of Diseases* (ICD-10), which is used throughout the world.

"No Wrong Door" Policy

The "no wrong door" policy means that wherever a person presents or when they pursue treatment, the entirety of what they need is addressed. If a program, practice, or agency is unable to meet that person's needs, referrals and linkages are made.

Beyond this initial point, "no wrong door" addresses the importance of integrating all phases of the assessment process and, where possible and practical, treatment. This means that in a predominantly substance abuse–centered program, it's the expected standard of care to screen for mental disorders, and the same holds true for assessing substance misuse in people who present for mental health services.

On a human level, it also acknowledges the courage it takes to reach out. "I'm so glad you came in today. Let's sit down and see how we can help."

Person-Centered

Person-centered treatment can be summed up with a slogan taken from the harm reduction movement: "Meet the person where they're at." Person-centered treatment cues the clinician to focus on the individual, what they want, and what they want to change now (i.e., goals/priorities and level of motivation/stage of change). Embedded within person-centered treatment are the following principles:

- Empowerment for the person seeking treatment/support for self-efficacy
- Treatment goals and intervention are based on a thorough understanding of the person in treatment, not a "cookie-cutter" approach to treatment (What does this person want? What are this person's goals? What are their priorities?)
- A nonjudgmental approach from clinicians
- Validation of all positive change
- Identification of the individual's strengths
- An understanding of the person's entire social, religious, and cultural context

Cultural Responsiveness and Humility

Throughout the assessment and treatment process, attention is paid to the entirety of the person. This includes ethnicity, race, country of origin, primary language, gender, gender identity/expression, faith, spiritual practices, sexual orientation, and identification with specific groups. A culturally responsive clinician is open and willing to learn from clients and, free from stereotypes and assumptions, to listen to and understand their perspectives.

For programs and agencies, achieving and enhancing cultural competence might include trainings and in-services regarding particular groups, the hiring of multicultural and bilingual staff at all levels of the organization (including leadership), access to interpreter services and teletypewriting devices for the deaf (TTD/TTY), the availability of brochures and forms in multiple languages, and attention to the choice of artwork in waiting areas and clinician offices.

Trauma-Informed

People with co-occurring disorders have rates of trauma and posttraumatic stress disorder (PTSD) far higher than that of the general population. Trauma-informed services:

- Actively assess for histories of trauma in all clients
- Avoid traumatization and triggering in the process of therapy
- Provide a safe and healing treatment environment
- Support a person's natural coping skills while helping them develop and enhance their ability to cope and to recover from the effects of trauma
- Support the person's sense of self-efficacy and empowerment
- Consider gender-specific groups (when appropriate), which is strongly recommended in trauma and trauma/substance use disorder group therapies

Gender Identity and Sexual Orientation Sensitivity

Part of the process of recovery involves rigorous honesty with oneself about personal matters, including the disclosure of information to both one's therapist and possibly to other group members. This requires trust and a sense that one has a safe place to bring up issues related to gender identity and sexuality. The following are important things to consider:

- Providers must understand the specific concerns of individuals who are LGBTQ+ (lesbian, gay, bisexual, transgender, or questioning) and how these concerns might be affected in various treatment settings. Being able to disclose—"come out"— about sexual orientation and/or gender identity/expression in any situation is a highly personal and at times stressful decision. Disclosures need to be met in a nonjudgmental and accepting manner. This level of acceptance cannot be assumed, especially in group settings. Just as gender-specific groups can provide a safe and supportive environment, having groups available to LGBTQ+ people can lessen one form of treatment-related anxiety.

- People who identify as being a gender other than that assigned at birth should be addressed with the pronouns of their choice. A good rule of thumb is, if you don't know, ask: "What pronouns would you like me to use to address you?"

- LGBTQ+ people are at an increased risk for traumatization (e.g., bullying, sexual and physical assault, rejection by caregivers).

- LGBTQ+ people, especially youth, carry a higher risk for suicide. This does not appear related to sexual orientation and/or gender identity but to stressors, such as bullying, family rejection, and social stigma and discrimination.

The Quadrants of Care

Co-occurring disorders represent a large and complex matrix. They range from people with mild bouts of anxiety and depression who also meet criteria for alcohol use disorders to people with severe and persistent psychotic symptoms or disabling panic and anxiety who have multiple substance use disorders. Services appropriate for one person won't make sense for another. Because of this vast heterogeneity, it can be helpful to think of the severity of each of the co-occurring disorders.

Developed in the 1990s, the quadrants of care is one way to conceptualize large groups of people with co-occurring disorders, based on the relative severity of their mental health and substance use problems, not their specific diagnoses. The intent was to identify groups of people and the likely levels of care and resources they might require. It was particularly useful when thinking about the creation of mental health systems and the allocation of substance use and mental health resources:

- **Quadrant I:** Mild substance use/mild mental illness
- **Quadrant II:** Mild substance use/severe mental illness
- **Quadrant III:** Severe substance use/mild mental illness
- **Quadrant IV:** Severe substance use/severe mental illness

The following two-by-two grid, where S stands for substance use disorder and M stands for mental disorder, provides some typical resources and levels of care for people in each of the quadrants. A lowercase letter indicates a lesser degree of severity and acuity (i.e., can be addressed as an outpatient, might or might not require medication), and a capital letter refers to a more longstanding and severe problem (i.e., might require inpatient resources, medication, specialized therapies).

Although these broad categories can help, it is important to remember that as people either improve or relapse, they change quadrants. That is, someone with schizophrenia and a severe alcohol use disorder (Quadrant IV) might initially require an inpatient co-occurring admission when they are psychotic and in alcohol withdrawal. After obtaining and maintaining abstinence from alcohol and achieving good symptom

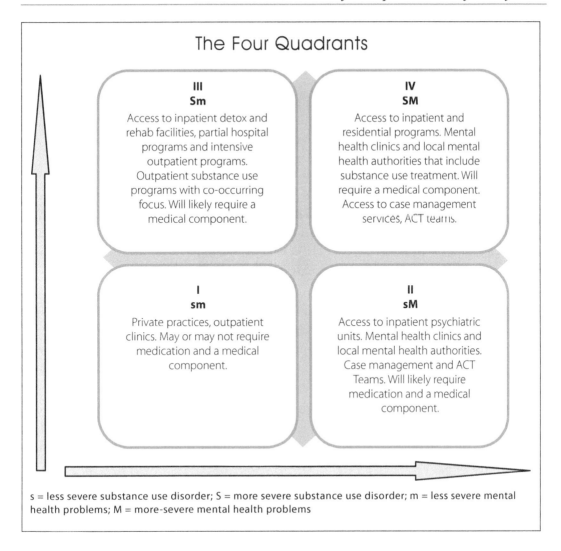

The Four Quadrants

III
Sm

Access to inpatient detox and rehab facilities, partial hospital programs and intensive outpatient programs. Outpatient substance use programs with co-occurring focus. Will likely require a medical component.

IV
SM

Access to inpatient and residential programs. Mental health clinics and local mental health authorities that include substance use treatment. Will require a medical component. Access to case management services, ACT teams.

I
sm

Private practices, outpatient clinics. May or may not require medication and a medical component.

II
sM

Access to inpatient psychiatric units. Mental health clinics and local mental health authorities. Case management and ACT Teams. Will likely require medication and a medical component.

s = less severe substance use disorder; S = more severe substance use disorder; m = less severe mental health problems; M = more-severe mental health problems

control of their psychiatric illness, they might require much less restrictive and intrusive treatment interventions (Quadrant II or possibly Quadrant I).

Evolution and Revision of the Four Quadrants: The four-quadrant system as it was initially configured is not widely used today. However, the underlying principle of characterizing the relative severity of the substance use and mental illness components is important when matching treatment to the person, including the level of care and clinical setting. Additionally, some state mental health and substance abuse systems continue to use the four-quadrant classifications when considering eligibility for resources (such as admission to state hospitals and state-operated substance use programs).

A more recent usage of the four-quadrant approach has been put forward by the National Council for Community Behavioral Health when looking at where to locate or co-locate medical services (primary care) for people with mental and substance use disorders. This has become increasingly relevant with the burgeoning expansion of the patient-centered medical home model and behavioral health home models, where the expectation is that an individual can have all of their health needs, including mental health and substance use, addressed in a single setting or integrated system. In this reworking of the four quadrants, substance use disorders and psychiatric disorders are lumped together and characterized as more severe or less severe, and they are then matched with more or less severe medical disorders and needs:

- **Quadrant I:** This category is for people with lower severity of both behavioral health and primary health care needs. People in this category could likely have their needs met in a typical primary care setting with access to coordinated behavioral health and psychiatric consultation. Behavioral health and substance use screenings would be included in the overall assessment.

- **Quadrant II:** For this population with higher-severity behavioral health and lower-severity primary health care needs, a full spectrum of behavioral health and substance use services needs to be available. One model for service delivery might include an embedded primary care physician and/or primary care nurse practitioner (APRN) in a more predominantly behavioral health clinic or behavioral health person-centered medical home.

- **Quadrant III:** This quadrant includes people with lower-severity behavioral health and substance use problems and higher-severity health issues. This population requires access to coordinated medical services, including access to specialty medical, surgical, and in-home services. Similar to Quadrant I, behavioral health assessment will be included in the overall processes, with the availability of behavioral health consultation, such as meeting with a psychiatrist or psychiatric nurse practitioner.

- **Quadrant IV:** This is for people with both medical needs and higher-severity behavioral health/substance use needs. One model for service delivery would be a person-centered medical home within a behavioral health setting. A full spectrum of both medical and behavioral health services would include access to specialty medical/surgical services.

Stages of Treatment

The stages of treatment derive from the stages of change model (see Chapter 4) developed by DiClemente and Prochaska. The stages of treatment provide a model by which a person becomes involved in and progresses through treatment. Each stage involves a particular goal—such as realizing that drinking has become a problem—that must be met prior to moving on.

Engagement: The engagement phase involves the initial steps in which an individual connects with a therapist or treatment program. Engagement strategies can be generated by the person seeking treatment or by a clinician or agency looking to offer services to an individual in need (i.e., outreach). During engagement the client may or may not be interested in addressing their substance use or other problem behavior. The goal of engagement is for the client to become connected to some form of treatment/therapist. It is crucial to establish a trusting relationship. Engagement strategies can include:

- Calls to 2-1-1 info line
- Searching available services via the internet
- Agency outreach to people with mental illness and substance use disorders to let them know about available services that may include homeless outreach and the use of peer-engagement specialists
- Attending an open 12-step meeting (e.g., AA, NA, SMART Recovery, Dual Diagnosis in Recovery, etc.)
- Signing up for an online self-help service and/or downloading apps

Persuasion: Persuasion is where the person begins to explore goals they might have around their mental health and substance use, and the clinician helps support them in the direction of their goals and aspirations, rather like a sales pitch: "I can see that you're living in a type of hell. What if I told you that this treatment could get you out of there? Would you be interested?" Persuasion strategies include:

- Motivational interviewing (see Chapter 4) to help the person review the pros and cons of various risk behaviors related to their substance use and mental illness, to establish goals, and to support all positive change in the direction of their goals
- Intervention strategies, such as a family coming together to express worry and concern to a specific family member with substance use and mental health problems and to request that they engage in treatment. Alternatively, a family member or concerned significant other could get trained in Community Reinforcement and Family Training for Treatment Retention (CRAFT-T), discussed in Chapter 8, to help connect their loved one to treatment
- Education about recommended therapies
- Generating pros and cons lists around targeted behaviors (e.g., drinking, gambling, internet porn, taking medication, etc.)

Active Treatment: Active treatment includes strategies that help the person move toward their goals. The list of potential treatments, interventions, and wellness strategies is long and can be tailored to the person's interests, resources, goals, and needs. Active treatment can include:

- Group and individual psychotherapies
- Education around substance use and mental disorders
- Medications that target specific disorders and symptoms, such as medications for opioid, alcohol, and tobacco use disorders

- Peer supports
- Self-help groups, such as 12-step programs, SMART Recovery, and others
- Development of positive support systems, including family, friends, and faith communities
- Wellness strategies, such as adequate restorative sleep, daily exercise, healthful nutrition, supportive positive relationships, and meaningful activities, including paid employment, volunteerism, hobbies, music, travel, and pleasurable pursuits
- Treatment of active medical and dental issues and follow-up as needed

Relapse Prevention: In the relapse prevention stage, the client has achieved their stated treatment goals and would like to decrease their risks for relapse. On the mental health side of the co-occurring equation, this includes those strategies, treatments, and possibly medications that help the individual remain in remission. Relapse prevention is the stage of treatment where efforts are directed at ways to maintain and expand upon healthy habits, wellness, recovery, meaning, and personal growth. Relapse prevention strategies might include:

- Ongoing involvement with mutual self-help and taking on commitments, such as leading or even starting a 12-step or other group
- Maintenance of healthy habits and attention to wellness, including:
    - Adequate restorative sleep
    - Daily exercise
    - Sound nutrition
    - Meaningful activities
    - Positive social activities
    - Safe, affordable, and hygienic housing
- Ongoing participation with mental health treatment as needed
- Ongoing attention to medical and dental issues

Sequential, Parallel, and Integrated Treatment

One way to conceptualize a person's overall treatment is with the terms *sequential*, *parallel*, and *integrated*. Even though organizations such as SAMHSA urge providers to fully integrate treatment for co-occurring disorders, it is not always possible, practical, or even desirable to do so. However, with the concepts of sequential, parallel, and integrated treatment, it is possible to address all active problems and needs.

Sequential Treatment and Interventions: These approaches address one of the major issues (substance use or mental illness) at a time. As an overall treatment philosophy, it embodies older approaches to the treatment of co-occurring disorders, where it was felt that the substance use problem needed to be treated before the mental disorder. Historically, this led to a segregation of services (different agencies, different settings) between those that focused on substance use disorders and those that focused on mental disorders.

Nowadays there will be times, often when there is a pressing safety issue, where sequential treatment is both desirable and necessary. Sequential treatment can be provided in separate settings or within a single agency, system, clinic, or private practice. Examples include:

- A woman in alcohol withdrawal who is also depressed. Here the most pressing concern is to first treat her withdrawal and ensure it doesn't progress to delirium tremens, a potentially life-threatening condition.

- Someone who has a moderate or severe opioid use disorder is going in and out of withdrawal and is anxious and depressed. That person would likely benefit from treatment with opioid replacement therapy (buprenorphine, methadone) before mood and anxiety symptoms can be adequately addressed. It's likely that some or even all of the depression and anxiety may be withdrawal symptoms.

- A teen with bipolar disorder who is manic and engaged in high-risk behaviors but who is also smoking cannabis and drinking daily may need an inpatient psychiatric hospitalization to treat the mania before the substance use problems can be addressed. With inpatient treatment, the alcohol and drug use will be curtailed, and hopefully addressed, in the supervised setting.

Parallel Treatment and Interventions: These happen simultaneously, but in different settings and with different providers. Examples include:

- A man with OCD and a moderate alcohol use disorder who is in early remission might engage in cognitive behavioral therapy (CBT) with a private therapist for the OCD, see a psychiatrist or APRN for medication for one or both conditions, and simultaneously attend AA and use online support groups.

- A woman with an opioid use disorder and schizophrenia might attend a methadone or buprenorphine program while obtaining psychiatric services from a local mental health authority, community mental health center, or clinic.

- A woman with PTSD might belong to a trauma survivor's group while concurrently attending a weekly relapse prevention group for her alcohol use disorder.

Integrated Treatment for Co-Occurring Disorders: This approach can be conceptualized along a continuum of "how integrated"? Are all things addressed within a program with a single therapist, or with specific therapies that target both/all problems?

Because of the interrelatedness of substance use and mental disorders, it can at times be useful to conceptualize a person's presenting issues as a single non-DSM diagnosis, such as "bipolar alcohol use disorder," "schizophrenia opioid use disorder," or "obsessive-compulsive alcohol use disorder." Although clearly not how one would document diagnoses, this approach can help clinicians and clients identify how the substance use impacts the mental illness and vice versa.

Additionally, by keeping the focus on all active issues, treatment can be individualized in meaningful ways. Despite the reality of few absolutes in the treatment of co-occurring disorders, it appears to be consistent that improvements in either the substance use or mental health problem typically lead to some progress in the other. Examples of integrated treatments include:

- Manual-driven therapies and adaptations of therapies that target both substance use and mental disorders, such as integrated group therapy (i.e., for bipolar and substance use disorders), dual diagnosis dialectical behavioral therapy (DBT), integrated CBT, and many others

- Co-occurring partial hospital programs (PHP) and intensive outpatient programs (IOP), where groups and other interventions focus on both or all disorders through the course of the treatment day. Often they emphasize one more than the other, depending on the group—for example, a relapse prevention group (substance use emphasis) versus a psychoeducation or managing-illness group (mental disorder emphasis)

- Mutual self-help groups that focus on both substance use and mental health

- Integrated assertive community treatment teams for people with severe and persistent mental health problems

- Case management and other community supports that help individuals with all aspects of their recovery

Integration of Primary Care with Mental Health and Substance Use Services: The Patient-Centered Medical Home Model

While this book focuses on the integration of mental health and substance abuse services, the current movement is toward the integration of all of a person's health care needs. This shift is embodied in the patient-centered medical home (PCMH) model.

The PCMH model, which evolved from a collaboration of the American Academy of Family Physicians, the American College of Physicians, the American Academy of Pediatrics, and the American Osteopathic Association, emphasizes the delivery of high-quality evidence-based care through the use of well-coordinated teams in primary care settings. Core components of the PCMH model include:

- A personal physician, nurse practitioner, or physician assistant with whom the patient can develop a relationship

- A team approach, with a physician leader

- Care management that represents a movement away from episodic and acute care to long-term views of illness management. This approach is especially important when thinking about chronic disorders, whether psychiatric, substance use, or medical. The care manager (typically a nurse, but in some instances a social worker, psychologist, or other health care professional) works directly with the client and is part of the treatment team. Clinical functions of the care manager include:

- o Maintaining a connection and collaborative relationship with the patient
- o Providing education to the patient and the family
- o Monitoring symptoms and communicating them to the person's primary care provider and the team
- o Enhancing and supporting self-efficacy and self-care
- o Problem-solving with the patient to ensure maximization of benefit from the treatment plan
- A whole-person (holistic) approach that includes all stages of life; attention to wellness and prevention strategies; in-home supports; community, family, and peer supports; and an overarching biopsychosocial approach
- Integration of behavioral health and substance use services
- Coordinated care through the medical home that enables the person to access and obtain linkages to necessary specialty services, acute care when needed, labs, procedures, etc.
- Quality and safety with an emphasis on "best practices" and the use of evidence-based medicine
- Enhanced access to care that may include open scheduling (where people are able to present for services without an appointment), clinic hours expanded to accommodate work schedules, on-site childcare, personal assistance in overcoming barriers to treatment (such as transportation), and telehealth options
- Reimbursement to the providers that reflects the added value of the PCMH model

The Behavioral Health Home Model

Similar to the PCMH model discussed above, the behavioral health home (BHH) model is geared toward individuals with higher mental health and/or substance-related needs. The BHH model begins with a premise that people with serious mental health and substance use needs may not be well serviced in traditional primary care settings. BHH-designated agencies may offer all services under one roof (primary care, mental health, substance use) or through formal linkages between providers. Core clinical features of the BHH include:

- **Self-Management Support:** An assessment is conducted regarding an individual's ability to get their clinical needs met and to educate, support, and provide resources to see that this happens.
- **Delivery System Design:** Multidisciplinary teams incorporate care management and a system to prevent people from "falling through the cracks." This often

comes in the form of regular team meetings where individual clients are discussed and barriers, unmet needs, and such can be problem solved.

- **Decision Support:** This is the deliberate focus on best practices and evidence-based/informed treatment options.

- **Clinical Information Systems:** This involves the use of health-outcomes data both to guide the treatment of an individual—such as when to get a colonoscopy—and to look at population data—such as indicators of metabolic syndrome, blood pressure, obesity, type 2 diabetes, and elevated cholesterol—that are a common risk for individuals on certain psychiatric medications.

- **Community Linkages:** This is to encourage and help consumers access available resources that can include peer supports, club houses, exercise, vocational and educational resources, housing assistance, meals on wheels, community pantries, senior centers, and more.

Understanding Behavioral Health Diagnoses and the DSM-5

The current system of diagnoses in the United States is the American Psychiatric Association's DSM-5. This manual contains more than 300 diagnoses and also includes the accompanying ICD-10 codes, which are used by all billing entities (e.g., insurance companies, Centers for Medicare and Medicaid Services [CMS], hospitals, and physicians' offices).

The DSM-5 utilizes clusters of symptoms that involve the patient's mood, perceptions, thought processes (cognitions), and behaviors to define diagnoses. Emotions, behaviors, and/or disturbances of thought are labeled as abnormal and considered a disorder when they cause significant impairment in the person's ability to function in one or more major aspects of their life (work, home, social, recreation) and/or cause significant distress.

To complicate matters, tremendous overlap occurs between many disorders. People can often meet criteria for multiple disorders, and/or their symptoms may not fit neatly into diagnostic categories. In these instances, diagnostic clarifiers, such as "other specified" or "unspecified," may be appropriate.

In the DSM-5, most behavioral health diagnoses are based on a collection of symptoms (anxiety, hearing voices, delusions, memory loss, suicidality, sadness, etc.) versus more objective findings seen in medical diagnoses, such as a tumor, infectious agents (bacteria, viruses) or abnormal physical symptoms (elevated blood pressure), abnormal lab values, and so forth.

This system has both merits and shortcomings, and its reliance on subjective findings reflects how much is still unknown about the human brain, as well as its complexity. But it does provide a common diagnostic language and conceptualization of mental disorders. Clinicians who work in behavioral health, substance use, and co-occurring arenas need to be familiar with the DSM-5, as it reflects a current standard of practice in the United States.

The DSM-5 replaced the DSM-IV-TR in May 2013. Major changes included:

- Elimination of the multiaxial system. All mental health and substance use diagnoses are now listed in the same manner as other medical diagnoses. In practical usage the diagnosis listed first is the one most addressed by the current service.

- Elimination of the Global Assessment of Functioning scale. Clinicians are now encouraged to use other measures of functioning and disability, such as the World Health Organization's Disability Assessment Schedule, version 2.0 (WHODAS 2.0).

- Several new diagnoses in the DSM-5 include disruptive mood dysregulation disorder, hoarding disorder, binge eating disorder, and premenstrual dysphoric disorder.

- Many diagnoses were renamed. For example, substance use and dependence are now "substance use disorders" that are rated on a continuum of mild, moderate, and severe.

- Criteria has been revised for some disorders.

- An increased reliance on specifiers has been incorporated, such as with anxious distress, mixed features, rapid cycling, panic attacks, and so on.

CHAPTER 2

....

The Comprehensive Assessment Part One:
Personal, Psychiatric, Family, and Social Histories, and the Mental Status Examination

OVERVIEW

The next three chapters cover the process of getting to know the person who is accessing, or receiving, services: your patient/client. A thorough assessment includes a tremendous amount of data that starts with the first phone contact or visit and

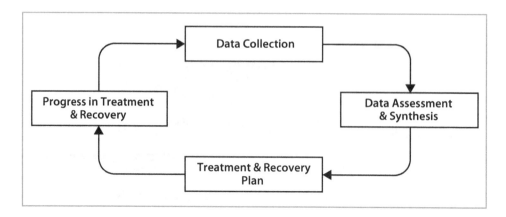

continues throughout treatment. The process of clinical assessment, data collection, and synthesis is continuous and specific to the person in treatment and their goals.

Beyond the generation of hundreds, if not thousands, of bits of information, the assessment process is where someone can tell their story and express how they might like to change it (their goals and priorities). For people with co-occurring disorders, one challenge is how to differentiate between symptoms due to the use of a substance versus what is caused by an underlying psychiatric disorder or even a medical one. It is the metaphor of trying to separate the forest from the trees. It is important to take in all the information and to not jump to conclusions. Are this person's voices a symptom of schizophrenia, the residual effects of phencyclidine (PCP) or synthetic cannabis, a brain tumor, or a belief that they have to appear "crazy" to diminish a possible legal consequence? What role does early trauma play in their current circumstances?

We must consider all possibilities based on the data and the person before us. This starts with the most common causes of a symptom or syndrome and moves to those that are less typical. In medical terms, this process is called *generating a differential*, and it is an important skill to cultivate. For example:

- Is the anxiety from an anxiety disorder, PTSD, or problems at work? Or is it a symptom of withdrawal from certain substances, such opioids, alcohol, benzodiazepines, nicotine, and others? Could it be both? Or something else entirely?

- Is someone manic or intoxicated with alcohol, PCP, stimulants, or a hallucinogen? Is the person both manic and using alcohol to try and calm down or get some sleep? Or is the substance use a symptom of the manic state (increased pleasure-seeking activity)?

- Are an adolescent's intense mood swings and angry outbursts a result of normal adolescence, the start of bipolar disorder, intermittent opioid withdrawal from an addiction to pain medications, or a side effect of stimulants prescribed for ADHD?

Split over three chapters, the comprehensive biopsychosocial assessment includes all aspects of a person's past and present history. Throughout assessment and treatment, the clinician, along with the client, weighs the information and uses it to clarify diagnoses, map out goals and objectives, and select interventions that make sense.

These chapters contain a series of handouts that can be completed by the person in treatment, completed collaboratively (i.e., the clinician and patient work on them together), or used as the basis for a structured interview (i.e., one where particular areas of information are addressed in a logical sequence). Taken together, these chapters comprise a comprehensive and integrated assessment of all areas of the person's life. Tools of this nature are typical in agencies accredited by the Joint Commission, as well as the Commission on Accreditation of Rehabilitation Facilities (CARF), and are the standard for facilities and practices that bill organizations such as CMS and most insurance companies and HMOs.

Personal/Identifying Information

Personal and identifying information includes the client's age, race, marital status, and other pieces of data the clinician has noted, such as the number of children, current living situation, and occupation. When presenting cases between clinicians, the identifying information is the opening line, for example: "This is a twenty-four-year-old never-married Caucasian father of two who presents with…"

Chief Complaint/Presenting Problem

The chief complaint contains the stated reason why this person is seeking treatment today:

- "I want to get clean."
- "I'm hearing voices that tell me to hurt myself."
- "My anxiety is through the roof."

Typically, although not always, the chief complaint is left in the person's own words. In some instances, the necessities of billing will require that the chief complaint also include more clinical language that will meet the payer's (e.g., insurance company, Medicare, Medicaid) medical-necessity criteria:

- John presents with an escalation in his alcohol consumption. "I've got to stop drinking. It's killing me."
- Client presents with a chief complaint of suicidal thoughts with command auditory hallucinations. "I hear a voice that tells me to jump in front of traffic."
- Client presents with disabling anxiety and agoraphobia. "My anxiety is through the roof. I'm too frightened to leave the house."

In case presentations, the chief complaint is clearly stated within the first or second sentence:

- Mrs. Anderson is a forty-seven-year-old married mother of four and a certified public accountant who seeks treatment for severe depression with anhedonia. "Nothing I do matters anymore. Everything is an effort."
- Karel Fried is a thirty-three-year-old never-married man who lives with his parents, has a history of schizophrenia, and presents to the open-access clinic today with a chief complaint of "I just got out of the hospital, and I need meds."

History of Presenting Problem

This portion of the evaluation allows the patient to tell their story. It's where the clinician gets a sense of how the person pieces together their current situation. How do they think things got to where they are? What are the different factors, both positive and negative, that led to today's visit?

It is common for first visits—regardless of location—to involve some element of a crisis, where active stressors contribute to the current difficulties. Well-written presenting problems begin to address the *who, what, when, where, why,* and *how much* of the current situation. The more specific, the better, and they might incorporate scales and the results of screening tools we'll cover. In the example below, I'll introduce a simple 10-point scale where you ask, "On a scale of 1 to 10, with 10 being the worst depression anyone could have, how would you rate yours now?"

> Case Example: Mrs. Jones states that she's been feeling depressed (8/10) and anxious (7–9/10) for the past three weeks. It started when her hours were reduced at work and she found herself unable to sleep at night, worrying about how she'd meet her mortgage and other financial responsibilities. "I can't get my mind to shut up so I can fall back asleep." She's also concerned about her increased use of alcohol, which has gone from two to four drinks per week, to consuming the better part of a 1.5-liter bottle of wine a night. For the past two weeks, she has drank earlier in the day, and she's noticed that her hands shake in the morning. She reports having a drink prior to today's evaluation to "steady my nerves."

The history of the presenting problem is also an ideal place to cover DSM-5 criteria that will format the diagnoses used later. If a person presents with a complaint of depression, now is a good time to describe any of the nine diagnostic criteria for that diagnosis. Or if someone says they've been "manic" in the past, have them give specifics: how long it lasted, their sleep patterns, their level of energy, and whether there was an increase in goal-directed activities, pressured speech, racing thoughts, and so forth.

PSYCHIATRIC HISTORY

Obtaining a thorough psychiatric history at the start of treatment is crucial. As with the substance use history in the next chapter, it's best to have multiple sources of information (e.g., the patient, past records, family, etc.). You want to know about past treatment, as well as when the person first began to notice a problem with mood, thoughts, and/or behavior. A clinician's access to prior records is often limited at a first meeting. Regardless, a good-faith effort should be made at the start to request records and to get releases of information signed for past treaters. This is part of the current standard of care, and to skimp on this leaves clinicians, agencies, and their clients open to unnecessary risk.

A thorough history helps decrease the likelihood of missed diagnoses and misdiagnoses, such as documentation of a prior manic episode, which is crucial to an accurate diagnosis of bipolar disorder. While this will be discussed later, it's not enough for someone to say, "I've been diagnosed with bipolar" and to carry it forward as a diagnosis, but it should prompt a careful exploration of whether or not that person has had a prior episode of mania or hypomania.

The past psychiatric history provides important information regarding the individual's relative risk of harm to self or others based on past behavior. Have there been hospitalizations for suicidal thoughts or behavior? Have there been episodes of violence toward property or others?

The clinician will learn about the individual's treatment preferences, past trials of medication, and other therapies that might or might not have been useful.

This is also a logical place in the evaluation to determine whether the person has completed a psychiatric advance directive or would like to do so. Psychiatric advance directives are documents the person completes that describe personal preferences for treatment. They are most frequently completed by individuals with a history of serious mental illness who may have had multiple prior treatments, including inpatient admissions. Psychiatric advance directives may include:

- Specifics about the individual's symptoms and diagnoses, as well as what the individual might experience during a crisis
- Who the individual does and does not want contacted and involved with their treatment
- Whether the individual has designated another person to make health care decisions on the individual's behalf, should the individual be unable to do so (often referred to as a "health care proxy")
- Preferred medications (e.g., "This is what works for me. This does not.")
- Preferred facilities
- Strategies that work best for the individual should that person be emotionally or behaviorally out of control

A useful resource that explains psychiatric advance directives, including a state-by-state guide, is the National Resource Center on Psychiatric Advance Directives (NRC-PAD) at www.nrc-pad.org/.

Family Psychiatric History

Most psychiatric and substance use disorders can have a genetic component. If mood disorders (depression, bipolar), anxiety disorders, or psychotic disorders (schizophrenia) run in a person's family, the likelihood of developing a disorder is increased. This risk increases the closer the relative is to the person and if multiple relatives are affected.

Handout 1 can be completed by the patient, completed collaboratively with the patient, and/or used in a structured interview by the clinician.

Psychiatric and Family
Psychiatric History

Please complete all questions thoroughly. If you require further space, feel free to write on the back and/or use additional pages.

1. How old were you when you first had any interaction with a mental health professional?
   a. Why did you see this clinician?

2. When you were a child or teenager, were you ever diagnosed with a mental disorder, including ADHD?
   a. How old were you at the time?
   b. What was the condition or disorder(s)?
   c. Did you take medications for this?

3. Have you ever been in outpatient psychiatric treatment or counseling? (If yes, complete question 4. If no, skip to question 5.)

4. Please list all past outpatient psychiatric or behavioral health or counseling treatments. If you can't remember the specifics, give as much detail as you can.

Who You Saw	Age at the Time	Reason for Going	Was it Helpful?	Type(s) of Treatment. (Individual, Group, or Family Therapy; Medication; Other)

5. Have you ever had psychological testing? If so, when and by whom?
   a. If yes, do you have a copy of the test results?

6. Have you ever been admitted to a psychiatric hospital/ward? (If yes, complete question 7. If no, skip to question 8. Do not include inpatient detoxification and drug rehabilitation stays here.)

7. Psychiatric admissions

Name of Facility	Your Age at the Time (or Dates)	Reason for Admission	Length of Admission	Type(s) of Treatment Received	Was it Helpful?

8. Have you ever been prescribed psychiatric medication(s)? (If no, skip to question 11.)

9. Are you currently on any psychiatric medications? (If yes, please fill out the following table.)

Name of Medication	Dose	Prescriber	Reason You Take It	Is It Helpful?	Do You Have Problems (Side Effects, Adverse Reactions)?

10. Medication history: Please list all psychiatric medications you have taken in the past.

Name of Medication	Your Age (or Dates) When You Were Taking It	Reason(s) It Was Prescribed	Dose(s)	Was It Helpful?	Reason(s) It Was Stopped

11. Who in your family has a psychiatric history or has been diagnosed with a disorder(s)? If you think someone has a psychiatric problem, but it's never been treated or diagnosed, describe what you think the problem is.

Family Member	Diagnosis/Problem	Treatment History (if any)

12. Has anyone in your family ever attempted or committed suicide? (If yes, please give details.)

13. Do you have a completed psychiatric advance directive? (This is a written document that describes your personal preferences for treatment, including who in your life you'd like to be involved in treatment and what works best for you in crisis situations.)

14. Would you like the opportunity to create a psychiatric advance directive?

15. What other information regarding your psychiatric history do you think is important for your clinician to know?

SOCIAL HISTORY

People are formed and shaped by their genetics, how and where they were raised, their religious and cultural beliefs, their sexual orientation, their gender identification, and the sum of their experiences. And like a good story, you want to know how things started, how they progressed, and how they got to the present point.

An individual's upbringing and background provide important clues into that person's current situation, aspirations, and difficulties. Often in the course of obtaining a person's story and family and personal history—how they did in school, what major losses and traumas/adverse events they might have suffered at an early age—one discovers the origins of various mental health and substance use problems. Likewise, family and cultural attitudes and practices can help clinicians understand their patients' frame of reference. For example:

- "Everyone in my family uses drugs and drinks. I thought that was normal."
- "Things went downhill when Dad left. Mom started drinking, and I was just angry all the time."
- "I was fine until everyone in my family dropped dead. I started to get panic attacks, and the only thing that helped was booze."
- "I could never sit still in school. I was always getting into trouble."
- "In my religion, we don't believe in psychiatry."
- "My mom killed herself, and I found the body."

As with the previous handout, Handout 2 can be completed by the person in treatment, completed collaboratively with the patient, or used as the basis for a structured interview.

Personal History

Please complete all questions thoroughly. If you require further space, feel free to write on the back and/or use additional pages.

1. Where were you born and raised?

2. How many times did you move before age eighteen?

3. Describe your parents' relationship.

4. If your parents got divorced or separated, how old were you at the time?
   a. Who did you live with then?

5. Describe your relationship with your mother.

6. Describe your relationship with your father.

7. How many brothers and sisters do/did you have?
   a. Where do you come in the birth order (i.e., oldest, youngest, in the middle)?
   b. Describe your relationship(s) with your siblings.

8. How did you do in school?
   a. Did you get in trouble in school (suspensions, detentions)?
   b. Were you bullied?
   c. How far did you go in school (highest grade completed and degree(s) obtained)?
   d. If you dropped out, why did that happen?
   e. If you attended college or trade school, what was your major?

9. Your sexual orientation is _____.
   (heterosexual/straight, gay, bisexual, other)

10. You identify as what gender? _____.
    (male, female, trans male, trans female, non-binary, other)

11. How old were you when you had your first romantic relationship?
    a. Describe your history of intimate relationships.
    b. Are you currently married?
    c. Have you been married?
    d. How many times have you been married?

TRAUMA HISTORY

Trauma, the experience of being in or witnessing life-threatening or catastrophic situations, can change a person. It is an area of behavioral science in which specific diagnoses, such as PTSD and acute stress reactions, become tied to life events.

It is important to understand a person's experiences of having been victimized, abused, and/or assaulted (physically and/or sexually). Were there other adverse childhood experiences, such as a parent or caregiver who was frequently drunk or high? Did the person go through devastating natural or human-made events, like floods, hurricanes, tornadoes, or fires? Have they witnessed others, especially people to whom they're close, being assaulted or killed? Has someone been involved in gang violence? Has someone been exposed to armed conflict, either as a civilian or as a member of the military?

In addition to a history of past discrete traumatic experiences, such as a sexual assault or history of combat-related duty, it is also important to assess for a history of recurrent and ongoing trauma (sociocultural trauma). This type of trauma might include being bullied at school or the workplace, being subjected to expressed racism or homophobia, or living in a setting that includes an ongoing threat of violence or terrorism. For some, conditions of poverty, malnourishment, and unstable/unsafe housing may also overwhelm their ability to cope.

Our responses to traumatic events can vary from intense fear, helplessness, anxiety, and depression to uncontrollable surges of anger and rage, often with increased reliance on alcohol and substance abuse. Other defenses that help people cope can include emotional numbness and a sense of walling out the memories of the event(s). Because of this tendency, the clinician needs to exercise great sensitivity so as not to unnecessarily open emotional wounds, especially in the early phases of treatment.

Screening questions, including how the client responds to these questions, will lay the groundwork for how this material is explored and treated. If the person describes a significant history of trauma, it is reasonable to also have them complete a more thorough assessment tool, such as the PTSD Checklist for DSM-5 (PCL-5). To specifically assess for adverse childhood experiences, or ACES, many agencies and practices use the "Know Your Aces Score" 10-item questionnaire.

Trauma Screening Questions

1. As a child, did you experience anything you would consider emotional abuse or neglect?
2. As a child, did you experience any physical abuse?
   a. Bullying at school or home (by others, siblings, relatives)?
3. As a child or adult, have you ever been physically assaulted?
4. As a child or adult, have you ever been in situations where you were coerced or forced into any kind of sexual act?
5. As a child or adult, have you directly (not through the media) witnessed or been involved in a natural or human-made disaster (fire, tornado, life-threatening flood, etc.)?

6. Have you been in a war zone, either as a combatant or civilian?
7. As a child or adult, have you ever felt overwhelmed by other life experiences, such as living in poverty, having inadequate food, or living in unsafe/unstable conditions?
8. Do you currently experience any symptoms that you believe are a result of the trauma you experienced?
    a. Nightmares?
    b. Panic attacks?
    c. Behavioral outbursts (rage attacks)?
    d. Flashbacks?
    e. Situations (people, places, things) you avoid for fear they will trigger symptoms?
    f. Physical or medical problems or symptoms that stem from the trauma?
    g. Other

LEGAL HISTORY

Substance use disorders and some mental disorders are associated with high rates of arrests and legal problems. It is an unfortunate truth that more than two million people with serious mental illness are currently incarcerated in this country. Prior arrests, periods of incarceration, and felony records can have a direct bearing on the person's treatment, as well as represent potential barriers to their life goals. For example, once someone has a felony record, their ability to apply for certain jobs and live in various housing settings may be hampered. Incarceration is associated with high rates of stress-related mental disorders, such as PTSD, and fatal overdoses are common in the weeks and months after release from a correctional facility.

Getting an accurate legal history often involves the use of multiple informants (i.e., sources of information) because individuals may be reluctant to divulge prior and current legal problems. Many states maintain searchable databases for prior offenses and pending charges, as well as lists of registered sex offenders. Unlike protected medical-health data, an adult's history of arrests and incarcerations is in the public record. If someone has a probation or parole officer, then the clinician will need to get written permission at the start of treatment to be able to communicate with that individual.

At times, a person's legal status may be why they have presented to treatment. This can range from court-mandated treatment to the advice of an attorney in the setting of pending legal problems, such as a driving-under-the-influence (DUI/DWI) arrest. It is important to know this from the outset and to not assume that someone will disclose the information. At a minimum you would like to know:

1. Do you have any current legal problems or involvement?
2. Have you ever had a DUI/DWI? If yes, ask how many, and get the details. Was time served? If a DUI/DWI case is pending, get the specifics and what the expected legal outcomes might be—suspension of license, jail time, mandated treatment?

3. Have you ever been arrested?

4. How many times have you been arrested?

5. What were you charged with?
    a. Do you have any felonies on your record? (If yes, get the details. It's important to know when the last one was and if the person is attempting to have their record expunged.)
    b. Have you ever been charged with a sex crime? (If yes, get the details, and ascertain whether the person is currently on a list of registered sex offenders.)

6. Have you ever been incarcerated?

7. How many times have you been incarcerated?
    a. How long were you incarcerated?
    b. Were you in the general population or a specialized (behavioral health) unit?
    c. How much of your original sentence did you serve?

8. Are you currently on probation or parole?
    a. Who is your probation or parole officer?
    b. Are you willing to sign a release of information so we can communicate with your probation or parole officer?

It's important to note that rates of substance use are high among people with criminal records. Those who have histories of opioid use disorders are the single-highest risk group for fatal overdose in the days and weeks after they are released from prisons and jails. The causes are multiple: loss of tolerance to opioids, profound psychosocial stress, return to environments that support drug use, comorbid depression, PTSD and anxiety, and a relative lack of adequate treatment while incarcerated. Agencies or individuals working with people as they are released from corrections need to provide ready access to medication for opioid use disorders or have linkages that can offer rapid intake.

THE MENTAL STATUS EVALUATION

The mental status evaluation is a systematic review of a person's thought processes, observable behaviors, and emotional state. It consists of standard elements, but they need not be obtained in a specific order. The evaluation has formal components but also includes information obtained throughout. It starts when you first see the person in your waiting room.

All significant findings in the mental status exam should be noted and explored. Here you will observe and record strengths and areas where the person may struggle. In the assessment phase, it is best to keep an open mind about the cause(s) of any symptom. For instance, if the person seems well composed and articulate but shows problems with tasks that involve memory and concentration, that could be an indicator of dementia (neurocognitive disorder), such as Alzheimer's Disease. It might also be a symptom of an attention problem or part of a hypomanic state where thoughts move so rapidly the individual struggles to focus and remember what you've just told them. It could also be due to intoxication or a drug withdrawal state, or it could be the anxiety of the assessment itself.

Elements of the Mental Status Exam

1. General appearance: How does the person look and act?
   a. Clothing: Are they dressed appropriately for the weather, time of year, situation, and age? Are their clothes clean and in good repair? How do they choose to present themself? Every article of clothing and jewelry represents a choice they made. A tie-dyed Grateful Dead T-shirt presents a very different image from a suit and tie and will likely have significance to that person.
   b. Hygiene, grooming, and distinguishing features: Is the person groomed? Do you notice tattoos or piercings? Do they appear to have a sense of personal style?
   c. Noticeable movements: Do they have tics or any physical mannerisms that seem excessive or draw your attention?
   d. Does the person have a distinctive smell? Are they malodorous? Do you detect the scent of alcohol or marijuana?
   e. Eye contact: When you greet this person and as you go through the evaluation, do they make a typical amount of eye contact? Do they stare excessively or avoid direct eye contact?

2. Level of alertness: Do they appear awake and well rested? Are they sleepy? Do they nod off? Do they appear intoxicated? Hyper?

3. Level of cooperation: Is the person generally forthcoming with personal information? Do they appear guarded, irritable, or suspicious? (e.g., "Why do you need to know that?")

4. Are they an accurate historian? Does the story they tell line up with what you know about them from other sources (e.g., old records, reports from family, information obtained from prescription monitoring systems, etc.)? Are there significant discrepancies?

5. Mood and affect:
   a. Mood: How does the person describe their current emotional state in response to: "How are you feeling today?" If they describe themself as feeling anxious, depressed, or some other emotion, see if you can get them to quantify the severity. Numeric scales can be useful here: "On a scale of 1 to 10, with 10 being the most severe, describe your current state of sadness, nervousness, anxiety, or anger."
   b. Affect: How do you read/perceive the person's emotional state(s) based on facial expression, tone of voice, and body language? How do they appear to you? Does their expression change fluidly in response to the material discussed?
   c. Does this person's stated mood and your observation of their emotional state match, or is there discordant mood and affect? An example would be when a woman tells you her depression is a 10 out of a possible 10, but she smiles, laughs, and makes jokes throughout the evaluation.

6. Speech, language, and tone of voice: What do you notice about the person's speech?

    a. Is English their first language? (If not, ascertain whether an interpreter is required.)

    b. Is the volume of their speech normal, too loud, or do you have to strain to hear them?

    c. Do they speak so rapidly that you have to interrupt them to ask questions, as is often seen in people who are manic, hypomanic, or under the effects of cocaine, other stimulants, and some hallucinogens?

    d. Do they stutter or slur their words?

    e. Do they struggle to find words?

    f. Is there a normal range of inflection in their speech, or is there a flatness and dullness of tone, as is sometimes seen in psychotic disorders, such as schizophrenia?

    g. Do they sound sluggish or intoxicated?

7. Thought processes: An assessment of thought processes is typically based on the flow of the conversation and speech but can also include the person's self-report on how they experience their thoughts.

    a. Do their thoughts flow one to the next in a logical sequence? Do conversations contain a natural back and forth, or do you struggle to understand what the person has just said? Does one thought seem disconnected from the next, as can occur in psychotic disorders, such as schizophrenia and various intoxication states?

    b. How does the person describe their own thinking? Do they experience their thoughts as racy or too slow? Do they ruminate on topics?

8. Are they able to interpret standard expressions, or do they struggle with metaphorical thought? This is assessed with the use of common sayings, such as "Tell me what it means when I say people in glass houses shouldn't throw stones." A correct answer might be "We all have our faults and shouldn't judge others." An indicator of more concrete thinking would be an answer like "Your windows would break."

9. Thought content: What topics occupy this person's thoughts?

    a. Stressors in their life?

    b. Do they repeat the same material over and over (perseverate or ruminate)?

    c. Do they focus on depressive themes, such as hopelessness, helplessness, and low self-esteem?

    d. Grandiosity: Do they have an inflated sense of their self-worth or abilities?

    e. Suspiciousness: Are they worried that people are out to harm them? This finding can be along a continuum from healthy wariness to unfounded paranoia.

    f. Do they experience delusions or hallucinations? (See item 11)

10. Cognitive style and cognitive distortions: How do they view their world, others, and themself? Do they use specific distortions, such as black-and-white thinking, catastrophizing, overgeneralization, labeling, and so on?

11. Delusions: Does the person experience delusions, which are fixed, false beliefs that, unlike cognitive distortions, leave the realm of reality? Some delusions can seem plausible, but on further investigation, turn out to be false, such as the unshakeable belief that a person's spouse is cheating when they are not. Or they can be markedly

odd and bizarre, such as the belief that someone is Napoleon Bonaparte or is taken by aliens every night to work in a factory making shampoo. Common delusional themes include:

    a. Paranoid and persecutory delusions: The unrealistic belief that others (possibly named individuals but could be unnamed persons or agencies, such as the IRS, the police, or the CIA) are out to harm the person. Such delusions can include the belief that the person is under surveillance or has been harmed or interfered with (physically, sexually, or emotionally) by the feared entity or individual.

    b. Grandiose delusions: These are exaggerated beliefs in a person's abilities, which can extend to the belief that they are a famous person, such as a prophet, messiah, ruler, political leader, or person of great wealth and power.

    c. Thought insertion and mind reading: Here the person believes others are putting thoughts into their head or that they can read other people's minds.

    d. Thoughts of reference: This is where someone perceives special messages where they don't exist. Examples include special messages in newspaper articles or on television or the belief that the serial numbers on dollar bills contain significance to the individual. For example: "The dollar's serial number starts with the letter A, and her name is Angie, and that means she loves me."

    e. Erotomanic delusions: The belief that another person, often a celebrity the individual has never met, is in love with them. These thoughts can progress to stalking behaviors and should be thoroughly explored.

    f. Other delusional themes can include the belief that someone is pregnant when they are not (pseudocyesis), that they have been replaced by aliens, or that their family has been replaced by imposters (Capgras delusion/syndrome).

12. Hallucinations:

    a. Auditory hallucinations: Does the person hear voices?

    b. Visual hallucinations: Do they see visions or things others don't?

    c. Tactile hallucinations: Do they have the experience of bugs crawling on their skin (formication) or other sensations that involve the sense of touch?

    d. Olfactory hallucinations: Do they smell things that aren't there? Do they believe they omit an odor that isn't reality based? Olfactory hallucinations most often involve unpleasant and noxious odors.

13. Orientation to person, place, and time (often noted as "orientation times three"):

    a. Does the person give their correct name?

    b. The correct day, date, and year?

    c. Can they tell you where they are currently? (often assessed by asking the person to tell you the name of the facility or address of where the assessment is taking place)

14. Level of literacy: This factor can be assessed by having the patient read a short paragraph and write out answers to related questions. Similarly, by using any of the handouts and worksheets in this book, you will quickly ascertain whether the person has difficulty with reading, writing, and comprehension.

a. Can the person read and write?

b. Is English their first language?

c. Can they read and write at a level consistent with their age and expected level of development and education?

d. Do they describe specific learning disabilities?

15. Focus and concentration: Are they able to perform tasks that involve concentration?

a. Serial sevens: Ask the person to subtract backward from 100 by 7. Have them do this for at least five sequential calculations: $100 - 7 = 93 - 7 = 86 - 7 = 79 - 7 = 72 - 7 = 65$. Prior to selecting this task, make certain they have an educational background that should allow them to do this.

b. An alternative task of concentration would be to have the person spell the word *world* forward and then backward.

16. Memory:

a. Immediate recall: Can the person repeat back three words immediately after you say them (door, ball, string)?

b. Short-term memory: Does the person report difficulty remembering things that happened in the last couple of minutes? Do they start to do something and completely forget what they were doing? A standard test for this capability would be to have them repeat three words (door, ball, string) and then ask the person to remember the words three to five minutes later.

c. Long-term memory: How well can they remember details of their personal history? Their childhood? Does what they tell you correspond with information you have from other sources? Is their story consistent, or does it change?

d. Do they describe gaps (amnestic periods) in their history?

- "I can't remember anything about my childhood."
- "Everything around the time of my motorcycle accident is a big blur."
- "I know I had electroconvulsive therapy. I just don't remember it."

ASSESSMENT OF DANGEROUSNESS (SUICIDALITY AND/OR HOMICIDALITY)

The National Vital Statistics from the Centers for Disease Control and Prevention (CDC) show that from 1999 through 2017, the age-adjusted suicide rate increased 33 percent, from 10.5 to 14 per 100,000. It is one of the ten leading causes of death in the United States. Globally, suicide accounts for approximately 800,000 deaths a year. And homicide in the United States is a leading cause of death in those under the age of forty-four.

Thoughts of wanting to kill oneself or others are an integral and vital part of the mental status evaluation, both at the initiation of treatment and throughout. These thoughts (ideation) and related behaviors can represent medical/behavioral health emergencies. It is crucial to thoroughly and frankly assess a person's current and past thoughts and actions of self-harm and/or harm to others.

At times, people will experience concurrent thoughts of wanting to kill both themselves and others. The direst outcome is a murder/suicide. High-risk scenarios for both suicide and violence toward others can include:

- Major life losses (e.g., job, marriage, home, health), especially when combined with depression and a sense of hopelessness

- A person with paranoid delusions who believes their spouse or significant other has been unfaithful. In general, paranoid delusions with a specific named individual, agency, or identified perceived aggressor or enemy must be taken seriously and thoroughly assessed.

- Marginalized teens, more commonly boys rather than girls, who fantasize about committing acts of violence and then taking their own lives

- Women with postpartum depression or psychosis must be carefully assessed, not just for suicidal thoughts and intent, but for thoughts of wanting to harm their children and infants.

- While not deemed a mental disorder, certain religious or ideological zealots can view murder or mass murder, combined with their own suicide, as being a sacrifice for a greater good.

If, in the course of the evaluation, you determine that this person is at imminent risk, every state has statutes around involuntary hospitalization (often starting with an emergency room evaluation) for people who are suicidal and/or homicidal. When in doubt, err on the side of safety, even if you're concerned that calling 9-1-1 will damage the therapeutic relationship. Remember, relationships can be repaired, but only if your patient is alive.

While there are no foolproof approaches to preventing suicide or aggressive acts, evidence supports the careful identification of risk factors and their treatment, when possible. One method is to identify specific risks and determine whether they are static (i.e., things that cannot be changed) or dynamic (i.e., things that can change and might become the focus of treatment interventions). This is often combined with an assessment of protective factors (i.e., those things that enhance resiliency and the ability to cope).

Static Risk Factors (Things That Cannot Be Changed)

1. Past behavior is the best predictor of future behavior. If a person has made serious suicide attempts in the past or has a history of violence toward others, this information should be given significant weight. How lethal were any attempts in the past? A person who required medical hospitalization or admission to an intensive care unit (ICU) demonstrates the potential for future lethal attempts. Have they killed or seriously hurt someone before? Did they go to prison for this? What were the circumstances behind their violent act(s)?

    a. Were they intoxicated?

    b. Psychotic?

2. Does the person have a mental disorder or more than one?

3. Is there a family history of completed suicide?

4. Gender: Even though women make more suicide attempts than men, men of all ages have higher rates of completed suicide and typically choose more lethal methods (79 percent of suicides are men). Men also have much higher rates of violence toward others (including homicide) than women.

5. Age: Older white men, especially in the setting of a major loss or illness, have high rates of suicide. More recently, this demographic has shifted down to middle-aged white men.

6. Race: Statistically, white non-Hispanics and American Indians/Alaskan Natives are at greater risk for suicide than nonwhite Hispanics and African Americans. African Americans, especially young men, are at the greatest risk for being victims of homicide.

7. Belonging to the LGBTQ+ community is associated with increased suicide risk.

8. Occupation: Clearly this can be considered both static and dynamic, but certain occupations are associated with higher rates of suicide. These include:

    a. First responders (firefighters, police, paramedics, and EMTs)

    b. Military personnel

    c. People who are incarcerated

    d. People who are homeless

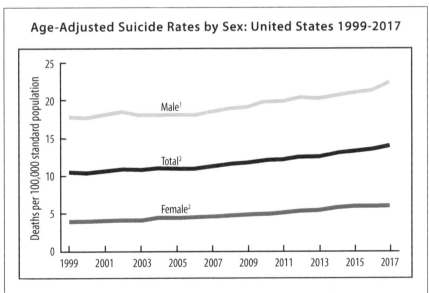

Age-Adjusted Suicide Rates by Sex: United States 1999-2017

[1]Stable trend from 1999 through 2006; significant increasing trend from 2006 through 2017, $p < 0.001$.

[2]Significant increasing trend from 1999 through 2017 with different rates of change over time, $p < 0.001$.

Source: National Center for Health Statistics, National Vital Statistics System

Dynamic Risk Factors (Things That Can Change and May Become a Focus of Treatment)

1. Lethal means: Does the person own a firearm? Guns are the most frequent means of suicide, especially among men (56 percent). Having access to a firearm increases the risk of suicide threefold and of being murdered twofold. Have they been stockpiling medication or accumulating street drugs for a fatal overdose? Poisoning/overdose is the most common form of suicide in women (37.4 percent).

2. Do they currently experience potentially treatable symptoms of mental illness?
   a. Are they depressed? Do they endorse symptoms of hopelessness (can't see a future)? Hopelessness is a significant finding that increases the risk for completed suicide.
   b. Are they manic or hypomanic? Do they have mixed features (symptoms of both mania and depression at the same time)?
   c. Are they delusional? Paranoid? Do they believe they are being threatened or are in danger? If they believe they're being persecuted, is it by a particular person or entity?
   d. Do they hear voices? Do the voices tell them to harm themself or anyone else (command auditory hallucinations)?
   e. Is the person experiencing a worsening of PTSD, OCD, or other mental disorder?

3. Have they recently been diagnosed with a major mental illness? The greatest risk of suicide for a person with schizophrenia occurs in the first year after diagnosis. Ten percent will have a suicide attempt during the first year.

4. Are they currently using drugs and/or alcohol? Rates of both completed suicide and violence toward others rise dramatically when drugs and/or alcohol are involved.

5. Do they have medical problems or a recent medical diagnosis?

6. Does the person have active legal problems? A high-risk period for suicide—especially among young men—is around the time of arrest.

7. Have they had any recent losses?
   a. Financial setbacks, such as the loss of a job or foreclosure on a home?
   b. Death in the family or loss of a close friend?
   c. Death of a significant other?

8. Have they experienced any relationship stressors?
   a. Breakup of a relationship (including divorce)?
   b. Marital or relationship discord?
   c. Custody battles?
   d. Problems on the job, such as conflicts with supervisor or co-workers, or disciplinary actions in the workplace, such as informal and written warnings or suspensions?

9. Planning and preparation: Have they recently purchased a firearm? Have they engaged in other practicing or preparatory behaviors (e.g., tying a noose, going on internet suicide sites, stalking an intended victim)?

Protective Factors

(Things That Help Prevent a Person from Engaging in Suicidal or Homicidal Behaviors)

Note: As with risk factors, some protective factors are static (unchangeable) and some are dynamic (can change).

1. Faith, religious beliefs, and spirituality
    a. "It's against my religion. I don't want to go to hell."
    b. An ability to draw strength from one's faith
2. Family ties and responsibilities
    a. "I couldn't do that to my children."
    b. Family members who display active concern and a willingness to help their distressed family member
3. Fear of the outcome of acting on their urges
    a. "Sure, I'd love to see him drop dead, but I'd never actually go through with it. I'd never survive prison."
4. A belief that the person will get through their current difficulties
    a. "I know I'll get through this."
    b. This is temporary. Suicide is permanent.

The Suicide Ladder

One approach to obtaining the suicide assessment is to start with open-ended questions that become increasingly specific. This is sometimes referred to as a suicide ladder:

1. Have you ever had thoughts of killing yourself?
2. Have you ever tried to kill yourself?
3. Tell me about the time(s) you tried to kill yourself.
    a. When was it? (If there are multiple times, you'll want to know about all of them. Were they in the distant past, within the last three months, or yesterday?)
    b. What led up to it (e.g., breakup, loss of a job, feelings of overwhelming depression and hopelessness, etc.)?
    c. How did you hurt yourself?
    d. Was the intent to die or something else? (Nonsuicidal self-injury, such as cutting, burning, and head banging, is a common feature in personality disorders, such as borderline personality disorder.)
    e. What happened afterward? Did you seek treatment? Did you require medical hospitalization? Psychiatric hospitalization?
    f. Did you sustain any lasting physical damage from the suicide attempt?
4. Do you currently have thoughts of killing or hurting yourself?
5. What way(s) are you thinking of hurting yourself? (Do they have a present plan? Most people who contemplate suicide have an idea of how they'd do it.)
    a. Do you have access to the means to carry out your plan (e.g., firearms, a lethal overdose)?

b. Have you made preparations or practiced the plan? (This can include identifying a beam or tree that could hold their weight if they tried to hang themself, the purchase of a gun, or changes in behavior around firearms they already own, such as taking a gun from the safe and loading it.)

c. Have you made other preparations?
   i. Updated a will?
   ii. Purchased an insurance policy?
   iii. Written a suicide note?
   iv. Given away possessions and/or returned things borrowed from others?

6. What's the likelihood that you'll carry out this plan?
7. What stops you from carrying through with your plan?

If the person is actively psychotic (hallucinating, delusional, and/or displaying grossly disorganized speech and/or behavior), the clinician will also want to assess for the presence and nature of any current delusions or hallucinations:

1. Are you hearing voices?
2. What do the voices say?
3. Do these voices ever tell you to hurt yourself or anyone else?
4. Have you ever done what these voices tell you to do?

The Columbia-Suicide Severity Rating Scale

The Columbia Protocol, also known as the Columbia-Suicide Severity Rating Scale (C-SSRS), developed by Kelly Posner, PhD, is the most widely used and evidence-supported suicide risk assessment tool. It is written in plain language, is easy to use, and is available free of charge from the Columbia Lighthouse Project (formerly the Center for Suicide Risk Assessment). Their website is: https://cssrs.columbia.edu. They offer free training to clinicians and researchers. The C-SSRS has been translated into numerous languages, and these are all available to download. It is listed by the Joint Commission as one of their approved tools to both assess and screen for suicide risk.

The C-SSRS assesses suicidal ideation and behaviors and can be worked into the policies and procedures of an agency or practice. For instance, a positive response on the screening questions would trigger a more thorough investigation of the person's current risk. This in turn will inform recommendations for treatment, which might include emergent assessment.

Assessment of Dangerousness to Others

As with suicidal thoughts and behaviors, a history of violence toward others is important data that can be a predictor of future risk behavior.

1. Have you ever gotten into physical fights?
2. Have you ever injured anyone?
   a. If yes, what did you do?
3. Have you ever been arrested for any kind of assault? (If yes, explore the specifics.)
   a. How badly injured was the other person?
   b. Did they require medical treatment?

      c. What charges were brought?

      d. Was jail time served?

4. Have you ever killed anyone? (If yes, explore the specifics.)

      a. What were the circumstances (military, gang involvement, while committing another crime, etc.)?

      b. Were charges brought?

      c. Was jail time served?

5. Do you currently have any thoughts of hurting another person? (If yes, explore the specifics.)

      a. Do you have a plan?

      b. Do you have the means to carry out this plan?

      c. What's the likelihood that you'll carry out your plan?

6. What stops you from carrying through with your plan?

If the person is actively psychotic (hallucinating, delusional, displaying grossly disorganized speech and/or behavior), the clinician will also want to assess for the presence and nature of current delusions, especially persecutory ones, or hallucinations:

1. Is there someone or something that wishes you harm?
2. How certain of this are you?
3. How often do you think about this?
4. Have you taken steps to protect yourself from this person(s) or thing(s)?
5. Are you currently hearing voices?
6. What do the voices say?
7. Do these voices ever tell you to hurt yourself or anyone else?
8. Have you ever done what these voices tell you to do?

ASSESSMENT OF STRENGTHS AND RESILIENCIES

Throughout the evaluation and ongoing treatment, you assess your client's abilities. What things does this person do well? What strengths do you identify, and what strengths/positive attributes can they see in themself? The ongoing assessment of strengths is useful for several reasons. It provides realistic points to validate your client when they struggle with negative thoughts about themself: "You may be having a hard time now, but no one can take away the fact that you went eight years without a drink."

A person's self-identified strengths let you know something about how they view themself and about the person they'd like to be. Strengths can also be called upon to help move the person toward stated goals: "You mentioned that your faith is especially important to you. Have you considered taking on some volunteer work at your church, especially on the weekend, when you struggle to not drink?"

From another perspective, a person's strengths frequently overlap with known resilience factors. These are discussed further in the chapter on wellness, but they include faith, humor, connections to others and positive relationships, a sense of meaning and purpose to one's life, and attention to the maintenance of physical, emotional, and spiritual balance. Areas to explore with regard to strengths include:

1. Relationships: Are they able to maintain close and loving relationships?
2. Do they have a strong social support network (family, friends, coworkers, faith community)?
3. Are they socially skillful?
4. Do they attend to adequate sleep and nutrition?
5. Do they get regular exercise?
6. Do they demonstrate an ability to get their needs met? How well do they navigate systems?
7. Assertiveness: Are they able to ask for what they want and effectively say no to unreasonable requests?
8. How well do they handle disappointment and frustration?
9. How motivated are they to work on their substance use and mental health problems?
    a. Have they had significant prior successes in treatment?
10. Ability to complete tasks and goals: What things do they do well and take pride and ownership in?
    a. Do they possess special skills and talents?
    b. Do they excel in school or the workplace?
    c. Are they athletic?
    d. Are they an involved parent?
11. What strategies have they used in the past to achieve success? This might include past periods of sustained abstinence or extended periods without emotional/ behavioral problems.
12. Do they have a strong work history and work ethic?

CHAPTER 3

The Comprehensive Assessment Part Two:
Substance Use, Medical Histories, and Collateral Sources of Information

OVERVIEW

It's no surprise that people with co-occurring disorders often receive wrong diagnoses. Withdrawal from alcohol or opioids or a crash from a cocaine binge can be confused with severe depression or anxiety. And things become murky when details of substance use, medical issues, or mental health problems go unreported, as they often do.

There is great potential for harm related to missed and wrong diagnoses. An unrecognized withdrawal from alcohol or Valium-type drugs (benzodiazepines) can lead to dangerous—even fatal—withdrawal syndromes. To treat the depressed half of bipolar disorder with antidepressants can precipitate mania and worsen irritability and agitation, which in turn can intensify a substance use problem(s): "I needed the booze to shut down my racing thoughts."

Accurate diagnostic assessments can be hindered by a person's minimization, lack of recognition, or concealment of substance use and/or mental health issues:

- "I just drink socially."
- "Cocaine's not a problem."
- "The pills are prescribed. I have pain. I'm not an addict."
- "I don't take Xanax all the time, just when I need it."
- "I don't have schizophrenia. That's for crazy people. I'm not crazy."

To tease apart a person's substance use and mental health diagnoses, we must take a careful history and look for objective data. We need to identify individual symptoms and put them together with the entirety of who the person is, where they come from, their genetics, epigenetics (i.e., those things that cause particular genes to be expressed or not), experience, culture, age, gender, gender identity, beliefs, spirituality, goals, and aspirations.

THE SUBSTANCE USE HISTORY

When did use of any substance—inclusive of alcohol, cannabis, and tobacco—first occur? How has it progressed? When did the person first identify it as a problem? Or perhaps they don't view their use as problematic.

For those who work in Joint Commission and CARF–accredited clinics and facilities, the patient history will be part of an intake assessment that maps out each substance used, the duration of the use, and the quantity consumed. It will include questions about legal, occupational, medical, and/or social consequences from the use, such as arrests for possession or DUIs/DWIs, work-related problems, negative health consequences, and damage to or loss of major relationships.

It is important to gather information about all aspects of substance use. Why does someone use cocaine versus marijuana or alcohol? Understanding a person's drug(s) of choice gives clues to other domains of their life and to the presence of co-occurring mental health problems. Is the primary goal in taking the substance to get high? To be social? Or is the goal to alleviate emotional or behavioral symptoms, such as depression, loneliness, boredom, or anxiety?

- "Pot's the only thing that makes me calm."
- "I know it sounds strange, but cocaine lets me focus."
- "If I don't drink, I don't sleep."
- "I like the buzz."
- "I can't stand parties, but if I throw a few back, I can have a good time."

It is interesting to note that, on average, women use substances to medicate away painful emotions, while men are more likely to use drugs and/or alcohol to get high.

The assessment process, which is ongoing, is similar to an investigative reporter trying to get the full and balanced story. This process uses the core questions behind any good mystery: who, what, when, where, why, and how.

The DSM-5 provides a checklist of ten to twelve common symptoms for each potential substance use disorder. The terms *abuse* and *dependence* have been eliminated and replaced by the severity modifiers of mild, moderate, or severe. The severity is assigned based on the number of symptoms present, as well as on clinical judgment. The "mild" diagnosis replaces the older DSM-IV-TR substance abuse diagnosis, and "moderate" and "severe" correspond to the older substance dependence diagnosis. Other notable changes in the DSM-5 include the elimination of recurrent legal problems as a criterion, the inclusion of cravings and strong urges to use, and an increase in the number of criteria required to make the lower level (mild) diagnosis (which was raised from one to two). Although the DSM-5 criteria are specific for each substance, the general approach is as follows:

Over a twelve-month period, a pattern of substance use leads to significant distress and/or impairment—this could be at work, at home, or in relationships and can involve neglecting important obligations, etc.—accompanied by two or more of the following:

1. Increased consumption of the substance over time

2. A desire to quit or cut down and/or unsuccessful attempts to do so

3. Considerable time spent trying to obtain the substance and/or recover from its effects

4. Cravings and urges to use the substance

5. Continued use of the substance results in failure to meet obligations at home, at work, or in other settings

6. Continued use of the substance results in social or relationship problems

7. Important activities—social, work, family—are given up as a result of the substance

8. Substance use in dangerous situations, such as driving while intoxicated

9. Continued use despite the realization that the substance causes health and/or emotional problems

10. Tolerance to the substance: Needing to take larger amounts to get the same effect or possibly no longer being able to achieve the same effect

11. Withdrawal symptoms: Specific to the substance in question, ranging from potentially life-threatening withdrawals, as can be seen with alcohol and Valium-type drugs (benzodiazepines), to more mild syndromes as seen with caffeine. This criterion is also met if the person takes the substance to avoid withdrawal symptoms, such as someone who is opioid dependent who may need to dose themself multiple times a day. Or a heavy drinker might need to consume alcohol throughout the day to prevent tremors or more severe withdrawal symptoms.

Exhibiting two to three of the preceding symptoms is considered mild, four to five is considered moderate, and greater than six is considered severe.

Once a problem with a substance has been identified, it is important to get the details. Handout 3, which can be completed with a client as a structured interview or given as a take-home or in-group/in-session assignment, helps flesh out the individual's relationship with their substance(s) of use. It can also be used to clarify the presence of a substance use disorder and its severity. Handout 3, along with other assessment tools and questionnaires, are discussed in the next section.

ASSESSMENT TOOLS AND QUESTIONNAIRES FOR SUBSTANCE USE

There are many screening and assessment questionnaires and tools that are helpful for assessing the presence and severity of substance use disorders.

The CAGE-AID Questionnaire

Perhaps the simplest is the widely used four-item CAGE Adapted to Include Drugs (AID) questionnaire for detecting alcohol and substance use problems. CAGE is an acronym, with each letter corresponding to one of the four questions.

The CAGE-AID Questionnaire

Instructions: Two or more yes answers indicate the possibility of a drug or alcohol problem and should be investigated further.

1. Have you ever felt you needed to **Cut** down on your drinking or drug use?

2. Have people **Annoyed** you by criticizing your drinking or drug use?

3. Have you ever felt **Guilty** about drinking or drug use?

4. Have you ever felt you needed a drink or used drugs first thing in the morning (**Eye-opener**) to steady your nerves or to get rid of a hangover?

Scoring the CAGE-AID is simple: Two or more positive answers correspond with a likely problem and the need for further evaluation. The fourth question—the eye-opener—speaks to the presence of physical dependence on a substance. The eye-opener question addresses many substances that cause physical dependence and withdrawal, such as alcohol, opioids (e.g., heroin, fentanyl, methadone, buprenorphine, pain pills, etc.) and benzodiazepines (e.g., Valium, Xanax, Librium, Ativan, etc.).

The Addictions Severity Index

The Addictions Severity Index (ASI), developed by Thomas McLellan, is a semi-structured interview that takes approximately one hour to complete. This is typically done at the start of treatment, such as admission to a rehabilitation facility or admission to an IOP. It focuses both on the historical use of substances over the person's life, as well as in the past thirty days. The final score is rated on a scale of 0–10, with 0 being no problem with no need for treatment and 10 being an extreme problem with treatment necessary. The ASI has been used as both an assessment and outcome measure in numerous studies.

The Alcohol Use Disorders Identification Test

Specific to alcohol, the Alcohol Use Disorders Identification Test (AUDIT) is a research-validated, ten-item questionnaire designed for primary care settings, although it is easily incorporated into evaluations in other settings. Copyright for the AUDIT is through the World Health Organization. It may be downloaded and reproduced without cost. Several full-text versions are available online. Links to the AUDIT include:

- pubs.niaaa.nih.gov/publications/Audit.pdf
- whqlibdoc.who.int/hq/2001/WHO_MSD_MSB_01.6a.pdf?ua=1 (This link includes both the screening tool and guidelines for its use and scoring.)
- pubs.niaaa.nih.gov/publications/arh28-2/78-79.htm

FAMILY SUBSTANCE USE HISTORY

Genetics and family history play important roles in the likelihood that someone will develop a substance use problem. Genetics (i.e., others in the family with substance use disorder) account for as much as 50 percent of the likelihood that someone will develop a problem.

Therefore, social and family factors help shape a person's understanding of their substance use. If drinking wine at a meal is the norm, it is good to know this, as it may create issues for a person in recovery from an alcohol use disorder. If the person's mother has/had problems with substance use, was she actively using when she was pregnant with the identified client?

In addition to obtaining the history of the person's family and identifying which members have had substance use problems, it is important to identify who in their life currently uses. Are others in the home drinking or drugging? Is a significant other currently using?

Core Questions on Substance Use and Abuse

Instructions: Please answer the following questions completely. If you require further space, feel free to write on the back and/or use additional pages.

1. What is/are your drug(s) of choice? (Please include all tobacco products, vaped products, alcohol, and cannabis.)

2. How much do you use?

Substance Used	Age of First Use	Amount Used/ Day	Last Used	Number of Days/ Weeks Used	Cost/ Day of Use	Method of Use (Smoked, Injected, Snorted, Drank)

3. What do you experience from each substance?

Substance	Effects

4. Write a brief description of how your use of substances has developed over your lifetime. (Write on the back if necessary.)

5. Has the amount you used changed over time? (Describe how your usage has changed over time.)

6. How do you obtain your alcohol and/or other drugs?

7. How much time do you spend obtaining mind-altering substances?

8. When do you use (times of day)?

9. Who is present when you use?

10. Where do you use?

11. Why do you use?

12. What are the consequences of your use?

    a. Financial

    b. Occupational

    c. Emotional

    d. Health

    e. Social

     f. Legal

     g. Recreational

     h. Other

13. How do you feel about your use?

14. What is the longest period you've gone without using substances?

15. What symptoms of withdrawal—if any—have you experienced when going without substances?

16. What is/are your current level(s) of craving for any drug and/or alcohol? (Use a 10-point scale, with 10 being the highest craving.)

17. What makes your craving increase or decrease?

18. Has anyone in your family (currently or in the past) had problems with drugs and/or alcohol?

19. Does anyone in your current household use drugs and/or alcohol?

20. If you have a significant other (husband, wife, partner), do they currently use drugs and/or alcohol?

     a. Has that use been an issue for them in the past?

21. If you have problems with your mood or behavior, including prior psychiatric diagnoses, did your emotional problems come before or after your drug and/or alcohol use?

22. Do you ever use substances to medicate away unwanted feelings or emotions, such as depression, anxiety, or shyness? If yes, please describe.

SEEING BEYOND DENIAL AND LIES: A BEHAVIORAL APPROACH

Honesty may be the best policy, but anyone familiar with the nature of substance use disorders knows that deception, denial, minimization, and lies—both to oneself and to others—are symptomatic of these disorders and not an indictment of the person. From sneaking cigarettes or hiding empty bottles to avoiding arrest when committing illegal acts to obtain the next fix of heroin, fentanyl, pain pills, or methamphetamine, lies and minimization often become part of life.

To complicate matters, an interesting equation around dishonesty and trust presents itself. People have both a natural tendency to believe one another and to get upset when they realize they've been lied to. Lies and secrets can destroy relationships, both in families and in clinical settings. The loss of trust is a source of pain for both the person with the substance use problem and those who care about them. Clinicians face the potential pitfall of labeling the person as a sociopath, incorrigible, or a lost cause.

- "He swore to me he'd stopped, and now I find he's hiding bottles in the woods."
- "I can smell it on her clothes."
- "His PlayStation® is missing. Last time this happened, he pawned it for drugs."
- "He's just here because it's court mandated. He's not really interested in getting sober."

A nonjudgmental attitude that views the words out of a person's mouth as merely one source of information is a useful stance. You want to listen to what the person says but also observe their behaviors and any signs or symptoms of heavy use, withdrawal, or intoxication. I find it useful to view words and actions through a behavioral lens: What are the functions of the denial and the lies? What are the related emotions?

On the surface, these questions might appear obvious, but understanding why someone engages in a behavior like lying to conceal or minimize drug use gives us insight into a person's view of the world, themselves, and others. The purpose (function) of the lie or minimization can provide clues to their level of motivation to do something about their substance use. If someone doesn't see or acknowledge the problem, it's likely that they are precontemplative.

The following table gives some common lies and minimization statements.

The Minimization and/or Lie	Related Emotion(s)	Function(s)
My drinking is not a problem.	Shame: "I don't want anyone to know." Fear: "I can't stop." Anger (irritation): "It's no one's business!"	To maintain the habit. To assure oneself and others that things aren't so bad.
Minimization of the amount of a substance used. • "It was just two beers." • "I'm a social drinker."	Annoyance Shame	To maintain the habit. To conceal the extent of the substance used. To reassure others that this is not a problem.
Hiding signs of drug or alcohol use.	Fear Shame Guilt	To maintain the habit. To avoid negative consequences of the behavior, such as arrest, loss of relationships, loss of job, loss of custodial rights.
Misrepresenting (exaggerating or outright lying about) the amount of a substance used or severity of psychiatric symptoms to gain access to treatment.	Cool detachment Desperation	To receive controlled substances (opioid replacement medication, benzodiazepines, stimulants) for personal use or for possible diversion (i.e., sale or use not intended by the prescriber).

MEDICAL HISTORY

A person's medical history often contains clues to current and past difficulties with substance use and psychiatric disorders. Negative health consequences can and do result from substance use disorders, as well as from the effects of many psychiatric medications. For example:

- Did a football injury, gynecological problem, migraines, or dental work lead to an addiction to painkillers (opioids)?
- Did recurrent childhood illnesses and surgeries lead to PTSD and recurrent depression?
- Did they develop diabetes after being on medication for bipolar disorder or schizophrenia?
- Did they contract hepatitis from intravenous drug use?
- Is this person's tremor related to the use of antipsychotic medication (tardive dyskinesia, drug-induced parkinsonism), alcohol withdrawal, or something else?

At a minimum, the following information should be gathered, either as part of a structured interview or by having the patient/client complete a health screening form. This is similar to information collected in most medical and dental offices and can be completed by a client in the waiting room or prior to the first visit.

HANDOUT 4
Health Screening Form

Name:_____ Date:_____

Date of Birth:_____

Please answer the following questions.

	Yes	No
Do you have a primary care physician, nurse practitioner, or physician assistant? Name of your primary care physician, nurse practitioner, or physician assistant:		
Have you seen your primary care physician or nurse practitioner in the last year?		
Do you have an obstetrician/gynecologist? Name of your obstetrician/gynecologist:		
Have you seen your obstetrician/gynecologist in the last year?		
Do you have a dentist? Name of your dentist:		
Have you seen your dentist in the last year?		

Please provide the names of any other health providers you are currently see.

Name of provider	Reason for seeing them

Please answer the following questions. For yes answers, please specify the nature of the problem.

	Yes	No
Do you have eye or vision problems?		
Have you had a vision exam within the past year?		
Do you have dental problems?		
Do you have nasal (nose) problems or any problems with breathing?		
Do you have problems with your hearing?		
Do you have any skin problems?		

	Yes	No
Do you have high blood pressure?		
Do you have high cholesterol?		
Do you have diabetes?		
Is there a family history of diabetes? (If yes, specify who.)		
Do you have heart disease?		
Is there a family history of heart disease? (If yes, specify who.)		
Do you have lung disease, such as asthma, emphysema, bronchitis, or chronic obstructive pulmonary disease (COPD)?		
Is there a family history of lung disease? (If yes, specify who.)		
Do you have stomach problems, such as constipation or diarrhea?		
Do you have problems with urination?		
Do you have neck or back problems?		
Have you ever had a seizure?		
Have you ever had a head injury?		
Have you ever had a head injury where you lost consciousness?		
Do you have thyroid problems?		
Do you have any gynecological problems?		
Are your periods regular?		
Are you currently pregnant?		
Have you ever had kidney disease?		
Do you have liver disease (cirrhosis)?		
Have you ever had Hepatitis A, B, and/or C? (If yes, specify which.)		
Do you have HIV or AIDS?		
Do you have a history of sexually transmitted diseases?		
Have you ever had tuberculosis?		
Have you been tested for tuberculosis in the past year?		
Other (Please fill in any additional information about your medical history you feel is important.):		

Please answer the following questions.

	Yes	No
Has your weight changed in the past six months? (If yes, complete the following questions.)		
Was the weight change intentional?		
How much weight have you lost or gained in the past six months?		

Medical/Surgical Hospitalizations: Please list all surgical procedures and inpatient medical hospitalizations you have had. If further space is required, write on the back.

Reason for Surgery or Inpatient Hospitalization	Age at the Time
1.	
2.	
3.	
4.	
5.	

Allergies Please list all known allergies to medications and/or other substances.

_____

_____

_____

Current Medications: Please provide a complete list of all your prescribed and over-the-counter medications, including nutritional supplements and herbs you are taking.

Medication	Dose	Times per Day	Reason Taken	Prescriber
1.				
2.				
3.				
4.				
5.				
6.				
7.				

PAIN ASSESSMENT

If your client has physical pain, it needs to be addressed. An assessment of pain should include:

- Location: Where does it hurt?
- Quality of the pain: Is it stabbing, crushing, or pins and needles?
- Duration: Does it come and go, or is it constant?
- Circumstances related to the pain: Do certain things or activities make the pain better or worse?
- Severity of the pain: Ask the individual to rate their pain using a 10-point scale, with 0 being no pain and 10 being the worst pain imaginable.

PHYSICAL EXAMINATION, REVIEW OF SYSTEMS, AND LAB WORK

Physical and laboratory findings can help support or rule out diagnoses, alert medical professionals to health concerns and medication side effects, and provide objective data in multiple domains (from pregnancy to blood sugar levels). Later in this book, specific results will be reviewed in detail for each of the major substances of misuse.

Objective physical and laboratory findings can serve many purposes. They can enhance motivation to curb or stop problem behaviors and substance use: "My doc told me my liver enzymes are high. I've got to ditch the booze." They can uncover active medical issues that need to be addressed (which may or may not be a direct consequence of substance use), ranging from common conditions, such as diabetes, high blood pressure, and thyroid problems, to an unplanned pregnancy. Laboratory and physical results can also help confirm the status of a person's substance use, such as fresh track marks from intravenous drug use or tremors from alcohol or benzodiazepine withdrawal. The medical workup is also an opportunity for people to assess their physical health goals and interact with a primary care specialist who can provide expertise and guidance.

Finally, a medical workup (history, physical, and lab work) is often a prerequisite to medication and is a Joint Commission requirement for certain higher levels of care (e.g., residential, inpatient, partial hospital programs). This allows you to obtain baseline information and helps to decrease the likelihood that the person will experience side effects and/or adverse reactions to medications. A standard medical assessment includes a physical examination and lab work.

Physical Examination with Review of Systems

- Vital signs (temperature, blood pressure, pulse, height, weight)
  - An elevated blood pressure or pulse could be a sign of withdrawal from alcohol or benzodiazepines.

○ Malnourishment can be associated with several drugs of abuse, including advanced alcohol disease and heavy methamphetamine use.

○ Central (i.e., abdominal) obesity is a common finding in people who have been on many psychiatric medications.

- Skin

  ○ Are there signs of intravenous drug use (track marks, scars left by abscesses)?

  ○ Psoriasis can be associated with long-term alcohol use. It can also be a side effect of lithium.

  ○ Sores and lesions from skin picking are common in people with stimulant (amphetamines, methamphetamine) use disorders and in individuals in withdrawal from opioids. Skin picking, or excoriation, can also be found with anxiety disorders, body dysmorphic disorder, and other conditions.

  ○ Old scars may indicate deliberate nonsuicidal self-injury (cutting, burning) or past suicide attempts.

  ○ Heavy smokers may have nicotine stains on their fingers and on facial hair in men.

  ○ Rashes and sores may be signs of allergic reactions to medications. These can range from mild to life-threatening.

- Head, eyes, ears, nose, throat

  ○ The size of the pupils can pinpoint when people are on opioids. (The pupils are wide when individuals are in withdrawal.)

  ○ Condition of the teeth

    - Teeth condition is often poor in people who have neglected their health due to substance use or social deprivation.

    - Erosion of tooth enamel, especially on the front teeth, can be associated with frequent vomiting (binge-purge behavior), as is seen in some with eating disorders (bulimia and certain forms of anorexia).

  ○ Nasal problems can be associated with use of inhaled/snorted drugs.

- Digestive system

  ○ Diarrhea can be a symptom of opioid withdrawal or a side effect of many medications.

  ○ Constipation is a common side effect of many medications, including opioids and some antipsychotics, such as a clozapine. It can become severe and lead to bowel obstruction, perforation, and death.

  ○ Frequent nausea and vomiting are common in advanced alcohol disease and may be a sign of pancreatitis, gallbladder disease, or liver disease. They can be symptoms of withdrawal states and many medical conditions.

  ○ A distended abdomen, with evidence of fluid in the abdominal cavity (ascites) can be a sign of serious liver disease and is often seen in late-stage alcohol disease.

- o Abnormal liver enzymes can indicate multiple conditions, from inflammation of the liver due to alcohol and certain medications to cirrhosis, certain cancers, and viral hepatitis (high rates especially in people who have injected drugs).

- Urinary system

  - o Difficulty urinating can be a sign of intoxication with opioids and some frequently abused over-the-counter cold medications, such as dextromethorphan.

  - o Increased urination is seen in certain medical conditions and with some medications, such as lithium.

- Cardiovascular system (heart and blood vessels)

  - o Heart murmurs can be a sign of endocarditis, an infection of the heart common in people who use intravenous drugs.

  - o Swollen ankles can be a sign of serious heart problems, some secondary to drugs of abuse.

  - o Abnormal findings on an electrocardiogram (ECG) can be related to medication side effects, evidence of past heart attacks (myocardial infarctions), and other conditions.

- Respiratory system (lungs)

  - o Abnormal breath sounds (wheezing) and restricted lung expansion are common in smokers of tobacco, cannabis, or cocaine (crack).

- Musculoskeletal system

  - o Cramping and flu-like symptoms may be signs of opioid withdrawal.

  - o Complaints of pain need to be carefully explored; they may provide information about the cause of a physical dependence on a substance.

- Nervous system

  - o Tremors and increased deep tendon reflexes can be signs of withdrawal from alcohol or benzodiazepines.

  - o Numbness, tingling, or pain in the extremities can be associated with diabetes.

Lab Work

- Drug screens

  - o Drug screening is to the treatment of substance use disorders what checking blood sugar is to the treatment of diabetes. Be aware that the manner in which drug tests are obtained needs to balance the individual's privacy with the need for accurate information.

  - o Supervised drug tests decrease the likelihood that samples will be tampered with.

  - o Urine is by far the most common means (matrix), and depending on the setting where you work, samples can be "dipped" with quick-read results and/or sent to a lab.

o In legal or forensic settings, where test results can be used as evidence, you will need to follow written policies to ensure chain-of-custody handling of the specimen.

o Drug tests need to be specific for the individual and the substances of abuse. For instance, a person who is opioid dependent and on replacement therapy, such as methadone or buprenorphine (Suboxone/Subutex/Zubsolv, Sublocade), needs to have screens that can detect both potential opioids of misuse (oxycodone, heroin, fentanyl), as well as confirm that the person is taking the prescribed medication.

- Blood work will be specific to the individual and their drugs of use, medications, and other medical problems. Typical screening lab studies might include:

  o Complete blood count (CBC)

    - Can detect anemia (abnormally low blood count) that is often found in long-term drinkers

    - Can indicate the presence of infections

    - Can reveal serious adverse reactions to medication, such as dangerously low white blood cells in people taking certain medications, such as clozapine (Clozaril) and carbamazepine (Tegretol)

  o Liver enzymes

    - Some enzymes (SGOT, SGPT) may be elevated in long-term drinkers.

    - Some enzymes may be elevated in intravenous drug users with hepatitis (liver inflammation).

    - Certain psychiatric medications carry a risk for liver disease.

  o Lipids (cholesterol, triglycerides, high-density and low-density lipoproteins) are often elevated in people with metabolic syndrome.

  o Amylase and lipase enzymes are typically elevated in people with alcoholic pancreatitis.

  o Pregnancy test

  o Hepatitis and HIV test

FAMILY AND OTHER SOURCES OF INFORMATION (COLLATERALS)

In addition to a careful medical history, important outside information can be obtained from family, a spouse, other health care providers, probation officers, and case workers. This needs to be done with the signed permission of the person in treatment and/or their legal guardian, if they have one.

It is best to have the person in treatment sign releases of information (i.e., forms that give specific permission for you to talk with others about the patient) at the first meeting. The rules around releases should be explained, and the person should be advised that they can revoke their permission either verbally or in writing at any time. Certain exceptions to that last statement may apply in forensic (legal) circumstances or when the individual has a court-appointed guardian or is a minor. The rules around when information can and cannot be obtained without an individual's permission vary by state.

The yield of information from family and others can help clarify not only the substance use history but can also provide clues to mental health problems, family histories of mental illness and substance use disorders, and potential barriers to successful treatment, such as a partner or family member who actively uses drugs and/or alcohol.

Outside sources of information are indispensable. In certain situations, not communicating with these sources can lead to serious problems later in treatment. Here are a few examples:

- Children and adolescents. Each state has specific statutes as to confidentiality of the patient health information of minors. Where a minor's privacy is protected, even from their parents, it may be broken in certain emergent situations (threatened suicide or other life-threatening circumstances). Also, while the information is protected if the child is on the parent's insurance, there may be disclosures on the claim forms, such as itemization of services, including drug tests.
- Young adults living with a parent(s)
- People involved with the criminal justice system who have been mandated for treatment
- Other situations where treatment is mandated by an outside entity, such as child protective services, department of public health, or employee assistance programs (EAP), where the person's ability to keep their job, professional license, or be a custodial parent is dependent on successful completion of a substance use and/or mental health program

PRIOR RECORDS

No evaluation is complete without a review of past treatment. Although they can be a challenge to obtain, prior records are important. As the assessment progresses, keep track of facilities and/or previous and current providers. Obtain releases of information so that you can talk to current providers and request records. Some individuals may have copies of their records. They should be encouraged to bring them to the evaluation. If it's a child or adolescent, request that the parent or guardian bring all related materials from past assessments.

If the person has been seen in your practice or agency, make sure you review earlier records. This includes material that might have been obtained before a change to an electronic record was made.

STATE-OPERATED PRESCRIPTION MONITORING PROGRAMS

All states now maintain prescription monitoring sites. At a minimum, these sites provide information on what controlled substances (opioids, benzodiazepines, certain sleeping medications, stimulant medication for ADHD, medical marijuana, certain hormones) the patient has been prescribed. Each state has rules about who can, and who must, access this information—typically prescribers, doctors (MDs and DOs), nurse practitioners (APRNs), physician assistants with prescriptive authority, and pharmacists. Many states now have requirements that the database must be checked prior to prescribing opioids and other controlled substances.

In addition to prescribers and pharmacists, different states have added others who can go into the database, typically under the auspices of a prescriber. This allows nurses, therapists, substance use counselors, and other members of a treatment team to access this important information.

Both at the beginning of and periodically throughout treatment, it's important to query the site. By doing so, you may see that a person's use of opioids and/or benzodiazepines is different than what you've been told. The data also provides information as to whether the person has been getting prescriptions from multiple prescribers and if they use multiple pharmacies.

In some instances, this information, when combined with drug testing, may increase your suspicion that some—or all—of these medications are being diverted. For instance, a person who is getting monthly prescriptions for diazepam (Valium) but has a negative drug screen for benzodiazepines should raise a concern.

Controlled Substances

What's a controlled substance? Controlled substances are drugs deemed by the federal government (Pure Food and Drug Act 1906, Controlled Substances Act 1978) to have significant potential to for abuse and dependence.

These are divided into five categories or schedules. The lower the number, the higher the perceived dangers for abuse, misuse, and/or dependence. Schedule I drugs are considered—by law—to have no legitimate medical use, which has implications for the legality to even study them. As a result, there has been limited research into cannabis in the United States, as it is still classified as a Schedule I substance.

- **Schedule I:** Heroin, cannabis/marijuana, lysergic acid (LSD), peyote, methaqualone
- **Schedule II:** Cocaine, methamphetamine, methadone, hydromorphone, hydrocodone (many prescription opioid pain medications), fentanyl, Dexedrine, amphetamines (Adderall and others), methylphenidate (Ritalin and others)
- **Schedule III:** Ketamine, steroids, codeine containing products with less than 90 mg/dose.
- **Schedule IV:** Benzodiazepines (lorazepam, diazepam, and many others), certain sleeping medications (Zolpidem/Ambien, and others)
- **Schedule V:** Medications containing lower amounts of codeine, certain opioid antidiarrheals (Lomotil), some central nervous system depressants (Lyrica)

CHAPTER 4

....

The Comprehensive Assessment Part Three:
Stages of Change and Level of Motivation for Change

Overview
Stages of Change Model
Assessment of Motivation for Change

OVERVIEW

From the early stages of treatment (engagement and persuasion), through the final phase (termination), it is important to understand your patient's readiness to address their substance use and other behaviors or situations they find problematic. Readiness for change and motivation to do so are fluid and influenced by many factors. I view them like the vital signs of blood pressure, pulse, weight, and temperature. They should be checked and nudged in the direction of ideal health and wellness.

- What is the person's current level of motivation?
- How does this level of motivation correspond to the person's current stage of change?

Readiness and motivation are moving targets and seldom progress in a straight line. When someone wakes up hungover, they might swear to never again drink. Come five o'clock and happy hour, the vice-like headache is forgotten, cravings and urges to drink take over, and thoughts of abstinence are but a memory. Alternatively, someone who never thought their alcohol use was a problem might quit drinking after being told they have hepatitis, cirrhosis, or serious alcohol-related heart disease (alcoholic cardiomyopathy).

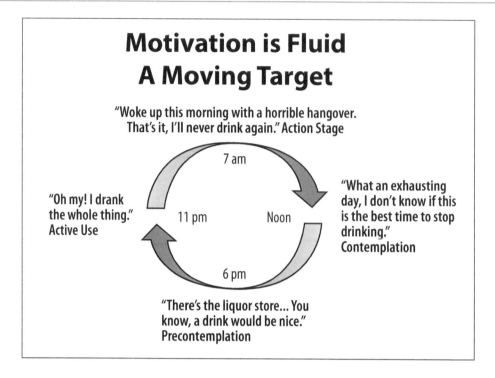

STAGES OF CHANGE MODEL

Developed by Prochaska and DiClemente, the stages of change provide a model to assess readiness for change. While first used with substance use and addictive disorders, a stage of change approach can be applied to any behavior or circumstance a person hopes to change, such as a problematic relationship, their fitness level, or the decision to take a new medication. The stages can be conceptualized as follows:

1. **Precontemplation:** The person is unaware a problem exists.
2. **Contemplation:** The person realizes there's a problem but is not ready to make a change.
3. **Preparation/Planning:** Plans are made to do something about the problem.
4. **Action:** Decisive action is taken to address the problem.
5. **Maintenance:** The problem has been fixed, and efforts are in place to not slip back.
6. **Relapse/Recycle:** A lapse and recurrence of the problem behavior or substance use requires a return to earlier stages to get things back on track. The severity of the lapse can be minor to extreme.
7. **Termination:** The problem no longer requires effort to maintain the change.

Stage of Change	Thoughts	Behaviors
Precontemplation The person is unaware a problem exists.	• My drinking is not a problem. • I have no interest in giving up cigarettes. • I just use cocaine socially. I could stop any time. • The pills are prescribed. I don't have a problem with them, and I'm certainly not addicted to them. • I don't have an eating disorder. • Nothing is wrong with my thoughts. So what that I hear voices? • It's just the way he is. It doesn't bother me when he gets in one of his moods.	Problem behavior continues without change.
Contemplation The person believes a problem is present but is not ready/willing to take action.	• I sometimes drink too much. • Cigarettes are expensive and they are not good for me. • I wish I could stop using cocaine, but the cravings are too strong. • I might be getting into trouble with the pills the doctor prescribed. Whenever I go without them, I feel sick. • It's not normal to make myself throw up every day. • The voices are real to me, but they make it hard to get stuff done. • When he yells and screams, it scares me. I know I shouldn't put up with this, but I can't leave him.	Problem behavior continues; some early, or tentative, attempts to change the behavior may be evident.
Planning/ Preparation The person makes plans to do something about the problem.	• I'll call the clinic to make an appointment. • I'll make a quit date and put it on the calendar. • I've got a friend in NA. I'll ask her to take me to a meeting. • I'll look up programs my insurance accepts to get off these pills. • I have to find someone who knows how to treat eating disorders. • I'll make an appointment to see a psychiatrist. • I've started to put together an escape plan. I'm worried he might hurt me if he finds out about it.	Problem behavior continues; some early attempts to change the behavior may be evident.

Stage of Change	Thoughts	Behaviors
Action Concrete steps to address are made to correct the problem.	• Today, I will not drink. • Today, I'll put on a patch and not smoke. • I've deleted the number of my drug dealer and have blocked her calls. I will not use. • I've started to taper off the pain meds, and I'm scheduled to start my medication-assisted treatment. • I've started CBT for my bulimia, and I might take medication as well. • I've started medication for the voices and have found an internet peer group of people who hear voices. • I moved out when he was at work and am in a safe house.	Plans are implemented. The problem behavior decreases or stops.
Maintenance The behavior has been changed, and the person engages in strategies to strengthen and reinforce the positive changes.	• I will attend AA for the foreseeable future to support my sobriety. • I've tossed all the ashtrays and am using the money I would have spent on cigarettes to take a vacation. • I no longer hang out with my old drug friends. • I know that I need to stay away from pain pills. If my doctor offers, I'll ask for alternatives. • I still see my therapist, but not as often, and I stay focused on healthy eating. • I take my medication daily, and when I feel like stopping it, I remind myself of how much more I'm able to get done without the voices. • The relationship is over. I don't take his calls and have blocked him from my Facebook page.	Strategies to maintain the new behavior are continued, although possibly at a diminished level.
Relapse/Recycle The person experiences a relapse and recurrence of the problem behavior or substance use and must renew efforts to get things back on track.	• Not good. I got myself in a situation where I _____ (drank, smoked a cigarette, did cocaine, took a pain pill). I thought I could handle it, and now the substance use is escalating back to where it was. I need to put a stop to this. • I can't believe I just made myself puke. I thought I had this under control. Apparently not. • I was out of meds and didn't fill them in time. I think on some level, I wanted to see what would happen if I just didn't take them because I've been doing so well. • He caught me in a moment of weakness, and now he thinks we're going to pick up right where we left off. I can't let that happen.	The person needs to reinvest in recovery and put plans into motion (action phase) that will get them back on track. Also, a careful examination of what led up to the relapse, possibly using a behavioral chain analysis (see Chapter 8), may yield areas for further work.

Stage of Change	Thoughts	Behaviors
Termination The changes, whether related to substances or other behaviors, are embedded, and the person no longer experiences cravings or urges.	• I'm someone who just can't drink. • I'm an ex-smoker. • I don't go near cocaine. • I'll only let them give me opiates if there's no other choice. • I haven't thought about making myself vomit in years. • Taking the medication is just a part of my daily routine. • I was once in an abusive relationship. That won't happen again.	No further actions are required. Changes have been incorporated into the person's daily life.

ASSESSMENT OF MOTIVATION FOR CHANGE

Along with understanding where a person is in the change process, it is important to understand what fuels their motivation. Is someone seeking substance use and/or mental health treatment on their own initiative (internal/intrinsic motivators), or are outside forces at play (external/extrinsic motivators)?

Although nothing is wrong with external motivators, their presence is important to note because treatment issues and willingness for change may be compromised in some circumstances, especially if the motivator has an end date. For example:

- "The minute I'm off probation, I'm out of here."
- "I'm just doing what I have to do to keep my job."
- "They wouldn't have let me out of the hospital if I wasn't taking the medication. Now that I'm out, I don't want it or need it."
- I don't want to hurt my unborn baby, so no booze, pills, or cigarettes until after she's born.
- "My parents gave me an ultimatum—either get off drugs or get out of the house."

Frequently, it's a combination of motivators that leads a person to treatment. You'll want to understand these: "What was it that made you decide to walk through the door today?"

Internal/Intrinsic Factors	External/Extrinsic Factors
"I'm sick and tired of feeling sick and tired."	Court-ordered mandate (drug court, jail diversion, mandated treatment following a DUI)
Health concerns: "My doctor told me I've damaged my liver from the drinking."	Family pressure/tough love: "My mom told me either I get clean or I find somewhere else to live."
"I don't want this lifestyle anymore."	Mandated by work—Get into treatment or risk losing the job.
"I want to be a better role model for my children."	Involuntary psychiatric commitment. In most states, this action centers around imminent risk of harm to self or others and possibly grave disability as well.
"I don't want to end up like my father."	Treatment mandated as part of divorce or custody proceedings.
"I don't want to be depressed anymore."	Treatment stipulated by a child-protective agency.
"I know I need help."	Treatment/assessment stipulated by another agency, such as the Department of Motor Vehicles.
"My substance use and the way I'm behaving go against my morals. I don't like the person this has made me."	I'm starting a new job, and they drug test. I've got to ditch the pot.

A person's level of motivation and where they are in the change process are closely linked. When motivation is high, a person is more likely to change, and when motivation is lacking, change is doubtful. This connection between motivation and change provides the underpinning for the therapeutic strategy of motivational interviewing.

CHAPTER 5

....

Creating a Problem/Need List and Setting Goals and Objectives

OVERVIEW

The prior three chapters focused on the collection of large amounts of information (data) about your patient. They covered what's found in standard assessment or intake tools in facilities and organizations that are accredited through the Joint Commission, CARF and other oversight agencies.

However, data that is collected and not interpreted or utilized serves no purpose. This chapter focuses on how to sift through the information collected and organize it into a workable problem/need list with meaningful goals and objectives for treatment. We will attend to the mechanics and requirements of good documentation and the construction of treatment-and-recovery plans, and two guiding principles will be stressed. They are:

1. Treatment is collaborative, and the treatment relationship is of primary importance. This is true even when outside forces, such as court, child protective services, or others, have mandated the person be in treatment.
2. A person's goals and priorities provide the rudder for treatment.

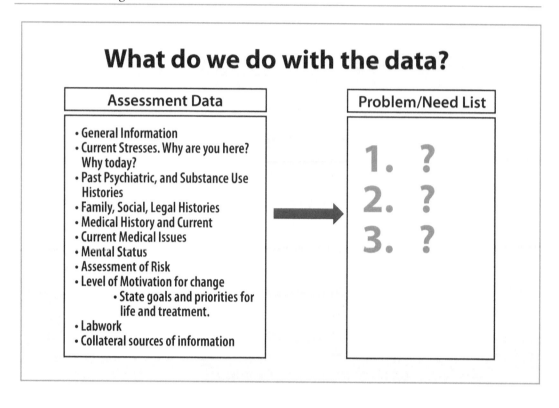

Problem/Need List

Problem/need lists serve multiple purposes:

- They help both the client and the clinician focus on the issues of greatest urgency and concern.

- They incorporate and reflect the client's aspirations and priorities.

- They serve as the backbone of treatment-and-recovery plans and guide the creation of specific goals and objectives.

- They will be used when providing services reimbursed by third-party payers (e.g., insurance companies, Medicare, Medicaid).

- They ensure that no active issues identified in the assessment are forgotten.

How to Generate a Problem/Need List

The simplest method to construct a problem/need list is to go through the data collected and identify anything significant. This includes things that are abnormal, out of range, a potential focus of treatment, barriers to treatment, client strengths, and so on. Then it is a matter of taking those bits of data, either lumping them together by themes or natural connections, or separating them to stand as their own problem or need. These two strategies can be summed up as "lump the data" or "list the data."

The problem/need list typically contains the criteria used to generate diagnoses, but it is not a reiteration of the diagnoses. Rather, the problem/need list is an articulation, based on the data, of what needs to be worked on, accompanied by some indication of the severity of the situation and the evidence to support the existence of the stated problem/need.

Problem/Need List Exercise

Instructions: Make a copy of the following case study (a referral to an outpatient mental health and substance abuse clinic) and highlight or circle every piece of information (data) that can be considered significant. Complete this exercise prior to continuing to the next section.

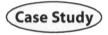

Brad Trainer

Identifying Information: Brad is a thirty-four-year-old divorced construction worker and father of two who presents to treatment following his second DUI/DWI arrest three weeks ago.

Chief Complaint: "My attorney said it would be good for me to get into a program for the weed and drinking, and maybe I need it. Though, to be honest, this whole thing is a crock. It's not like I hurt anyone."

History of Presenting Problem: "So, I was drinking with some buddies after work, like we always do, and there was a cop waiting outside the bar. It was like shooting fish in a barrel. I know you're supposed to say, 'No officer, I haven't had a drop,' but he'd been watching. My lawyer says we could maybe sue for entrapment. But this is bad, like they could lock me up. They pulled my license, and I'm getting rides to work, but you can only do that for so long, and... sometimes you've got to do what you've got to do, and if I get pulled over for driving without a license, I'm totally screwed. If I can't drive, I can't work. I can't pay child support. My ex will be all over me for that. And now I'm not supposed to drink or smoke weed, which are the only things that chill me out. My nerves are shot. I can't sleep thinking about this stuff, like my mind won't shut up."

Appetite is good. He reports his current alcohol consumption as a six-pack per night in bars with friends after work Monday through Thursday, with larger amounts on the weekend. He smokes one to two joints a day, but at the advice of his attorney, he stopped four weeks ago. He admits to "two beers with the guys" last night.

Past Psychiatric History: "I saw the school shrink a few times when I was little. They said I had ADHD. I probably did, could never sit still, always running my mouth. Got detentions like once a week." At age nine, he was prescribed methylphenidate (Ritalin) by his pediatrician. "I took them a few times, think they helped, but my dad would take the bottle, so I hardly ever got them."

Family Psychiatric and Substance Use History: His mother has been treated for depression and anxiety; he does not know if she's on medication. He describes his father as an alcoholic who is currently sober. His younger sister is in a methadone program and struggles with depression.

Substance Use History: He first smoked cigarettes at ten, marijuana at twelve, and began to drink beer and hard liquor with his friends by fourteen when they could get it. He's tried cocaine: "I like it way too much, and I know I need to stay away from it." He's used pain pills and benzodiazepines but states these are not an active issue for him. He denies intravenous drug use and has never been in treatment. He currently smokes a half-pack/day of cigarettes.

Medical History: He admits to no active medical problems. His blood pressure is mildly elevated at 150/90, and his pulse is rapid at 110.

Social History: Brad grew up in a semi-rural Connecticut town. He is the second of three children. His parents separated and then divorced when he was twelve. "I didn't see my dad much after that, probably a good thing. He was not a happy drunk, and you knew to stay out of his way. If you didn't move fast, you'd get hit, and he didn't pull his punches. He does the AA thing now, tells me I should go with him. Maybe I will. But all that higher power stuff… not for me." Brad's mother is a retired elementary schoolteacher who is on her third marriage. "My stepdad died from a heart attack, and the new bum she's with is a drunk like Dad. At least this one doesn't hit her." He reports extensive fights between his biological parents that often became physical. "A couple times the cops got called, and once they hauled Dad away for the night." His older brother is married with children and lives in California. "We don't talk much. He was the smart one, got his stuff together and got out." His younger sister has ongoing mental health and substance use problems and lives in a sober house. "She goes to a methadone clinic."

Brad reports being good at sports and having friends growing up. He graduated from a technical high school where he studied carpentry. "I wanted to go on for plumbing, but too much course work. I'm not good with book stuff. But give me a weird angle to figure out, or how to make a roof line work, and I've got it."

Brad met his ex-wife, Tiffany, in elementary school. "Childhood sweethearts." She became pregnant at seventeen. "I figured we had to get married. I did love her… still do." The marriage lasted ten years, and they have two children: Trent, seventeen, and Ashley, ten. "I turned into my Dad, and when protective services got involved, she told me it was her and the kids or the booze. I tried to stop, and I'd go a few months… I guess I picked the booze." He describes his relationship with Tiffany as volatile, and there was a period after the divorce where she had a restraining order against him. "I couldn't stand the guy she was dating. Total creep." At present they talk once or twice a week. "I still have feelings for her, and it kills me what I've done to my kids."

Legal History (confirmed via the state's Department of Justice website): Two DUIs, one breach of peace and disorderly conduct ten years ago. He has never served jail time.

Mental Status Examination: Brad is a well-developed man, dressed in jeans, a button-down flannel shirt, and work boots. His hair is combed. He makes good eye contact, is animated, and appears mildly tremulous. His speech is rapid, though he can be interrupted. "Yeah, I've always been a fast talker. When I was in school, it got me into constant trouble. Teachers said I could not shut up. Probably true." He admits to daily struggles with intense anxiety, which he rates as a 9 out of 10 today. "It gets bad. Sometimes it's like I can't breathe. Always been like that. Work helps, like when I'm in the zone, booze helps and so does weed." A depression screen—the Patient Health Questionnaire-9 (PHQ-9)— is mildly positive with a score of 12. There is no evidence of psychotic symptoms. He denies any thoughts to harm himself or anyone else.

Labs: A urine toxicology at today's appointment is positive for cannabis (THC). His breathalyzer is mildly positive at .02. He states his last drink was at 11 p.m.

Prescription Drug Monitoring Database: No prescriptions for controlled substances are noted for the past three years.

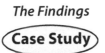

Brad Trainer

Identifying Information: Brad is a thirty-four-year-old divorced construction worker and father of two who presents to treatment following his second DUI/DWI arrest three weeks ago.

Chief Complaint: "My attorney said it would be good for me to get into a program for the weed and drinking, and maybe I need it. Though, to be honest, this whole thing is a crock. It's not like I hurt anyone."

History of Presenting Problem: "So, I was drinking with some buddies after work, like we always do, and there was a cop waiting outside the bar. It was like shooting fish in a barrel. I know you're supposed to say, 'No officer, I haven't had a drop,' but he'd been watching. My lawyer says we could maybe sue for entrapment. But this is bad, like they could lock me up. They pulled my license, and I'm getting rides to work, but you can only do that for so long, and... sometimes you've got to do what you've got to do, and if I get pulled over for driving without a license, I'm totally screwed. If I can't drive, I can't work. I can't pay child support. My ex will be all over me for that. And now I'm not supposed to drink or smoke weed, which are the only things that chill me out. My nerves are shot. I can't sleep thinking about this stuff, like my mind won't shut up."

Appetite is good. He reports his current alcohol consumption as a six-pack per night in bars with friends after work Monday through Thursday, with larger amounts on the weekend. He smokes one to two joints a day, but at the advice of his attorney stopped four weeks ago. He admits to "two beers with the guys" last night.

Past Psychiatric History: "I saw the school shrink a few times when I was little. They said I had ADHD. I probably did, could never sit still, always running my mouth. Got detentions like once a week." At age nine, he was prescribed methylphenidate (Ritalin) by his pediatrician. "I took them a few times, think they helped, but my dad would take the bottle, so I hardly ever got them."

Family Psychiatric and Substance Use History: His mother has been treated for depression and anxiety; he does not know if she's on medication. He describes his father as an alcoholic who is currently sober. His younger sister is in a methadone program and struggles with depression.

Substance Use History: He first smoked cigarettes at ten, marijuana at twelve, and began to drink beer and hard liquor with his friends by fourteen when they could get it. He's tried cocaine: "I like it way too much and I know I need to stay away from it." He's used pain pills and benzodiazepines but states these are not an active issue for him. He denies intravenous drug use and has never been in treatment. He currently smokes a half-pack/day of cigarettes.

Medical History: He admits to no active medical problems. His blood pressure is mildly elevated at 150/90, and his pulse is rapid at 110.

Social History: Brad grew up in a semi-rural Connecticut town. He is the second of three children. His parents separated and then divorced when he was twelve. "I didn't see my dad much after that, probably a good thing. He was not a happy drunk, and you knew to stay out of his way. If you didn't move fast, you'd get hit, and he didn't pull his punches. He does the AA thing now, tells me I should go with him. Maybe I will. But all that higher power stuff... not for me." Brad's mother is a retired elementary schoolteacher who is on her third marriage. "My stepdad died from a heart attack, and the new bum she's with is a drunk like Dad. At least this one doesn't hit her." He reports extensive fights between his biological parents that often became physical. "A couple times the cops got called, and once they hauled Dad away for the night." His older brother is married with children and lives in California. "We don't talk much. He was the smart one, got his stuff together and got out." His younger sister has ongoing mental health and substance use problems and lives in a sober house. "She goes to a methadone clinic."

Brad reports being good at sports and having friends growing up. He graduated from a technical high school where he studied carpentry. "I wanted to go on for plumbing, but too much course work. I'm not good with book stuff. But give me a weird angle to figure out, or how to make a roof line work, and I've got it."

Brad met his ex-wife, Tiffany, in elementary school, "Childhood sweethearts." She became pregnant at seventeen. "I figured we had to get married. I did love her... still do." The marriage lasted ten years, and they have two children: Trent, seventeen, and Ashley, ten. "I turned into my Dad, and when protective services got involved, she told me it was her and the kids or the booze. I tried to stop, and I'd go a few months... I guess I picked the booze." He describes his relationship with Tiffany as volatile, and there was a period after the divorce where she had a restraining order against him. "I couldn't stand the guy she was dating. Total creep." At present they talk once or twice a week. "I still have feelings for her, and it kills me what I've done to my kids."

Legal History (confirmed via the state's Department of Justice website): Two DUIs, one breach of peace and disorderly conduct ten years ago. He has never served jail time.

Mental Status Examination: Brad is a well-developed man, dressed in jeans, a button-down flannel shirt, and work boots. His hair is combed. He makes good eye contact, is animated, and appears mildly tremulous. His speech is rapid, though he can be interrupted. "Yeah, I've always been a fast talker. When I was in school, it got me into constant trouble. Teachers said I could not shut up. Probably true." He admits to daily struggles with intense anxiety, which he rates as a 9 out of 10 today. "It gets bad. Sometimes it's like I can't breathe. Always been like that. Work helps, like when I'm in the zone, booze helps and so does weed." A depression screen—the Patient Health Questionnaire-9 (PHQ-9)—is mildly positive with a score of 12. There is no evidence of psychotic symptoms. He denies any thoughts to harm himself or anyone else.

Labs: A urine toxicology at today's appointment is positive for cannabis (THC). His breathalyzer is mildly positive at .02. He states his last drink was at 11 p.m.

Prescription Drug Monitoring Database: No prescriptions for controlled substances are noted for the past three years.

Construct the List

In the example of Brad Trainer, one can identify more than forty individual bits of significant data. Most of this information can be divided into two large categories: those related to his substance use and those related to his current and past difficulties with his mood.

Substance Use–Related Data	Mental Health–Related Data
Pending DWI/DUI charges (Second DWI/DUI)	"Nerves are shot."
Identified substances of alcohol and marijuana	Can't sleep: "Mind won't shut up."
Drinks after work daily with friends/co-workers; Six beers Mon–Thurs; More on the weekends	ADHD diagnosis as a child; Ritalin at age nine; Thinks it helped: "I could never sit still"; Father diverted his medication
One to two joints/day; Says he stopped four weeks ago	Mother treated for anxiety and depression
Fears jail	Witnessed domestic violence between his parents
Fears loss of driver's license	Sister with depression
Fears loss of job	Parents divorced when he was twelve; Little subsequent contact with his father
Fears being unable to meet child-support obligations	Completed a technical high school
Father with an alcohol use disorder who is currently sober	Currently employed
Sister in treatment with methadone	Volatile relationship with ex-wife; History of a restraining order against him; Talks with her on a regular basis; "I still have feelings for her"
Cigarettes at age ten; Smokes a half-pack per day	Intense anxiety 9 out of 10: "Sometimes it's like I can't breathe."
Has tried cocaine; Never used intravenous drugs	Positive depression screen: PHQ-9 score of 12 (mild)
Marijuana use and alcohol started in early teens	Uses cannabis and alcohol to decrease anxious symptoms
Toxicology screen is positive for cannabis	
Breathalyzer mildly positive at .02	
Never been in substance use treatment	
Slight tremor	
Mild elevations in blood pressure and pulse	

While most of the information fits into one of these two large topics, some pertains to both. It is not clear how much of his depression and anxiety are related to his current stressors: threat of jail, loss of his license and/or job, financial pressures, and relationship worries. And other pieces of information, such as his slight elevations in blood pressure and pulse, could be due to the stress of the evaluation, alcohol withdrawal, underlying hypertension, or other causes.

Medical Issues
Mild elevations in blood pressure and pulse
Slight tremor

Moving forward into treatment, this information must be captured, and the problem/need list is one way to start. That said, it is not necessary or desirable to relist information you've already collected. Rather, the goal is to distill the material into succinct statements around which you and your client will construct treatment.

Problem/need statements should be complete and understandable by the clinician, the patient, and quite possibly the insurance reviewer, who will need to know that the stated problem is something for which reimbursement can be authorized. Finally, the order in which the problem/need statements are listed should be based on what you and your client view as the most pressing concern.

Continuing with the example of Mr. Trainer, an initial problem/need list might look as follows:

Problem/Need List

1. **Active and severe substance use**, as evidenced by (AEB) increased use of alcohol and daily cannabis, DUI and pending legal issues, threat of license and job loss, loss of a major relationship secondary to alcohol, signs of possible alcohol withdrawal, and cigarette smoking
2. **Severe anxiety and mild depressive symptoms** with disturbances in sleep, anxious ruminations, problems with attention and focus, and a childhood history of ADHD; Significant history of adverse childhood experiences, including domestic violence and physical and emotional abuse; probable panic attacks
3. **Active and past medical problems:** mild elevations in blood pressure and pulse, tremor of unknown cause (possible alcohol withdrawal)

ESTABLISH TREATMENT GOALS AND OBJECTIVES

The goals, objectives, and priorities you set with your client provide the treatment rudder. Whether or not you are headed in the right direction—accomplishing the goals—will help you evaluate the interventions and strategies you have selected. In my experience, the rushed or cookie-cutter establishment of goals and priorities hampers treatment, as there will not be clarity around the purpose of therapy. Why are we here today? What is it we/you hope to accomplish? Some people will struggle to identify meaningful goals and priorities for themselves. At the end of this chapter, I've included a worksheet that can help.

Organizations and agencies such as CMS and the Joint Commission define goals and objectives differently. For the sake of this book they will be as follows:

- *Goals* are considered the product or finish line of a course of treatment, such as a lasting sobriety or remission of depression.
- *Objectives* (short-term goals) are the stepping stones on the way toward the bigger goal, such as making it through an alcohol detoxification program and starting therapy and possibly medication for anxiety and/or depression.

When establishing goals and objectives, keep the following five points in mind:

1. They are specific to the individual.
2. They are realistic.
3. They are measurable.
4. They are behaviorally based (something is being done).
5. They are desirable.

Goals and Objectives Are Specific to the Individual

All treatment starts and ends with your client. What does this person hope to achieve over the course of treatment? Outside of your office, what things matter to them, and how have those been affected by their current and past circumstances?

Your client's treatment plan needs to reflect who they are, their aspirations, and their priorities. Programs and practices with prescriptive "cookie-cutter" treatment plans will fall short of this and of the standards and policies set forward by the Joint Commission, CMS, and others.

When setting goals with your patient, it's important to hear what they want from treatment and from life. The simplest approach is to ask, "What is it you'd like from treatment?" or "Where would you like things to be six months from now? A year from now?" or "What would you like to work on?"

When eliciting a person's aspirations, it's possible that their goals might differ from what you want them to be. For instance, someone who presents with depression and heavy alcohol use might not have abstinence from alcohol as a goal. Or someone in an abusive relationship that fuels their anxiety and depression might not view leaving their significant other as desirable, safe, and/or financially realistic. In these examples, it is important to understand the client's perspective and to consider a strategy that meets that person where they are. This doesn't mean their goals won't change in the future, but right now, this is where the client is.

To demonstrate that all goals are in fact the client's, some organizations, including the Joint Commission, want to see goals in the client's own words, or at least that their ideas are clearly represented. This creates a level of complexity when combined with the other necessary components of goals (i.e., measurable, realistic, behaviorally based, and desirable). In order to achieve this, clinicians will sometimes need to construct goal statements that incorporate the client's own words and ideas with terms that fulfill the requirements of an acceptable goal statement.

- Example: "I want to stop using drugs and alcohol."

In this instance, the client's statement fulfills all requirements. The measurement is 100 percent abstinence.

- Example: "I want to be less depressed and anxious."

In this case, measurable outcomes need to be added to the client's expressed goals: "Client will experience a 30 percent or greater decrease in depression and anxiety as measured on a 10-point scale."

An approach used throughout this manual is to capture the client's goals in their own words and then develop them with language that is measurable, behavioral, and so forth in the body of the treatment-and-recovery plan.

Goals and Objectives Are Realistic

When constructing treatment, keep track of what can reasonably be accomplished with the specific individual. This varies depending on the setting, the client, and their needs.

A realistic goal for a brief inpatient hospitalization might be elimination of the suicidal thoughts and behavior that precipitated the current admission. In contrast, the goals for a six-week outpatient co-occurring program, such as an IOP, might be a 50 percent decrease in depressive symptoms and forty-two days without the use of illegal drugs or alcohol. In ongoing individual outpatient therapy for co-occurring anxiety and cocaine use, realistic goals might include sustained abstinence and a 50 percent reduction in anxiety as measured on a metric such as the Generalized Anxiety Disorder 7-Item Scale (GAD-7).

As you work with clients to create their goals and objectives, think about what they might be able to do easily, and then push a bit further. For an adolescent who dropped out of school as a result of emotional, behavioral, and drug problems, what would it take for that teen to go back or to get their equivalency diploma? Is this goal realistic? For someone with frequent relapses with drugs and alcohol, what are some changes that person can make to decrease the likelihood and/or severity of a next relapse? If they are someone who never went to 12-step or other peer-based groups, maybe that's a change they can make. To push further, can you get them to commit to seven meetings in seven days or thirty in thirty? The harm reduction mantra of "Meet the person where they're at" can help. Maybe they're not ready to walk through the door of a 12-step meeting, but what about joining one online? Or ditch the meeting idea altogether and see what they, and you, can come up with.

Goals and Objectives Are Measurable

The Joint Commission, CMS, and others have policies and/or standards that require treatment goals and objectives be measurable and specific. Beyond this, being able to quantify progress helps both the client and the clinician by allowing you to look back and see what has been achieved and what remains to be done.

The use of scales and measurements (metrics) can provide a useful language between the clinician and their client as they progress through treatment: "So how's the anxiety today?" "It's good, no more than a 2 out of 10."

The following list contains practical strategies to ensure that your treatment goals and objectives are measurable.

1. **Absolutes:** Words such as *all, none, yes,* and *no.* Or the person *will* or *will not* do something. Here the measurement is either 0 or 100.

    Example: Caleb <u>will</u> obtain affordable housing by the end of the month.

    Example: "I <u>will</u> be abstinent from alcohol."

    Example: The client will take <u>all</u> medication as prescribed.

    Example: "I want to stop cutting." Margaret will engage in <u>no</u> self-injurious behaviors.

2. **Use of numerical scales**

    a. **Likert scales:** These include 5-point scales where 1 is typically never or none and 5 is all the time or extreme.

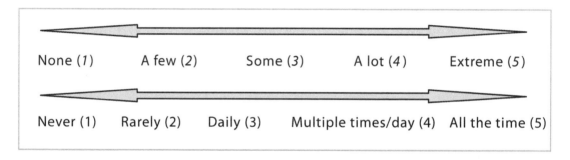

None (*1*)   A few (*2*)   Some (*3*)   A lot (*4*)   Extreme (*5*)

Never (1)   Rarely (2)   Daily (3)   Multiple times/day (4)   All the time (5)

    Example: "I want to be less anxious." Using a 5-point scale, the patient will report anxiety as being no greater than a 2.

    Example: The client will report a decrease in the frequency of panic attacks from a 4 (multiple times/day) to a 2 (rarely/less than one per week).

    b. **Subjective units of distress (SUDs):** A 100-point scale that is defined by the client. Zero is usually no distress, and 100 is the most distress possible. SUDs are often used when doing cognitive behavioral and other related therapies.

    Example: "I want to be less depressed." Using a 100-point scale (100 being the worst), the patient will report depression no greater than a 30.

    c. **Other scales,** such as a 10-point scale, are often used to rate the severity of pain, with 0 being no pain and 10 being the worst imaginable.

Example: Using a 10-point scale (10 being the worst), Sheila will report that her anxiety never goes above a 4.

Example: "I want my drug cravings to go away." Using a 10-point scale, the client's craving for heroin will never go above a 2.

3. **Standardized screening tools and assessment scales**

   a. **Tools to measure signs and symptoms of drug and alcohol withdrawal,** such as the Clinical Institute Withdrawal Assessment (CIWA) and the Clinical Opioid Withdrawal Scale (COWS)

   Example: The patient's symptoms of alcohol withdrawal will be managed so that she scores no greater than a 2 on the CIWA.

   b. **Tools to measure mood and anxiety symptoms,** such as the Beck Depression Inventory-II, Patient Health Questionnaire-9 (PHQ-9), PTSD Checklist for DSM-5 (PCL-5), Yale-Brown Obsessive-Compulsive Scale (Y-BOC), and World Health Organization's Disability Assessment Schedule (WHODAS 2.0)

   Example: "I don't want to be depressed." The patient's depression will be no higher than a 7 on the PHQ-9.

   Example: Lorna will exhibit a 30 percent or greater decrease in her obsessive-compulsive symptoms as measured with the Y-BOC.

4. **Parameters and specific amounts:** The use of *less* or *more* <u>accompanied by specific amounts.</u>

   Example: Frank will attend <u>three</u> or <u>more</u> AA meetings per week.

   Example: Carla will utilize <u>three</u> or <u>more</u> DBT coping skills and record them on her weekly diary card.

   Example: "I've got to stop washing my hands a hundred times a day." Jean will decrease her hand washing behavior to <u>less than five times/day</u>.

Goals and Objectives Are Behaviorally Based

Goals and objectives imply something will be achieved by the patient. To do this, they require an action word (verb). Useful examples include *achieve, apply, demonstrate, experience, identify, maintain, master, obtain, show, understand,* and *utilize.*

Example: Carl will <u>achieve</u> abstinence from cocaine.

Example: "I want to be less anxious." The client will <u>experience</u> a 30 percent decrease in anxious symptoms as measured using a 10-point scale.

Example: Carl will <u>attend</u> a SMART Recovery meeting daily for the next four weeks.

Goals and Objectives Are Desirable

Having desirable goals seems obvious, but sometimes getting you and your client to agree on what is desirable will be a challenge. This often happens when the clinician or the program has a goal that differs from the patient's.

- "I'm not ready to stop drinking. I want to be able to keep drinking socially."
- "I plan to use synthetic cannabis because I know my probation officer doesn't test for it."
- "I'm just here for court. The second that's done, I'm out of here."
- "I've always been depressed. I always will be depressed. I'm not interested in doing anything about that."
- "They told me I have schizophrenia and need to take these pills. I think they're idiots, and if the pills are so great, they can take them."

In these instances, the challenge is to arrive at mutually acceptable goals and objectives. This might involve the use of a harm reduction and motivational approach where you start where the client is now.

- "I'm not ready to stop using." The client will attend three or more substance use groups per week and complete a pros and cons list around her current usage.
- The client will attend weekly substance use education and weekly motivational interviewing sessions, with a focus on cannabis.
- "I don't want to go to jail because of pot." The client will attend program with the goal of being substance free, at least until his legal issues have resolved.
- The client's level of depression will be assessed, and at least two treatment options that she has not previously tried will be made available to her.

Your Goals & Priorities

The following pages contain lists of things many people find important. Next to each is a place for you to check those that matter to you. Check as many as you like. If you think of something not on these pages, write it down. Remember, these are your goals and priorities and not what you think others might want for you.

Relationships
- I want to be in a committed/romantic relationship. _____
- I want to improve my relationship with my partner. _____
- I want more/better physical intimacy and/or sex. _____
- I want to improve my relationship with my children. _____
- I want to improve my relationship with my parents. _____
- I want good relationships with other family members. _____
    - o Be specific and write in whom: _____
- I want to have lots of friends. _____
- I want one or two good friends. _____
- I like to be around people. _____
- I like a lot of time alone. _____
- Other: _____

Health
- My health is important. _____
- I need to work on my health. _____
    - o Be specific: _____
- Exercise is important to me. _____
- I want to exercise more and/or more regularly. _____
    - o Write in how much and what type: _____
- Sleep is important to me. _____
- I want to sleep more. _____
- I want to sleep less. _____
- I want to watch what I eat. _____
- I want to lose weight. _____
- I want to gain weight. _____
- I want to take medication as prescribed. _____
- Other: _____

Drug and Alcohol Use
- I want to stop using (write in the drug/drugs here): _____
- I want to cut down (write in the drug/drugs here): _____
- My recovery from drugs and/or alcohol is important to me. _____

- I want to stop smoking cigarettes. _____
- My continued abstinence from cigarettes is important. _____
- Other: _____

Gambling and Online Activities
- I want to work on how much time/money I spend gambling (write down how much time/money you currently spend): _____ _____
- I want to change my online behavior. (Be specific: Is this related to time or more related to the kind of activities you participate in online, such as shopping, gambling, pornography, social networking?): _____ _____

Emotions
- I want to be more emotionally stable. _____
- I want to be less depressed. _____
- I want to be less anxious. _____
- I want inner peace. _____
- Other: _____

Money
- I want to have a lot of money. _____
- Money is not so important to me. _____
- I want enough money to be comfortable. _____
- I want enough money to retire and not have to worry about paying the bills. _____
- Other: _____

Spirituality
- Being a part of a church/temple/synagogue is important to me. _____
- I don't like to be a part of organized religion. _____
- My spirituality is important. _____
- My faith in God is important. _____
- Giving back to others is important to me. _____
- Meditation is important to me. _____
- Prayer is important to me. _____
- Other: _____

Creativity
- Being creative is important to me. _____
- I like to make stuff. (Be specific): _____
- Playing music is important to me. _____

- I want to learn some kind of creative skill. _____
- Other: _____

Work
- I want a full-time job. _____
- I want a part-time job. _____
- My current job is important. _____
- Any job is important. _____
- I don't want to go to work. _____
- I want to do volunteer work. _____
- Other: _____

School
- School is important to me. _____
- I want to go back to school. _____
- These are my school goals (be specific): _____

Home
- My home is important. _____
- Where I live is important. _____
- I like to spend most of my time at home. _____
- I like to spend most of my time out of my house/apartment. _____
- I want to find a stable place to live. _____
- Other: _____

Hobbies & Fun Activities
- Spending time on my hobbies is important. _____
- I want to have more fun. _____
- Scheduling time for activities and/or hobbies is important. _____
- I want to spend time on fun things. (List at least three.)
    - o _____
    - o _____
    - o _____
- I want to travel. _____
    - o Here are some places I'd like to go: _____
    _____
    _____
- Other: _____

Pets
- My pets are important. _____
- I would like to have an animal(s). _____
- Other: _____

Step Two

Go back through the items you identified as important, and circle up to three that are extremely important and that you want to work on now. Write them here.

1. _____

2. _____

3. _____

Step Three

Of the two or three things you identified as most important, rank them in order: first, second, and third. Put a star next to the one that you want/need to address right away, which may or may not be number one. Look at what you've written down and see if these are indeed your most important goals/ priorities. If not, make necessary adjustments.

1. _____

2. _____

3. _____

CHAPTER 6

....

Treatment-and-Recovery Plans

Overview

Principles of Treatment-and-Recovery Planning

Interventions

Structure of Treatment-and-Recovery Plans

Sample Treatment-and-Recovery Plan

Dynamic Aspects of Assessment and Treatment

OVERVIEW

Clinicians who treat substance use and mental health disorders are often faced with a difficult dichotomy when it comes to documentation and treatment planning. On the one hand, it is crucial to identify your client's strengths, dreams, and aspirations and to build on those elements. But the realities of insurance reimbursement are such that what needs to be recorded focuses on deficits, or what is wrong, diagnosable, and disordered. If you cannot document the medical necessity for your services, you will not get paid.

This split between what must be recorded so that services can be reimbursed and the benefits of strength-based assessments and treatment planning have led some organizations and providers to create two sets of treatment plans: one that demonstrates medical necessity and the other that is a more client-friendly document, sometimes referred to as a recovery or wellness plan.

While there are merits to having both the medical-model treatment plan and the client-friendly recovery plan, there are also potential pitfalls, such as overvaluing one and undervaluing the other. There's an increased paperwork burden and the risk that the focus will become less about the relationship and work with the client and more about the thorough completion of forms.

For the sake of this text, both halves of this equation—the need for strength-based treatment *and* documentation of medical necessity—will be included in a single treatment-and-recovery plan. Beyond forms, the important point is that treatment planning is a process with real clinical value. It's the blueprint for treatment.

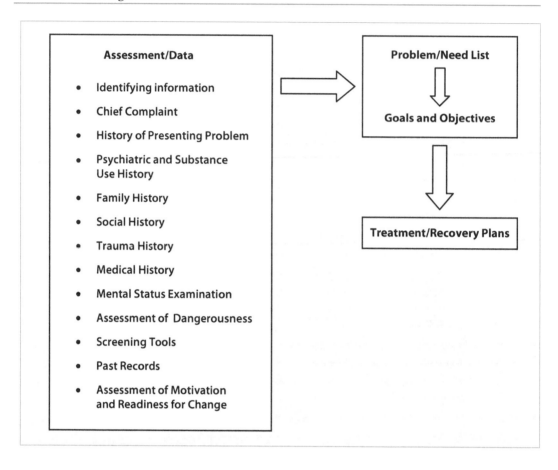

Treatment-and-recovery plans flow naturally from the ongoing distillation of information you get from your patient, the problem/need list, and the goals and objectives you've established.

Principles of Treatment-and-Recovery Planning

Treatment-and-recovery plans will include the following aspects:

1. Plans are developed collaboratively between the client and the clinician.
2. Plans center around the client's needs, aspirations, challenges, and problems. One approach is for clinicians to view themselves as a consultant to their client.
3. Treatment-and-recovery plans are process driven. They are not set in stone but are constantly reassessed and revised based on the client's circumstances.
4. All potential resources for positive change—not just interventions that are considered clinical—can be incorporated into plans. For example:

    a. Take the dog for a daily walk.

    b. Go to the gym three times a week.

    c. Have lunch with a sober friend.

    d. Volunteer at my church's food pantry.

e. Enroll in one course at the community college.

f. Download and use a meditation app three times a week for at least fifteen minutes.

INTERVENTIONS

Interventions are the specific strategies, treatments, skills acquisition, utilizations of peer-support systems, faith-based activities, family, friends, and other resources that will be used to help the person move toward their goals and objectives. Interventions are tools in your client's and your respective toolkits. And like hammers and screwdrivers, you need the right tool for the right job. Just as you wouldn't try to hammer a screw into drywall, mismatched or one-size-fits-all treatment strategies won't get the job done. The toolbox analogy also works to see what is needed to help the client progress. Do they have the necessary tools, or is part of the work of treatment to help them expand what's in their toolkit (skills acquisition)?

INTERVENTIONS SHOULD

1. Relate to the client's goals and objectives
2. Relate to the problem/need list
3. Have ownership. Someone is responsible for seeing that they get done. (This might be more than one person, especially where the clinician or other member of the multidisciplinary team and the client have roles to get the intervention accomplished.)
4. Have defined parameters. Just as all the goals and objectives need to be measurable, so too interventions should have specific parameters—how many sessions, of what length, over what period, and so forth. If there is an anticipation that an intervention will continue indefinitely, such as taking medications for persistent conditions, that should be noted.
5. Be realistic. Goals and objectives are in the realm of what can be accomplished by the client and the clinician.

STRUCTURE OF TREATMENT-AND-RECOVERY PLANS

At a minimum, treatment-and-recovery plans contain the following:

1. The active problems/needs that are the focus of treatment
2. The specific goals and objectives tied to the problems and needs
3. Interventions (treatments, strategies, family, peer and community resources, etc.) that will be employed in the interest of moving the person closer to their goals

The following form, which can be used as is or adapted to your organization, incorporates Joint Commission and CARF standards for treatment planning, as well as those required for most insurers, including CMS. In addition, specifics related to peer activities and a strength-based recovery philosophy have been incorporated into the form.

Treatment-and-Recovery Plan

Patient's Name:	
Date of Birth:	
Medical Record #:	

Level of Care: _____

ICD-10 Codes	DSM-5 Diagnoses

The individual's stated goal(s): _____

1. Problem/Need Statement:
Long-Term Goal:
Short-Term Goals/Objectives (with target date):
1.
2.

2. Problem/Need Statement:
Long-Term Goal:
Short-Term Goals/Objectives (with target date):
1.
2.

3. Problem/Need Statement:
Long-Term Goal:
Short-Term Goals/Objectives (with target date):
1.
2.

Interventions					
Treatment Modality	Specific Type	Frequency	Duration	Problem Number	Responsible Person(s)

Identification of strengths: _____

_____

Peer/family/community supports to assist: _____

_____

Barriers to treatment: _____

_____

Staff/client-identified education/teaching needs:

_____

Assessment of discharge needs/discharge planning:

_____

Completion of this treatment-and-recovery plan was a collaborative effort between the client and the treatment team members:

SIGNATURES		Date/Time:
Client:		
Physician:		
Treatment Plan Completed By:		
Primary Clinician:		
Other Team Members:		

SAMPLE TREATMENT-AND-RECOVERY PLAN

Using the case study, the related problem/need list, and goals and objectives of Brad Trainer in the previous chapter, the following treatment-and-recovery plan can be assembled.

Treatment-and-Recovery Plan

Patient's Name: **Brad Trainer**

Date of Birth: **2/12/1987**

Medical Record #: **XXX-XX-XXXX**

Level of Care: Intensive Outpatient (IOP)

ICD-10 Codes	DSM-5 Diagnoses
F10.20	Alcohol use disorder, moderate
F12.10	Cannabis use disorder, mild
F41.1	Generalized anxiety disorder, with panic

The individual's stated goal(s): "I don't want to lose my license or my job. I really don't want to go to jail."

1. Problem/Need Statement: Active and severe substance use, as evidenced by (AEB) increased use of alcohol and daily cannabis, DUI and pending legal issues, threat of license and job loss, loss of a major relationship secondary to alcohol, signs of possible alcohol withdrawal, and cigarette smoking.
Long-Term Goal(s): Achieve lasting sobriety from alcohol and tobacco; Discontinue cannabis while under any legal oversight.
Short-Term Goals/Objectives (with target date): 1. Successfully discontinue all alcohol (starting today) 2. Continue to abstain from cannabis (starting today) 3. Attend 90 percent, or more, of scheduled IOP days (starting today)

2. Problem/Need Statement: Severe anxiety and mild depressive symptoms with disturbances in sleep, anxious ruminations, problems with attention and focus, and a childhood history of ADHD; Significant history of adverse childhood experiences, including domestic violence and physical and emotional abuse; Probable panic attacks.
Long-Term Goal(s):
1. Achieve a 50 percent or greater decrease in anxious symptoms as measured with the GAD-7
2. Improve focus and concentration by at least 20 percent using a 10-point rating scale
3. Be free from panic attacks
Short-Term Goals/Objectives (with target date):
1. Clarify the psychiatric diagnoses (two weeks from today)
2. Achieve a 20 percent reduction in anxious and depressive symptoms using a 10-point scale (four weeks from today)
3. Problem/Need Statement: Active and past medical problems: mild elevations in blood pressure and pulse, tremor of unknown cause (possible alcohol withdrawal).
Long-Term Goal(s): Obtain a yearly physical and maintain blood pressure within a healthy range.
Short-Term Goals/Objectives (with target date):
1. Obtain a primary care physician or nurse practitioner and have a first appointment (one week from today).

Interventions					
Treatment Modality	**Specific Type**	**Frequency**	**Duration**	**Problem Number**	**Responsible Person(s)**
Group Therapy	CBT with co-occurring focus	3x/week	50 minutes/ group for 1 month	1,2	Mr. Trainer, primary clinician, or designee
	Chemical dependence education and relapse prevention	3x/week	50 minutes/ group for 1 month	1	Mr. Trainer, primary clinician, or designee
	Multiple family meeting	1x/week	1 hour	1,2	Mr. Trainer, identified family member(s) or S.O.
Individual Therapy	CBT individual therapy with co-occurring focus	2x/week	50 minutes/ for one month	1,2	Mr. Trainer, primary clinician

Nursing Assessment	Nursing assessment	Once and as needed	1 hour	1,2,3	RN
Initial Psychiatric Assessment	MD/Nurse practitioner assessment	Once	1 hour	1,2,3	MD/APRN
Psychopharmacology	Medication evaluation	Weekly	15–20 minutes	1,2,3	MD/APRN
Lab Work	Blood work/ other labs as indicated	Upon admission and as needed	N/A	1,2,3	MD/APRN
Specimen Collection	Breath analysis/ urine drug screen	As ordered	1 month	1,2	Clinician or designee
Peer Support	12-step group	2–3 meetings/ week	1 month	1	Mr. Trainer
Other	Obtain medical referral	Once	Brief	3	Mr. Trainer, program, MD/APRN

Identification of strengths: Strong work ethic, highly motivated to achieve abstinence and to not lose his job. Takes his role of being a father as a top priority and wishes to be more involved in his children's lives. He views himself as a moral person.

Peer/family/community supports to assist: Mr. Trainer views his mother as a significant support. She has been in recovery for more than ten years and has offered to go with him to NA meetings. She has also expressed willingness to attend multiple family meetings at the IOP. Mr. Trainer says he will obtain a sponsor through NA. He also identifies supports through his work but is cautious about what he divulges to coworkers.

Barriers to treatment: Mr. Trainer identifies the financial burden of being on leave from work. He hopes to return to work as soon as possible but realizes it may create scheduling difficulties with treatment.

Staff/client-identified education/teaching needs: To better understand the nature of his substance use and to identify specific triggers and vulnerabilities. To identify and understand possible connections between his depressive and anxious symptoms and his substance use.

Assessment of discharge needs/discharge planning: Mr. Trainer will be free from illicit drug use, and follow-up treatment will address both relapse prevention and ongoing assessment and treatment of any residual mood or anxiety symptoms.

Completion of this treatment-and-recovery plan was a collaborative effort between the client and the following treatment team members:

SIGNATURES		Date/Time:
Client:	Brad Trainer	3/15/2021, 2:00 p.m.
Physician:	Charles Atkins, MD	3/15/2021, 3:15 p.m.
Primary Clinician:	Gloria Anderson, LCSW	3/15/2021, 2:00 p.m.
Other Team Members:	Peter Green, CADAC	3/15/2021, 4:00 p.m.
	Lois White, RN	3/15/2021, 4:00 p.m.

DYNAMIC ASPECTS OF ASSESSMENT AND TREATMENT

A final point to make is that assessment and treatment are fluid processes. When we work with people who have complex lives, circumstances change, and treatment needs to reflect that. Substance use and mental health problems are not static. People will have lapses and periods of growth. Sometimes symptoms of one condition may obscure and confuse another.

Someone who presents in opioid withdrawal, complaining of severe depression and anxiety, may be depression free once they are out of withdrawal and on medication. However, you may now notice that they fidget throughout sessions and groups and are easily distracted. Both they and their mothers tell you these problems have been present since they were young. Suddenly the initial problem/need list, which included depression and anxiety, needs to be revised to address the emerging presentation of ADHD, which is common in people with substance use disorders (see Chapter 10).

Or even someone you have had in treatment for years, with a diagnosis of a depressive disorder, may suddenly come to your office manic or hypomanic: "Dr. Atkins, I haven't slept in three days, and I feel great! Here's a sweater I knitted you last night." The earlier diagnosis of unipolar depression, along with aspects of the treatment, need to be changed to account for what is likely bipolar disorder.

And with effective treatment, people improve. This needs to be reflected in the problem/need list, treatment-and-recovery plans, and the treatment itself. If a problem has resolved, that should be indicated, and plans should be updated and reworked based on changing levels of care, changes in the clinical focus, clarification of diagnoses, and so on. For those who bill Medicare and Medicaid, and/or are Joint Commission or CARF accredited, additional standards will mandate how frequently and under what circumstances plans need to be revised or rewritten.

CHAPTER 7

....

Levels of Care

LEVELS OF CARE

One early slogan of co-occurring treatment was and is "There is no wrong door." The intent of this statement is correct. When someone reaches out for help, that person needs to be met with open arms… and a correct level of care. For instance, it would be dangerous to attempt to treat a manic individual in serious alcohol or benzodiazepine withdrawal in an outpatient clinic. However, should such a person walk in, you wouldn't turn them away. What you would do is attempt to keep them calm while making the necessary arrangements, which might include calling 9-1-1 to get an ambulance to transport them to an emergency room. Similarly, someone with mild depression and anxiety who smokes cannabis daily is unlikely to require an inpatient stay, and their insurance company is unlikely to agree to reimburse that level of service.

In addition to safety concerns, other factors need to be considered when matching a person to a correct level of care, a treatment setting, and specific interventions. It won't just be a question of what is the best fit, although that is important. You need to take into account the real-world circumstances of community resources, the person's insurance or lack thereof, family resources, peer supports, active medical problems, level of motivation, personal preference, and so forth.

Levels of care can be thought of as a continuum that extends from inpatient settings—such as detoxification, medical and psychiatric units in hospitals, and freestanding substance use facilities—through residential programs, to a broad array of outpatient treatment options, both those run by professionals, as well as by peer and mutual self-help groups.

In some instances, level-of-care decisions will need to consider legal difficulties individuals might have. If they are incarcerated and require acute psychiatric or substance use treatment, then transfer to a hospital or specialty behavioral health unit will need to occur. Correctional systems are required to address the behavioral health and substance use needs of inmates, so even when people are incarcerated, these principles of best fit can be applied.

Another concept to keep in mind is that both substance use and mental disorders respond well to treatment but are also subject to lapses and clinical setbacks. Inpatient settings are reserved for individuals in high-risk situations who require acute and intense—possibly lifesaving—treatment. When the acute need has passed, it is appropriate for that person to step down to a less intense level of care, such as a residential rehabilitation program, PHP, IOP, or other form(s) of less restrictive outpatient treatment.

When to Use an Inpatient Option

When deciding on what is the most appropriate level of care, the first question is: Does this person require—or desire—an inpatient option, such as a medical detoxification unit or psychiatric unit? Key issues include the following:

1. **Safety and medical concerns:** All states have statutes that address imminent risk and that dictate when and how a person can be hospitalized involuntarily. These guidelines focus on the person being at imminent risk of harm to self or others and often include language that extends to extremely disordered and dangerous behaviors.

   a. Active suicidal or homicidal behavior

   b. Serious and active medical issues, such as alcohol or benzodiazepine withdrawal

   c. A person who requires detoxification who has co-occurring serious medical issues and/or a history of severe withdrawal syndromes in the past, such as alcohol or benzodiazepine withdrawal seizures and/or delirium tremens

   d. Grossly disorganized and dangerous behaviors (including substance-induced manic and psychotic states, as can be seen with PCP, synthetic cannabis, hallucinogens, amphetamines, bath salts, etc.)

e. Grave disability that results from the substance use and/or mental disorder (which can involve the person's behavior deteriorating to the point where they can no longer manage basic self-care, such as adequate nutrition, shelter, and clothing)

2. **Need for a higher level of care than what the person is currently receiving:** It is often the case that someone initiates treatment as an outpatient, but circumstances require a move to a higher level of care, such as a medically monitored drug detoxification for alcohol, a residential program, or a psychiatric inpatient unit, for a period of time. Reasons for this include:

   a. The emergence or reemergence of serious safety issues, as spelled out previously

   b. An inability to achieve specific treatment goals as an outpatient

   c. Recurrent serious lapses with drugs and/or alcohol where the individual is unable to achieve their stated goals

3. **Personal preference:** It might be that someone has the resources and the willingness to begin treatment on an inpatient basis. For them this might be the most efficient way to start a course of treatment.

   a. "I know myself. If there's even a chance I can get near booze, I'm going to drink. I need to break the cycle by getting into a rehab program for a few weeks."

4. **Mandated reasons for inpatient:** Circumstances where the individual has no choice but to be admitted to an inpatient unit, such as a court mandate for evaluation and treatment

INPATIENT OPTIONS

The selection of an inpatient setting will be driven by the individual's needs, preferences, and to some extent, personal resources (e.g., insurance, entitlements, transportation, available facilities, access to family and other supports, etc.). The two most important questions when selecting an inpatient option are:

1. What is/are the goal(s) for this admission? For the person with co-occurring disorders, this takes on added significance, as many inpatient facilities specialize in psychiatric disorders or substance use disorders but not both. That leads to the next question:

2. Can this facility meet the specific need(s)/goal(s) that drive this admission?

The following sections describe the major types of inpatient facilities. Within each, there will be variability in terms of quality of care, affordability, specialized services, and such.

Medical Hospital/Acute Medical Unit

The current standard of care for severe alcohol and benzodiazepine withdrawal involves management on medical units. This is on account of the potentially life-threatening nature of these conditions and the need to access a broad range of medical interventions, from intravenous medications to, in severe situations, the use of intensive care units.

Access to behavioral health services, both to assist in the assessment and management of delirium and other psychiatric co-occurring conditions, is through consultation with either the hospital's psychiatric service (psychiatrist, APRN, physician assistant, social worker) or the person's treating psychiatrist if they have privileges (i.e., are approved to see patients) at the hospital.

Medical units are typically unlocked, and if there is a need for suicide precautions or the individual is confused and at risk for self-harm, sitters or other interventions will be required to monitor them. Length of stay is driven by the need for ongoing acute medical hospitalization. At the point the active medical concern has been safely addressed, the person will be discharged or transferred to the next appropriate level of care.

Community Hospital Behavioral Health (Psychiatric) Units

These units are typically locked (with some exceptions) and are part of a larger medical hospital or system. Increasingly, psychiatric units have protocols to handle mild to moderate cases of alcohol and benzodiazepine withdrawal while addressing severe psychiatric symptoms (mania, psychosis, suicidality). Amid the opioid epidemic, more are also able to initiate medications for opioid use disorders and to continue treatment with those already on them. A potential advantage to hospital-based units is the access to medical care and ancillary hospital services, such as radiology and laboratory.

On average, inpatient admissions are brief (four to ten days), and at the point the person no longer meets criteria for an inpatient admission (i.e., is no longer suicidal, homicidal, gravely disabled, and/or in withdrawal), the patient is discharged and referred to a less restrictive level of care.

Freestanding Private Psychiatric Hospitals

These facilities are separate from medical hospitals, although they typically have formal agreements (i.e., memorandums of understanding) with area hospitals should a patient require transfer to an acute medical setting. Many freestanding hospitals have areas of expertise that might make one of them a best fit for a particular individual, such as specialized treatments for eating disorders, personality disorders, psychotic disorders, and so on.

Each facility's ability and willingness to work with co-occurring substance use disorders vary and should be assessed prior to admission. Concerns about the potential for a dangerous withdrawal needs to be clarified at the onset: "Do you treat alcohol withdrawal? If the person goes into serious withdrawal (has a seizure, delirium tremens, hallucinosis), how do you handle those situations?" and "Do you work with people who are opioid dependent? Do you provide opioid replacement therapy?"

Veterans Affairs Hospitals

There are Veterans Affairs (VA) Hospitals and Clinics throughout the United States, the Philippines, Guam, and the Virgin Islands. Services are available to active service members, their families, and some veterans with service-connected benefits. There are available substance use disorder services, as well as mental health services, and these vary by state and location. Admission to a VA inpatient detoxification unit, general psychiatric unit, or specialty unit (such as a PTSD or co-occurring disorder unit) will be based on the same symptom acuity that would necessitate admission to a community, state, or freestanding unit or facility. A central point of contact and information can be obtained through the Bureau of Veterans Affairs at www.va.gov or by calling the VA crisis line at 1-800-273-TALK/8255. You can also text at 838255 to speak with a VA responder.

State-Run Psychiatric and Substance Treatment Facilities

While the availability of state psychiatric hospitals has diminished greatly nationwide, most states still maintain facilities for individuals who meet their "target population criteria." These are typically people with histories of severe and persistent mental illness, often accompanied by substance use disorders.

Each state will have admission criteria that will include the presence of acute and severe psychiatric symptoms. In the case of substance use disorders, state-operated detoxification facilities will use criteria based on historical information (e.g., history of seizures, delirium tremens, etc.), as well as current presentation (e.g., acutely intoxicated or actively in withdrawal). Many states rely on the American Society of Addiction Medicine (ASAM) Criteria, described at the end of this chapter, when making level-of-care decisions, especially as they pertain to accessing state beds.

The length of stay in state hospitals varies, but they are typically reserved for longer lengths of stay. In some cases, it can be months and even a year or more.

Detoxification Units

Detoxification units specialize in safely managing withdrawal, mostly from alcohol and benzodiazepines. Detoxification admissions for alcohol range from a few days to a week or more, depending on the severity of symptoms. A complete and safe detoxification from high benzodiazepine doses can take on the order of weeks, although the latter stages can be managed in a rehab setting with adequate medical oversight.

Some detoxification units offer treatment for opioid use disorders. This should include the use of opioid replacement therapy with methadone or buprenorphine (Suboxone, Subutex, and available generics) or the opioid blocker naltrexone XR (Vivitrol).

Specialized detoxification units can be found in various settings, from general medical hospitals, state psychiatric hospitals, VA hospitals, and freestanding psychiatric hospitals to residential substance use programs and centers with integrated detoxification and rehabilitation programs. Things to consider when selecting an inpatient option might include the following:

- If the person requires a medically supervised detoxification from alcohol or benzodiazepines, does this facility have a record for successfully providing that treatment (i.e., does it have a medical detoxification unit)?

- If the person is manic, psychotic, or suicidal and misuses opioids, will the facility be able to handle both the psychiatric component and the substance use component, which may require opioid replacement, such as buprenorphine or methadone (i.e., does it have inpatient psychiatric unit with co-occurring capacity)?

- In addition to acute psychiatric and/or substance use symptoms, does this person also have serious and active medical issues that need to be addressed (i.e., is it a hospital-based psychiatric unit)?

- If the person is suicidal, is this facility prepared to safely monitor and treat them (i.e., is it an inpatient psychiatric unit, a freestanding psychiatric hospital, or a medical unit with 24/7 sitters)?

RESIDENTIAL TREATMENT

The option to use a residential program, frequently after a medically monitored detoxification, can be a useful strategy to break a pattern of compulsive substance use. In residential programs, the structure and therapy allow the individual to lay the groundwork for healthier habits and provide a physical separation from triggers and cues that exist at home and in community settings.

Residential options include standard four-week (twenty-eight-day) rehabilitation programs to lengthier residential settings, some of which include options for the individual to obtain work either within the facility's campus or in the outside community. Once the mainstay of both substance use and mental health treatment (like acute inpatient stays), residential treatment options are now reserved for individuals who cannot get their needs adequately met in a less restrictive setting.

For people with co-occurring disorders, it is important to evaluate prior to admission whether a residential program can meet both their substance use and mental health needs. It was once the norm that residential programs would not admit people with significant mental disorders. While this has changed somewhat, residential programs can be lumped into three broad categories:

1. **Substance use disorders only:** These programs only address the substance use issues. They will likely exclude individuals who have active mental health problems. Psychiatric services and mental health services are not provided.
2. **Co-occurring (dual diagnosis) capable:** These programs have some mental health services available but are focused on the substance use issues. Available mental health services will include access to a psychiatrist or psychiatric APRN and some attention to the interplay between mental health and substance use.
3. **Co-occurring (dual diagnosis) enhanced:** These facilities assess and treat both the substance use and mental health disorders. They are better able to manage the needs of people with active emotional, behavioral, and cognitive symptomatology. Some will specialize in particular diagnoses, such as schizophrenia spectrum disorders, severe personality disorders, affective disorders, PTSD, etc.

Partial Hospital Programs

Partial hospital programs (PHPs) were developed both as a step down from inpatient hospitalization, as well as a strategy to prevent inpatient hospitalization. The basic idea of a PHP is that a person can access an almost inpatient level of multidisciplinary services but be able to go home at night. PHPs run five to seven days per week, for four or more hours per day, and provide a multidisciplinary approach, which includes a psychiatrist/psychiatric APRN, nursing, some medical services (such as laboratory services), and a range of group, individual, and family therapies. To meet the Medicare requirement for a PHP, there must be at least twenty hours per week of programming.

PHPs are often specialized (e.g., programs might focus on geriatric populations, adolescents, personality disorders, general adults, eating disorders, co-occurring disorders, substance use, etc.). PHP treatment is largely group based but may include individual therapy as well, based on the person's goals and preferences. Medication management and psychiatric oversight by a psychiatrist and/or APRN are integral elements of PHPs.

Admission criteria for PHPs center on the likelihood that the person would require an inpatient hospitalization without this level of care, and most insurers, including Medicare, require the admitting physician to sign an attestation statement to this effect. For insurance purposes, PHP is most often billed through an individual's inpatient benefit. Length of stay in PHP is typically on the order of a few days to a few weeks.

Some substance use and co-occurring PHPs include ambulatory detoxification services, which might be appropriate for a person with mild alcohol withdrawal. Others offer services that include the use of medication (buprenorphine, methadone, naltrexone) for opioid-dependent individuals.

Intensive Outpatient Programs

Similar to PHP, intensive outpatient programs (IOPs) involve treatment on multiple days per week (three to five) for at least three hours per day. IOPs are also often specialized and utilize a multidisciplinary treatment team, including a psychiatrist/ APRN, social workers, other clinicians, nursing staff, possibly occupational and other rehabilitative therapists, psychologists, etc.

Admission criteria to IOPs include symptom acuity below the level of inpatient or PHP severity. This might entail moderate to severe depression, some suicidal thinking without plan or intent, some self-injurious behavior, psychosis, hypomania (and even mania if the person is not engaged in dangerous behaviors), moderate to severe anxiety symptoms, and active substance use disorders. Lengths of stay in IOPs range from a few weeks to a couple of months.

Assertive Community Treatment Teams

Assertive community treatment teams (ACTT) are community-based services largely reserved for people with severe and persistent mental illness, including those with co-occurring substance use disorders. Historically, ACTT services and community mental health centers/local mental health authorities developed as large state hospitals downsized and closed. The intent was to create wraparound community-based services for those with the greatest need.

ACT teams, which are often housed in community mental health centers or other state-run or state-funded mental health clinics, provide an intensive level of multidisciplinary support. ACTT services are community based, with an emphasis on working with people in their own home and in the community. Treatment is guided by the individual's needs and can include daily and sometimes multiple daily visits from a case manager and/or peer specialist.

Core Components of an ACT Team

- Case managers have small caseloads (10:1 ratio).
- Nurses and physicians/APRNs are a part of the team and have relatively small caseloads in order to address the needs of the clients served.
- The ACT team works collaboratively. All clients belong to the team and vice versa. There are frequent team meetings to review treatment and progress toward goals.
- ACTT services are not time limited. Once enrolled, clients may continue with ACTT for as long as the services are required.
- Continuity of staffing is encouraged so that clients are familiar with the ACT team members and are able to develop relationships.
- The team includes peer specialists (i.e., people with lived experience).
- Clients are a part of the team.
- The team includes a substance use specialist.
- The team includes a vocational specialist.
- The team includes a housing specialist.
- Crisis service is available 24/7.
- Any inpatient admissions and discharges are coordinated with the ACT team.
- The emphasis is on providing services and supports in the community versus in clinics or offices.
- Outreach and engagement strategies are emphasized.
- An integrated dual-diagnosis approach is used with clients who have co-occurring disorders. This includes motivational strategies, mutual-aid groups, and an emphasis on matching the level of service/treatment to the individual's level of motivation. The overall goal is abstinence from problem substance use, but there is a willingness to work with clients at all stages of change.

CASE MANAGEMENT AND TARGETED CASE MANAGEMENT

Case management and targeted case management are community-based programs that work with the person in their home and in the community. They are much less intensive than ACT teams, with visits from a case manager occurring a couple of times per week or less. Case managers may also not be a part of a larger multidisciplinary clinical team. For instance, some case management services, such as vocational or housing assistance, may have no clinical component.

ACTT and case management/targeted case management are often funded through a state's department of social services or mental health agency. In some states, these are run by a state agency and in others, by a variety of nonprofit providers, including some in-home nursing agencies.

Recent trends have seen some insurance companies provide case management, typically under the direction of a nurse care coordinator for clients with high needs, such as those with frequent emergency room visits and inpatient hospitalizations.

Outpatient Therapy Delivered by Professionals

There is a spectrum of effective outpatient treatments. This runs from individual therapy with a licensed psychologist, social worker, psychiatrist, or other professional licensed by your state to groups held in mental health clinics, in private practices, via telehealth, and in many other settings. For people with co-occurring disorders, the selection of a therapist, modes of therapy, and settings for treatment will be driven by the person's goals, clinical needs, preferences, and resources. The diagnosis-specific chapters of this handbook include recommendations for types of therapy.

Some points to consider when constructing an outpatient treatment-and-recovery plan include the following:

- If psychiatric medications are involved, can they be safely managed by the person's primary care physician or medical nurse practitioner? If not, ensure that the person has regular follow-up with a psychiatrist or psychiatric nurse practitioner. If this person is not also providing the therapy component, make sure that there is communication between the prescriber and the therapist.
    - o If medications are to be used for the treatment of substance use disorders, does this provider have the expertise and interest to provide them?
- Therapy should be specific to the person's goals, needs, and preferences. This customization might include specialized/diagnosis-driven therapies, such as those available for trauma, borderline personality disorder, OCD, depression, anxiety disorders, psychotic disorders, eating disorders, and so forth.
- A positive relationship with a therapist corresponds to overall better treatment outcomes. It is important that, whatever form(s) of therapy the person selects, they trust and feel comfortable with their therapist. A critical question is: Do you like your therapist?
- Are all the person's therapeutic needs and goals being met by the particular form(s) of therapy? For people with co-occurring disorders, answering this question will mean that the mental health components and the substance use disorder(s) are both addressed.

MATCHING TREATMENT AND SETTING TO THE PERSON AND DIAGNOSES

Does the level of care provide all or most of the services this person requires? For a person with co-occurring disorders, that means their substance use and mental health needs can be attended to in the same location (i.e., fully integrated treatment). If this is not possible—and it frequently isn't—it becomes a matter of putting together a treatment-and-recovery plan that fills in the missing pieces. Examples include the following:

- A woman who has both an opioid use disorder and schizophrenia. She might need to get her mental health services at an outpatient clinic or private practice while getting opioid replacement treatment through either a methadone clinic or practitioner who prescribes buprenorphine (Suboxone, Subutex, Zubsolv, generics) for opioid maintenance.

- A man who has severe problems with emotion regulation, as is seen in borderline personality disorder, and who also has an alcohol use disorder. An ideal program might be one where he can participate in DBT with a dual-diagnosis focus.

- A woman with both a severe eating disorder, such as anorexia, and moderate amphetamine use disorder will need treatment that addresses both, including medical monitoring with contingencies in place should her weight drop below a critical point or other medical complications develop.

- A man with moderate to severe OCD and alcohol use disorder will do best with a program or provider(s) that offers CBT and specific medication(s) for his OCD, as well as treatment for his alcohol problem.

RESOURCE ISSUES AND BARRIERS TO TREATMENT

A person's resources—ranging from family and friends to finances, job, housing, and more—need to be considered when creating realistic treatment-and-recovery plans and accessing services. As you evaluate resources, barriers to treatment will emerge and need to be addressed. Factors to consider include:

- **Personal preference:** Does the person agree with the recommended course of treatment?
  - o "I don't think I need inpatient. Could we try outpatient first?"
  - o "I'm not a group person. What about one-to-one therapy?"
- **Motivation:** Does the person's level of motivation match the recommended treatment?
- **Access to treatment:** Does the person have access to transportation or adequate technology (and know-how) to use telehealth?

- **Payment issues:** Are they able to pay for the recommended services? Do they have insurance limitations that affect their ability to afford prescribed medication, co-pays, and deductibles?

- **Employment constraints:** Will this person need to take time off from work? How will they manage this? Can treatment be provided in such a way or at such times where there is minimal disruption to their work life?

- **Housing:** Do they have stable housing? If someone is homeless, or in jeopardy of homelessness, this creates a front-burner issue that must be addressed as soon as possible.

- **Sober supports:** Does this person live in an environment where others use drugs and alcohol? This decreases the likelihood that someone will be successful in stopping their drug and/or alcohol use. Conversely, friends and family who are involved in recovery can provide everything from an understanding ear to a ride to a mutual-support group, with coffee and a piece of pie afterward.

- **Friends and family:** Who in this person's life do they want to be involved in their treatment? In what ways can those others help support the person in their recovery?

- **Availability of specialty services:** Is this someone who requires or would benefit from diagnosis-specific treatment, such as for trauma, eating disorders, or borderline personality disorder?

- **Medical barriers to treatment:** Is the person physically well enough to participate in therapy? Will they require special accommodations to make that possible?

AMERICAN SOCIETY OF ADDICTION MEDICINE (ASAM) CRITERIA

First developed in the 1980s to help providers determine a best level of care for individuals with substance use disorders, the ASAM Criteria (formerly the ASAM Patient Placement Criteria) have gone through revisions with increased attention to people with co-occurring disorders. The criteria, along with clinical judgment, help clinicians and organizations, such as state agencies and insurance companies, look at an individual and their circumstances and assess what would be the best fit at this point in treatment. This evaluation is done with the use of a multidimensional (six dimensions) assessment:

1. **Acute intoxication/withdrawal potential:** Is this person at risk for a serious withdrawal based on either current presentation or history?
2. **Biomedical condition and complications:** What factors need to be considered with this person's current and/or historical medical history and conditions?
3. **Emotional, behavioral, or cognitive conditions and complications:** What are this person's emotional, cognitive, and mental health needs and issues?
4. **Readiness to change:** What is the person's current level of motivation to change?
5. **Relapse, continued use, or continued problem potential:** What is this person's history of relapse? Do they continue to use despite negative consequences of that use?

6. **Recovery/living environment:** What is the status of the living situation? Do they have sober supports, or is their current home situation one that presents challenges and barriers to recovery?

The ASAM Criteria look at levels of care along a numerical continuum, from 0 = no treatment required to 4 = medically managed intensive inpatient treatment. It utilizes five levels of care that are further articulated based on program focus, intensity, and capacity for managing co-occurring mental, social, and medical needs. The five levels are:

- 0.5: Early intervention
- 1: Outpatient treatment
- 2: Intensive outpatient/partial hospitalization
- 3: Residential/inpatient treatment
- 4: Medically managed intensive inpatient treatment

Each level is further articulated with the use of decimal points for ranges of services within. The higher the number, the greater the intensity, such as:

- 2.1 Intensive outpatient program (IOP)
- 2.5 Partial hospital programs (PHP)
- 3.1 Low-intensity clinical residential
- 3.7 Intensive medically monitored inpatient

The ASAM Criteria are an industry standard, and over thirty states utilize them when making determinations about placement in state-funded treatment facilities and programs. An updated version of this manual was published in October 2013. The ASAM Criteria website is: https://www.asam.org/resources/the-asam-criteria/about.

CHAPTER 8

....

Key Psychotherapies, Mutual Self-Help, and Natural and Peer Supports

OVERVIEW

Throughout this book, specific social, therapeutic, and medication strategies will be discussed in each of the major diagnostic categories. Certain therapies and approaches—such as mutual self-help groups (AA, NA, SMART Recovery, All Recovery, etc.), CBT, motivational interviewing, peer-based interventions and supports, wellness management, and mindfulness training—have benefits that cut across diagnostic boundaries and can be used as building blocks in treatment.

Motivational Interviewing

Developed by William Miller, PhD, and Stephen Rollnick, PhD, motivational interviewing is a therapeutic approach that helps people make positive changes around problem behaviors. While initially studied in substance use, motivational techniques can be applied to a broad range of behaviors, from cigarette smoking and lifestyle/wellness choices (exercise, nutrition, adequate sleep) to adherence with medication regimens.

Motivational interviewing is change based and empowers people to make their own decisions. It steps back from a traditional advice-and-consent model ("I'm the doctor and this is what you must do") to one where you weigh the pros and cons of your own actions ("I've got to stop doing this; it's hurting me"). The basic approach to motivational interviewing is to let the person explore and resolve their ambivalence (conflicted feelings) around a problem behavior. It starts with an assessment of the pros and cons—"Do I get out of bed and go to work? Or do I sleep in and call out sick? Let's look at the advantages and disadvantages of both"—which we'll explore further. In the process, the therapist helps the person heighten the internal discomfort (dissonance) around the behavior to the point where they are more likely to change it in line with their goals.

In motivational therapy, it's the therapist's task to engage the client, to help them focus and articulate the area for change, as well as why the change might be important. Finally, the therapist helps the person plan and implement the steps needed to realize the desired change.

In the most-recent version of MI (Miller and Rollnick 2013) four key processes have been outlined as the basis of MI:

Engaging: to build and sustain the relationship.

Focusing: to set the agenda and behavior(s) to change.

Evoking: Use MI skills discussed below to help the client move towards their change goals.

Planning: How the person will move towards the desired change(s).

Techniques used in motivational interviewing include:

- **Express empathy through reflective listening:** The clinician listens closely to what the individual says and then reflects back the material to see if they have it right. This should not turn into parroting the person's words but should assure the client that they have been understood. For example:

    Client: "I really don't want to stop the booze. It's the only thing that calms me down at night. But if I don't, my girlfriend says she's going to leave me."

    Therapist: "So you don't want to stop drinking because you like the way it calms you down, but it sounds like you're worried that if you don't, your girlfriend will leave. Is that correct?"

- **Maintain a nonjudgmental stance:** This includes maintaining a neutral stance in both verbal and nonverbal expression. It's important that the clinician not step in and take on either side of the person's struggle with the behavior, as this may push them away from their goals.

- **Be nonconfrontational and noncoercive:** The therapist does not challenge the person's behaviors, attitudes, or beliefs but helps them look at their concerns regarding the behavior(s). It's the difference between saying, "Can't you see your drinking is killing you and destroying your relationship?" and "You seem conflicted about the effect your drinking has on your relationship with your girlfriend and on those elevated liver enzymes. Am I getting that right?"

- **Roll with resistance:** When looking at long-held behaviors, it's natural to not want to give them up. There are important reasons why people engage in harmful behavior. These must not be ignored or discounted. For therapists who practice motivational interviewing, it can be a challenge to not step in on the side of the behavior you are trying to support. The following is an **incorrect** example that is judgmental and blaming:

  Client: "I'm just not ready to give up the drinking."

  Therapist: "But if you don't, your wife is going to leave you. Is that what you want? Do you want your drinking to be the reason your marriage falls apart?"

  The following is a **correct** example that involves reflective listening with neutral stance:

  Client: "I'm just not ready to give up the drinking."

  Therapist: "I can see you're struggling with it. Tell me about that. Maybe do a pros and cons list about the drinking."

- **Heighten the internal dissonance (discomfort):** This is where the therapist serves as a repository of the pros and cons the client has presented about their behavior and strategically feeds them back. The challenge is to do this in such a way that you support the person's forward movement with change.

  Therapist: "I think I see your dilemma. On the one hand, you like the way alcohol makes it possible for you to feel comfortable in social situations. Yet on the other hand, you say things have gotten to the point where you can no longer control how much you drink, and it's resulted in some really bad consequences. How do you think you can resolve this?"

Other strategies employed in a motivational approach might include the following:

- **Use of pros and cons (decisional balance):** Have the individual write down all the things they like and dislike about a targeted behavior, such as substance use.

- **Use of scales to assess readiness for change:** "On a 10-point scale, with 10 being ready to do it today, how primed are you to stop using alcohol?"

- **Guiding questions around preparation for change:** "How do you plan to quit your smoking?"

- **Validate and acknowledge *all* positive change:** "Three 12-step groups last week? Well done!" "You're down to ten cigarettes…excellent! What are the reasons you cut down? How did you do it?"

COGNITIVE BEHAVIORAL THERAPY

CBT is a present-focused therapy that has its roots in behaviorism and cognitive therapy and was pioneered by Drs. Aaron Beck and Albert Ellis. The connections between what we think, feel, and do provide the framework of CBT.

CBT has been studied extensively as a research model and has a large body of evidence to support its usefulness in the treatment of anxiety disorders, depression, and a broad range of mental disorders, from ADHD to schizophrenia. It is one of the building blocks of numerous important therapies, which include evidence-based manualized treatments for trauma, therapies for working with people with bipolar spectrum and schizophrenia spectrum disorders, and it is one of the foundations of DBT.

CBT requires that someone learn techniques in therapy and then practice those techniques in the real world. To help solidify material learned in session, homework assignments are a component of CBT-based therapies.

In the CBT model, a thought—whether accurate or distorted—leads to an emotional response, which prompts the doing of a related behavior.

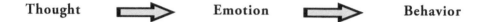

Thought ⟹ **Emotion** ⟹ **Behavior**

In some cases, the emotion may precede the thought, such as the surge of panic when an eighteen-wheeler cuts you off on the highway and you swerve out of the way. The corresponding rush of adrenaline leads to the catastrophic thought "I could have been killed." Regardless of the order, CBT provides the linkages between what we think, feel, and do.

As a therapy, CBT helps the client identify and then challenge distorted thoughts that lead to painful emotions and ineffective behaviors. The approach of the therapist is to help their client see how these present-day distortions are based on deeper-held beliefs that may or may not be accurate or fully accurate. As therapy progresses, these beliefs are challenged and reframed with accurate appraisals.

The identification of distorted thoughts, of which we are often unaware, requires tremendous attention to the specifics of the situation. A truism of CBT is that all emotional changes are preceded by a triggering or automatic thought: "What were you thinking right before you slammed down the phone on your mother?"

In CBT, it is important to become familiar with common forms of cognitive distortions and ways to challenge them. The style of therapy is conversational, directive, and frequently didactic, as skills and techniques are taught by the therapist. When homework is assigned, it must be reviewed at the next session to ensure that the material was understood and practiced. Homework review also provides an opportunity to fine-tune skills and coach the client to use them more effectively.

Common Cognitive (Thought) Distortions and
Approaches to Challenge and Reframe

- **Black-and-white thinking:** This is where people or situations are perceived as all one way or another. Someone is their friend or their enemy. There is no gray area.

  Example: "I can't do anything right."

  Challenge: "Well, as I look at things objectively, I do some things well, and others are a challenge. And when I struggle or do something incorrectly, it brings up these feelings of frustration and failure."

- **Catastrophic thinking:** Here, a small setback is magnified into something larger.

  Example: "I just know this headache is the sign of some horrible medical problem. It's probably a tumor."

  Challenge: See a doctor, get objective data. Maybe it's a brain tumor, but probably not.

- **Emotional reasoning:** Taking an emotional state to be a factual truth.

  Example: "I feel unlovable. Therefore, I am unlovable."

  Challenge: "Everyone is lovable. But when I feel blue, I think it makes me less of a person that someone could love."

- **Generalization:** A portion of something is taken to represent the whole.

  Example: A nurse with a difficult patient says, "The entire unit is out of control."

  Challenge: "No, it's really just this one person who's taking most of my time and energy. It makes me anxious because it's impacting my ability to care for my other patients and get my work done."

- **Labeling (judging):** A pattern of reducing people and situations to a single attribute or descriptor.

  Example: "My mother is a control freak."

  Challenge: "At times, my mother's insistence that things be done her way really annoys me. But there's much more to her than that."

- **Mind reading:** The belief that you know what others are thinking. Typically, this involves inaccurate interpretation of facial cues, body language, tone of voice, and so on. The distortion often centers on the belief that the other person thinks negatively about you. This distortion is common in people with social anxiety disorder.

  Example: "You can tell he hates me."

  Challenge: Strike up a conversation and try to get a more accurate read on what the other person thinks. "You seem upset. Is everything okay?"

- **Blaming:** Other people are responsible for your actions. One place this occurs is in abusive relationships and interactions: "Don't make me hit you."

  Example: "You made me mad."

  Challenge: Other people don't have the power to change our emotions. It is something we do with our own thoughts.

- **Shoulds:** An unrealistic expectation of being able to do everything perfectly

  Example: "I should be able to make the ten types of Christmas cookies my mother did while taking care of the kids and working a full-time job. Why can't I? What's wrong with me?"

  Challenge: "That's unrealistic. My mom stayed at home and didn't have to pay the kinds of bills I do. That said, I wish I had time to do more of that holiday stuff. I really miss it."

- **Fallacy of fairness:** A misplaced belief in some universal sense of fairness. Fairness is a human construct. Nature does not operate with a sense of fairness.

  Example: "After all I did for her, the least she could do is show me some respect."

  Challenge: There is no universal code of fairness. What one person thinks is fair, another might not agree with.

- **Fallacy of change:** A belief that wanting another person to change or trying to make them change will make it so. An elegant challenge to this distortion is found in the Al-Anon literature and is referred to as the three C's: "I didn't cause this, I can't control it, and I can't cure it."

  Example: "If he really loved me, he'd stop drinking."

  Challenge: It's impossible to make someone else change. It's something they must do themself.

Behavioral Chain Analysis

CBT, which has been adapted and incorporated into many therapeutic models, helps us understand and piece together the events that surround problem behaviors, from a suicide attempt to a lapse with cocaine. This can be done with a technique called behavioral chain analysis, which requires going into exquisite detail over what happened, what led up to it, what the person thought and felt, and what other factors contributed to the undesired outcome. The therapist and client identify causes, which become the focus of problem solving, cognitive challenges, and skills building to lessen the likelihood that the behavior and related negative emotions will reoccur.

How to Construct a Behavioral Chain Analysis

One way to construct a behavioral chain analysis is to begin with the problem behavior or emotion. From there, clarify everything that led up to the event. Help the client focus on what they thought and felt. Ask them what other factors might have contributed (vulnerabilities), such as being too tired, hungry, already upset over something, bored, or in physical or emotional pain.

At first, behavioral chain analyses may meet with some resistance because it takes time and effort. When you ask someone what led up to the relapse or overdose, it's common to get a response like "It just happened, I don't know what I was thinking." Be diligent, it may take several prompts and some encouragement to flesh out the particulars. In some ways, behavioral chain analysis is like being a detective or a reporter—you want to know the who, what, when, where, and why. But it is time well spent, as what emerges will help you and your client understand the behaviors and emotional states that the person wants to get a handle on. Beyond that, identifying where things got off track provides the information needed to strategically teach skills to help them through future situations.

In books, behavioral chain analyses are tidy and organized. In real life, mine are messy. As the person remembers more details, bubbles get added into any bit of blank space. At times, an important bit of information might trigger a mini separate chain analysis. While I've provided examples and worksheets, all you need is a piece of paper and something to write with.

The following is an example of a completed behavioral chain analysis.

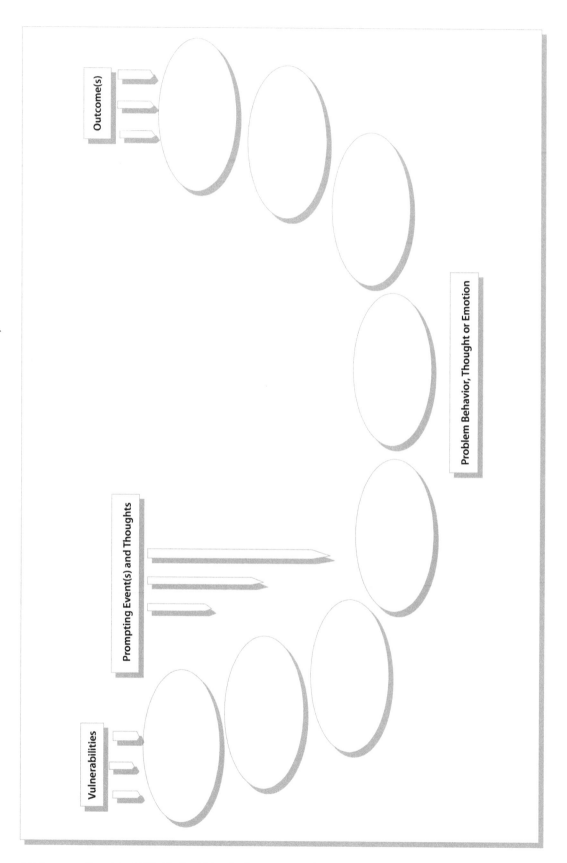

Example: A chain analysis for a woman following a serious relapse with alcohol.

Therapist: "Let's work backward from your lapse with alcohol and go through everything you thought, felt, and did beforehand."

Vulnerabilities

Didn't sleep well the night before. Skipped breakfast. Didn't go to the gym. Fighting with boyfriend.

Felt upset for not going to the gym. I feel fat and disgusting.

Co-workers talking about going to bar after work. They invite me.

Prompting Event(s) and Thoughts

Got a case of the "f" its. Why shouldn't I be able to have a drink now and then?

Problem Behavior, Thought or Emotion

Drank after work--three martinis in the bar.

Bought a bottle of vodka on the way home from the bar.

Got into fight with boyfriend who called me a drunk and walked out.

Drank half the bottle, called out sick to work. No more time off left for the year. I feel like a loser.

Outcome(s)

Discussion: In the completed behavioral chain analysis, the therapist and client will be able to identify areas to work on. These include:

Cognitive distortions

- Emotional reasoning: "I feel fat and disgusting."

- Naming/labeling/judging: "I'm nothing but a drunk."

- Catastrophizing: "I don't think I'm ever going to get better."

- Black-and-white thinking: "It's like the last four months without a drink are just gone, and I'm back to step one."

Skills deficits

- How to practice drug/drink refusal

- How to reduce emotional vulnerability and practice self-care (e.g., need to focus and problem solve how to get adequate sleep, exercise, and nutrition)

Applications of Cognitive Behavioral Therapy

CBT connects the dots between thoughts, emotions, and behaviors, and as a result, has nearly limitless applications. With CBT, the therapist and client identify targets, such as painful and excessive emotions, distorted thinking, and/or problematic behavior. Strategies, such as the behavioral chain analysis, help clarify the connections and point out areas for specific interventions, such as cognitive reframing and skills training and application. As a stand-alone therapy, CBT is considered an evidence-based practice for the treatment of:

- OCD
- Panic disorder
- Generalized anxiety
- Specific phobias
- Depressive disorders
- Personality disorders
- PTSD

When combined with other modalities, such as psychopharmacology, traditional substance use treatment, motivational interviewing, and mindfulness, CBT provides an important component of many new and emerging best practices that include the treatment of:

- Substance use disorders
- Bipolar spectrum disorders
- Attentional disorders
- Schizophrenia spectrum disorders

MINDFULNESS TRAINING

Founded in Zen and other ancient Eastern traditions, mindfulness-based techniques, used alone and combined with other therapies, have demonstrated robust benefits in a broad range of conditions, from pain, depression, and anxiety to substance misuse. Studies that include brain imaging before and after mindfulness training reveal interesting and exciting changes—among them, enhanced connectivity between areas of the brain associated with arousal and attention and increased gray matter.

Mindfulness can be taught and practiced free from any religious connotation. While its origins are in the contemplative religious practices of the East, mindfulness practice is fully compatible with Judeo-Christian and other religious and secular practices.

Mindfulness involves bringing one's attention to the present moment. Fundamentals of mindfulness include:

- Complete attention to the moment
- A nonjudgmental awareness of thoughts, sensations, and feelings
- Fluid awareness. One does not hold onto thoughts and feelings but lets them pass through consciousness like clouds that move across the sky.

One approach to teaching mindfulness begins with a focus on the breath, which then expands to include an awareness of thoughts, feelings, and sensations as they pass through the mind and the body. The breath, like our senses (sight, hearing, taste, proprioception, physical sensations, smell), can provide anchors to the present moment. These are things we do or experience that never shut off, though we may not notice them.

There are many ways to develop and teach mindfulness. Like any skill, it's best practiced daily. Common mindfulness exercises include the following:

- **Seated meditation:** With the legs comfortably crossed, focus on the breath as it enters and leaves the body. Observe the feeling of the breath as it passes in and out of the nostrils. Observe your thoughts without becoming fixed or attached to them. Let them come and go like cars on a moving train.
- **Walking mindfulness:** Take a walk and focus on each footstep as it connects to the ground. Observe what you see, feel, and think.
- **Count the breath:** While seated, lying down, or walking, count your breaths. On the inhalation, think the number one, and on the exhalation the number two. Get to ten and start again. If you lose count, gently remind yourself of the instruction and start at one. If you get to thirteen, observe that and start at one again, without judgment.
- **Mindfulness with daily activities:** Identify things you do each day and commit to doing them with total awareness. This could include mindful eating, brushing your teeth, shaving, gardening, etc.
- **Mindfulness of others**
    o Make a commitment to pay total attention when you are on the phone with a friend or family member.
    o When having lunch with a colleague, be present and focused just on them.
    o Take the opportunity to be present and in the moment when you interact with friends and family.
- **Mind-body practices,** such as yoga, qigong, tai chi, and others

A few global points to make here include:

- The goal of mindfulness is to be present in the moment. Many people believe they are supposed to achieve a calm nirvana-like state. That might happen, but it's not the objective. If the moment is an anxious, chatty one and the brain will not shut up, that's what it is. But if you observe that chattiness and can focus on the moment and the task—such as counting the breath—you have been mindful.

- Check in after every exercise. Mindfulness exercises are incorporated into many therapies (DBT, Seeking Safety, and others). Therapists must never assume that an individual has had a particular experience. Rather, allow time for people to discuss what an exercise was like for them. While one person's guided meditation might bring them to a floaty, happy state, someone else in the same group may have verged on a panic attack. The check-in also allows the leader to gently correct mistakes a person might have made during the activity.

- The length of activities will be based on the experience your clients have had with meditative practices and their willingness to engage. There is no correct answer. While mindfulness-based stress reduction (MBSR), a well-studied eight-week course, uses a daily practice of thirty to forty-five minutes, DBT starts with much briefer meditative practices (one to five minutes at a time) and also has a strong evidence base to back it. This latter approach, especially with people who have intense emotional dysregulation and problems with attention and focus, may be a gentler way in.

PSYCHOEDUCATION

"Knowledge is power" (Francis Bacon), and "The beginning of wisdom is the definition of terms" (Socrates). Throughout treatment, we want to teach and empower our clients about their options, how therapy works, what medications do and don't do, the principles of wellness, and so forth.

Methods to provide psychoeducation are both formal—such as specific groups and courses—and informal, as can occur in many professional and even nonprofessional interactions—such as within the peer support communities. With the availability of information through the internet, psychoeducation is often self-directed, and clinicians need to be aware and comfortable with perspectives and information that may be unfamiliar or may conflict with their treatment beliefs and approaches.

As a building block of treatment, psychoeducation is woven into therapeutic themes. This includes learning about the brain's reward system and how this may create challenges, especially during early recovery, and understanding the potential benefits and risks of specific therapies, including medications.

Education plays an important role in wellness and illness management. Topics are tailored to the specific needs, diagnoses, and cognitive abilities of the individual, as well as their interest level. One cautionary note: Be aware that some people can become triggered by graphic depictions of drug use, such as those found in popular movies and TV shows.

For prescribers, psychoeducation around medication may include the following:

- Verbal and written material on any medications prescribed or recommended. This includes the potential risks and benefits of any medication, as well as what to do should they have questions or problems.

- Time to ask questions about medications, as well as to ask about options, including the option to not take medication. For clinicians, it can be as simple as asking, "Do you have any questions? And if you don't have any now, and some occur to you, write them down and we'll talk about them next time."

- The prescriber asking the client questions about their medications to ascertain whether they fully understand what they're taking, why they're taking it, and how they're supposed to take it.

FAMILY INTERVENTIONS

Numerous studies have shown that including family, significant others, and key friends and supports in therapy is beneficial and improves outcomes. The type of interventions that make sense will be specific to the person in treatment and the constellation of that person's friends and family. Common approaches to family work include the following:

- **Individual family therapy:** Here the goals are often centered around enhanced communication and decreased conflict.

- **Family education:** Often conducted in a multifamily format. Here information around mental and substance use disorders is provided and discussed. This can be with or without the presence of the person in treatment.

- **Diagnosis-specific family work:** There are specific treatments, such as the family-focused therapy for bipolar disorder (Chapter 12), which provide psychoeducation and skills training to help improve outcomes and prevent relapse.

- **Community Reinforcement and Family Training for Treatment Retention (CRAFT-T):** This intervention involves the identified client/patient and a concerned significant other, such as a family member, partner/spouse, or friend. Developed by Robert Meyers, CRAFT-T teaches the concerned significant other techniques so they can help motivate the person with the substance use disorder to start treatment. It has also been studied with people already in treatment, where the concerned significant other works to help them stay motivated. Results for CRAFT-T are positive for both helping to get people into treatment and for treatment retention.

- **Mutual self-aid for family/friends** where the person in treatment may not be present. Among these self-help groups are those that specifically address substance use problems, such as Al-Anon and Adult Children of Alcoholics and those that focus more on mental disorders, such as support groups through the National Alliance on Mental Illness (NAMI).

NAMI (www.nami.org) is the largest grassroots advocacy and education organization, and it offers a variety of support groups, both for family members and for people with mental illness. NAMI also funds research and broad-reaching campaigns to raise awareness and understanding about mental illness. In addition to support groups, which are free, NAMI offers low-cost, up-to-date trainings, such as family-to-family trainings (twelve weeks) and a peer-to-peer training (ten weeks).

RELAPSE PREVENTION

Relapse prevention typically involves consolidating gains people have made in their recovery with substance use disorders. It can be provided in both group and individual sessions. Twelve-step and other mutual-aid programs, which include many online options, are often included when thinking about how to construct strong relapse prevention programs.

In a broader sense, relapse prevention can also be applied to mental disorders. Here the emphasis is on maintaining and practicing skills and overall attention to wellness so that relapses can be prevented or caught before they become severe. Specific approaches to relapse prevention include:

- **Avoidance of high-risk situations:** In 12-step lingo, this becomes, "people, places, and things" associated with past substance use behaviors.
- **Strengthening of sober supports:** This can include friends and family, as well as involvement with mutual self-help groups, such as AA and NA.
- **Maintenance of physical and emotional health:** This involves getting adequate sleep, exercise, and good nutrition, and attending to physical and emotional problems.
- **Education** around the risks of relapse and the nature of addictive disorders.
- **Filling the time:** Boredom and too much unstructured time can increase cravings. Part of a recovery plan can be the development of new sober activities, which might include hobbies, social activities, or learning new skills.
- **Avoidance of triggering materials** that show graphic depictions of substance use.

SKILLS TRAINING

CBT helps people understand the connections between dysfunctional emotions, thoughts, and behaviors. And skills training provides the tools to develop healthier ways to manage emotions, relationships, and life's challenges, large and small. Skills training can include broad-based strategies (such as engaging in a daily mindfulness practice and achieving competence at recognizing and reframing distorted thinking) and specific tasks (such as effectively turning down alcohol or drugs in a social setting or using repeated exposure techniques to lessen the anxiety associated with phobias, anxious avoidance, or OCD).

Skills training can be done in group and individual settings and uses an educational model (i.e., something is taught and then practiced). Manualized therapies use skills training as a core component, where a typical session includes discussion of the day's topic and some degree of related psychoeducation followed by the teaching of skills and the assignment of practice homework. Effective skills training typically involves:

- Presentation of information in a way that helps the client understand the task at hand, through readings, focused discussion, and handouts

- In-session practice of new skills

- Assignment of at-home practice to help generalize the skill to the real world

- Homework review to see if the skill is practiced correctly and effectively: "Did you try the new skill? Did it work?"

DBT is a prime example of an evidenced-based therapy that uses skills training (see Chapter 16). DBT breaks down a comprehensive array of skills into four modules: mindfulness, distress tolerance, emotion regulation, and interpersonal effectiveness.

Mutual Self-Help

On the substance misuse side of the co-occurring equation is an established track record for the usefulness of self-help groups, both 12-step and non-12-step. Mutual self-help 12-step groups, such as AA and NA, are the oldest and largest peer-support networks for people with substance use disorders. They have in-person meetings, and now online meetings, across the United States, Canada, and most other countries. For many, 12-step meetings provide the tools necessary to achieve and to maintain sobriety.

It is of prime importance to match the person to a mutual self-help group where they will feel comfortable, supported, and part of a community. A Buddhist recovery group may be ideal for one person, while someone else will feel more at home in an LGBTQ+ group with a 12-step focus. For people with co-occurring substance use and serious and persistent mental disorders, mutual-aid groups, such as Double Trouble in Recovery and Dual Diagnosis 12-step, can provide greater freedom to talk about medications, as well as psychiatric symptoms and syndromes.

The benefits to mutual-aid groups include:

- Sober support

- Sober setting

- No cost (sometimes a donation is requested for coffee and snacks)

- Connection with others who have similar concerns and struggles

- Access to mentors and possibly sponsors with more experience and time in recovery

- Freedom from the power structure of traditional treatment settings, where there is a designated expert/professional

- Validation for efforts in recovery

- Availability

The following section provides several examples of available mutual-aid programs.

Alcoholics Anonymous

Founded in 1935, AA (www.aa.org) is the original 12-step program and has an estimated membership of well over one million in the United States alone. Membership is based solely on a shared desire to stop drinking. Groups are apolitical, peer/nonprofessional run, and free. (Donations may be accepted to keep the meetings self-sufficient and to pay for snacks.)

While the prime focus of AA is abstinence from alcohol, people with other substance use problems are welcome. AA is open to all, and people with co-occurring mental disorders can benefit from the meetings. The 12-steps, which utilize introspection and changing of problem behaviors and patterns of thought, are compatible with other psychotherapies, such as CBT, DBT, and many others.

One potential barrier with AA involves the use of God and giving over control to a "Higher Power." Even the Serenity Prayer, by American theologian Reinhold Niebuhr, which has been adopted by AA, NA, and other 12-step groups, involves the use of a deity. "God grant me the serenity to accept the things I cannot change, the courage to change the things I can, and the wisdom to know the difference."

Another concern with 12-step groups that are focused on alcohol and/or drugs is that individuals with co-occurring mental disorders may experience pushback from other group members about the need for psychiatric medications or maintenance medications, such as methadone or buprenorphine. Both AA and NA have literature that specifically addresses the need for appropriate medication.

AA and NA are both abstinence-based programs. Individuals who do not have total abstinence from alcohol and other psychoactive substances (caffeine and tobacco are excluded) as a goal may find this creates conflict.

In order to be familiar with 12-step programs and their format, it is recommended that all clinicians attend several open meetings.

Narcotics Anonymous

NA (www.na.org) grew out of AA in the 1940s. The program is similar to AA, and the goal is for people who have used substances to come together with a common goal of getting and staying abstinent.

Al-Anon and Nar-Anon

These are 12-step programs to support family and friends of people with substance use disorders. In certain locations, simultaneous AA and Al-anon (or NA and Nar-Anon) meetings are held.

Adult Children of Alcoholics

This 12-step program is geared to help individuals raised in alcoholic and otherwise dysfunctional households to overcome problems rooted in their childhoods. It emphasizes the shedding of passivity and victimhood in pursuit of happy and healthy adult relationships.

Double Trouble in Recovery and Dual Diagnosis Recovery Groups

These 12-step format groups are geared for individuals who have both substance use and significant mental disorders. They are peer run, and while they do not have a national organization, they are frequently hosted/located in mental health clinics or are affiliated with outpatient hospital clinics.

Self-Management and Recovery Training (SMART Recovery)

SMART Recovery is an inclusive and nonreligious program that promotes autonomy and self-management in the face of addictive behaviors. It contrasts with 12-step models that maintain individuals are "helpless" in the face of addiction. The program is founded on Albert Ellis's rational emotive behavioral therapy (REBT), a type of CBT that emphasizes four points:

- Building and maintaining motivation
- Managing cravings and urges to use
- Understanding the connections between thoughts, emotions, and behavior
- Developing a full and balanced life

The SMART recovery website, which includes information and a meeting finder, is: https://www.smartrecovery.org.

Online Groups and Communities

Increasingly, online recovery groups, communities, and apps provide viable and reliable resources for people in recovery. There are both established resources and many new additions. What follows are a few of many:

- **In The Rooms:** The largest global network of online self-help/mutual-support groups—www.InTheRooms.com—this robust and free website asks for minimal information (which is kept confidential) and helps people in recovery find in-person, online, and video meetings 24/7. There are resources and meetings for friends and family, and it is not restricted to 12-step AA/NA-style groups. In addition to self-help/mutual-support resources, the website has searchable links to a broad array of treatment facilities.
- **Mystrength.com:** This app-based and online environment uses CBT and other approaches to help people manage depression, anxiety, chronic pain, insomnia, and substance use problems.
- **Reddit stop drinking group:** This online community is a place where individuals can motivate one another to control or stop their drinking: https://www.reddit.com/r/stopdrinking.
- **Soberistas:** This is a worldwide online community with a focus on women helping other women with their recovery: https://soberistas.com.

CHAPTER 9

....

Wellness and Resilience

Overview: The Pillars of Wellness

Sleep

Nutrition

Exercise

Social Connections and Supportive Relationships

A Sense of Purpose and Meaning

Attention to Acute and Chronic Medical Problems

Resilience

Hygiene and Sanitation

OVERVIEW: THE PILLARS OF WELLNESS

Just as there are strong connections between illness and early death with protracted stress, trauma, and adverse childhood experiences, there is an equally robust literature that demonstrates the benefits of healthful activities, habits, and attitudes. Lumped under the term *wellness* are core lifestyle components that are key to the development and maintenance of full, healthy, and meaningful lives. In effect, the pillars of wellness discussed in this chapter are a kind of owner's manual to healthier and fuller lives. The pillars of wellness include:

- Sleep (enough and of good quality)
- Nutrition
- Supportive relationships (friends, family, coworkers)
- Meaningful activity (work, hobbies, volunteerism)
- Connection(s) to the greater community, including faith communities
- Regular exercise
- Attention to acute and chronic medical problems
- Positive outlook (optimism)
- Hygiene and sanitation

This chapter also discusses resilience, which refers to those skills, attitudes, and circumstances that allow us to manage and overcome adversity and provide clues as to why one person may emerge from tremendous hardship unscathed and even stronger while someone else will be destroyed by it. We've come to learn about the life-shortening impact of recurrent trauma, especially childhood trauma and protracted stress. But there is a silver lining: We can do a lot to change that. And finally, I've included hygiene, which in the wake of the COVID-19 pandemic, we've been reminded that more than any other medical or public health advance has a direct bearing on health and longevity.

SLEEP

Research into the importance of restorative sleep is abundant and has ballooned over the past two decades. Large studies show that inadequate sleep correlates with early death from all causes. Some rather cruel experiments with rodents reveal that we die sooner from a total lack of sleep than from starvation. There are established connections between insufficient sleep and increased risks for Alzheimer's, obesity, hypertension, depression, substance use problems, heart disease, stroke, anxiety, and many other ills. From a clinical perspective, when someone does not get restorative sleep, one of the most important tools for emotional and physical health has been taken off the playing field. And even if the problem with sleep doesn't cause the person's emotional and physical problems, it makes things worse.

As researchers delve into the stages of sleep (non-REM and REM), what emerges is that all are important. Some key functions that occur while we sleep include:

- Memory incorporation and consolidation
- Immune processes, cellular repair, and removal of waste products from the brain, such as amyloid, during deep sleep
- Important anti-inflammatory processes
- Hormone regulation (a broad category that involves a wide range of substances and processes)
- Appetite regulation and glucose metabolism/insulin sensitivity
- Emotion regulation

There is much that clinicians can do to help, and it's important to know when to refer to a sleep specialist, such as with clients who present with symptoms of sleep apnea (i.e., inadequate airflow during sleep).

> **How much sleep is enough?** For most adults, an adequate night's sleep is at least six and a half to eight hours. Most studies of inadequate sleep look at people who habitually get six hours or less. Teens, children, toddlers, and infants require greater amounts.

The brain is the organ that regulates sleep. A basic understanding of the three processes that influence sleep's start and stop will help you strategize ways to help people optimize their sleep quality and quantity:

- **Sleep pressure (Process S):** Throughout the day, a product of metabolic/glucose metabolism accumulates (adenosine). As it does, we experience the need to sleep, which eventually becomes irresistible. As we sleep, adenosine levels fall, and we wake refreshed. Caffeine and other stimulants occupy the receptor adenosine uses. When the caffeine leaves the receptor, adenosine rushes in and we nod off. This is the causative factor in many highway and other accidents.

- **The circadian sleep/wake cycle (Process C):** We have an internal clock that cycles roughly every twenty-four hours. It's set by blue-green light that streams in through our eyeballs to the suprachiasmatic nucleus in the brain and lets us know it's morning. As night falls, this clock signals for the release of the pituitary hormone melatonin, which prepares the brain for sleep.

- **Activation hormones (Process A):** Many chemical messengers, hormones, and neurotransmitters rise and fall over the twenty-four-hour circadian cycle. As night passes, there is a steady increase of substances involved with arousal, most notably adrenaline (epinephrine) and cortisol.

While Americans consume billions of dollars in sleep aids, they are not the first recommendation for insomnia or sleep apneas—the two most common complaints. Especially with chronic use, sedative hypnotics can increase the risk for accidental and fatal overdoses in people with opioid used disorders who also have central sleep apnea.

> **Opioids depress respiration in three ways:** They decrease the number of breaths per minute, and they diminish the body's ability to sense lowered levels of oxygen and elevated levels of carbon dioxide.

What follows are two evidence-based and somewhat overlapping approaches to improve sleep and address insomnia. The first is a sleep hygiene handout containing twelve tips for better sleep, which can be reviewed and given to clients. And the second is a discussion of CBT for Insomnia (CBT-I), which has been shown to be as or more effective than sedatives in promoting sleep, without the side effects and risks.

Twelve Tips for Better Sleep

The following techniques can improve sleep quality and quantity, especially for those with insomnia. While some may help right away, others involve retraining the brain to connect the bed with sleep and may take two weeks or longer to achieve their full benefit.

1. Keep the bed for sleep and intimacy. If you read, watch TV, play video games, or check email and social media in bed, stop it. Your brain has come to associate the bed with things other than sleep. To retrain it, you must connect the bed to sleep and nothing else.

2. Set a regular wake-up time and bedtime. This will set and maintain your internal twenty-four-hour clock (circadian cycle).

3. Avoid caffeine after noon or altogether. Caffeine decreases both sleep quality and quantity. It takes hours to leave the body and should be avoided in people with insomnia.

4. Ditch the tobacco. Nicotine is a stimulant and decreases both sleep quality and quantity.

5. Turn your electronic screens (readers, TVs, smart phones) to nighttime mode after dark. That will block the blue-green light that prevents the release of the hormone melatonin. Consider finding lightbulbs that also do this for the bathroom and lamps you use at night.

6. Make the bedroom a sleep haven. Get a mattress you find supportive and comfortable, have the right pillow for you, and control the noise. Some people like total silence, but others prefer background white noise, such as waves, other nature sounds, and even a dishwasher, and there are many apps that can help.

7. Eliminate disturbances. If your bed partner or pets wake you up at night, address that. While we all love our animals, it may be in everyone's interest to have them sleep outside the bedroom or to train them to not interrupt your sleep.

8. Empty your bladder before bed to decrease unnecessary nighttime waking.

9. Get daily exercise. Among its many benefits, regular exercise increases the amount of a substance (adenosine) that promotes sleep.

10. If you can't fall asleep after twenty minutes, get out of bed and do something dull. Get back into bed when you feel tired and ready to nod off.

11. Avoid alcohol. Alcohol decreases sleep quantity and increases the number of times you'll wake at night. It also damages the natural stages of sleep.

12. Stay cool. Our bodies have a natural dip in temperature when asleep. Keep the bedroom cool and wear minimal bed clothes. Wash your hands and face, or take a bath or shower. The water does not have to be cool to achieve the desired effect.

Cognitive Behavioral Therapy for Insomnia

The American Academy of Sleep Medicine (AASM) and others place cognitive behavioral therapy for insomnia (CBT-I) as the first-line approach to address insomnia. This therapy, which has been manualized, includes three core components:

1. **Stimulus control:** This involves many of the techniques in the previous handout. You want to train the brain to learn that when the head hits the pillow, it's time to fall asleep, and to do that, you need to eliminate all factors that can interfere with sleep.
2. **Sleep restriction:** This technique involves calculating how much time a person is asleep and then only allowing them that much time in bed. If they only get five hours, that's how long they can stay in bed. Once sleep efficiency improves, the duration lengthens in fifteen-minute increments. Note: This is not recommended for people with bipolar disorder.
3. **Stress management and relaxation training:** Specific strategies are taught and practiced to decrease the hormones associated with activation and arousal (adrenaline/epinephrine, cortisol). This may include progressive muscle relaxation, body scans, breathing techniques, scheduled worry time, and many other strategies.

There is an excellent and free app from the VA and Stanford University that contains a wealth of useful skills and techniques: CBT-i Coach. It is meant to be used in conjunction with a professional, and it is available here: https://apps.apple.com/gb/app/cbt-i-coach/id655918660.

It's also important to know when to refer clients to a sleep specialist. The most common reasons will involve sleep apnea, whether obstructive (i.e., the problem results from diminished airflow due to structural issues) or central (i.e., the problem originates in the brain). Signs of apnea may include:

- Heavy snoring
- Gasping or gurgling while asleep
- Frequent awakenings
- Daytime tiredness and nodding off

NUTRITION

Here we hit a few general nutrition topics and then some specific ones that relate to people with mental health and substance use problems. To begin, we must eat. It's the fuel we burn, and the kilocalorie, a unit of heat, is the measurement. On the surface, it's a simple equation: To maintain a stable weight, calories taken in must equal those burned through metabolic processes. The more active the person, the more fuel they need. Should you wish to lose weight, you need to take in fewer calories and burn off more. But other factors, such as hormones, sleep, activity level, mental health, finances, medications, and even cultural influences, have brought Americans to our current overweight and obese predicament. In 2018, obesity rates ranged from 23 percent in Colorado to 39.5 percent in Mississippi and West Virginia. When we add in those who are overweight, the numbers balloon, and roughly two-thirds of Americans weigh too much. Negative health consequences include increased risks for heart disease, hypertension, stroke, cancer, sleep apnea, depression, anxiety, type 2 diabetes, and increased rates of early death from all causes.

While the above statistics are grim, they trend higher for people with serious mental health problems, such as schizophrenia and bipolar disorder, with rates of obesity and overweight at or above 80 percent. This brings greater risks for cardiovascular disease, type 2 diabetes, and hypertension and contribute to the overall lowered life expectancy for people with serious mental illness (between eighteen and twenty-five years). Although sedentary lifestyle and poor nutrition have been proposed as causes for our weight problems, people with mental health issues have to contend with antipsychotic and other psychiatric medications, many of which can cause profound weight gain—on the order of a half-pound to a pound per week.

Metabolic Syndrome

The term *metabolic syndrome* applies to a configuration of connected negative health factors that increase the risk for heart attack and stroke. Rates in the general public run around 23 percent and are substantially higher among those with serious mental illness. The symptoms include:

- High blood sugar (hyperglycemia)
- Insulin resistance and type 2 diabetes
- Elevated lipids (dyslipidemia), most notably cholesterol and low-density lipoproteins (LDL)
- Hypertension
- Obesity, especially truncal or central obesity (belly fat)

While the World Health Organization, American Heart Association, and others provide slightly varied criteria for metabolic syndrome, three or more of the above symptoms is indicative of the condition.

Adult Body Mass Index

Body mass index (BMI) is a simple measurement of a person's weight divided by kilograms. It is often used to screen and to follow weight status. There are many free apps and websites that will calculate BMI, including this one from the CDC: https://www.cdc.gov/healthyweight/assessing/bmi/adult_bmi/english_bmi_calculator/bmi_calculator.html.

BMI is one of many measurements, such as waist circumference and the use of calipers to measure fat, and needs to be interpreted along with other factors. For instance, a muscular individual may have a BMI over 25 but not be considered overweight. And an individual with anorexia who has water loaded to achieve a BMI over 18.5 is still underweight. Maintaining familiarity with BMI is important, as it is used as a DSM-5 criterion for the severity of anorexia and is a monitor for metabolic syndrome.

- 18.5 and below is underweight.
- 18.5 to 24.9 falls within the normal range.
- 25.0 to 29.9 is overweight.
- 30–35 is obese (class 1 obesity).
- 35–40 is obese (class 2 obesity).
- 40 or higher is considered severe or "morbid" obesity (class 3 obesity).

Food Choices

Our food choices and beliefs about what constitutes a healthy diet are diverse and based upon myriad factors. Friends, the internet, health professionals, and talk-show hosts provide a constant stream of information, often based on questionable evidence and pseudoscience. Research on specific diets and nutrients is complicated because of the number of variables involved, such as the many ways a nutrient can be eaten, whether or not it is attached to other molecules, and the complexities of ensuring that your control/placebo group has not inadvertently eaten some of the item being studied.

The truth is, as omnivores, we can process both plant and animal food sources and do well with a caloric intake that matches our daily metabolic needs—about 2500 kcal/day for men and 2000 kcal/day for women—with variations based on size and activity level. It is this daily caloric intake, as well as the habits we and our clients develop, that we can influence. Where so many of us need to be mindful to not overeat and put on unwanted weight, behavioral approaches toward food and activity level provide the greatest degree of evidence for success. An example of one such well-established program would be Weight Watchers. Examples of behavioral interventions might include:

- Identification of high-calorie foods, such as full-sugar sodas, and elimination or replacement with lower calorie options, such as a squirt of fruit juice into unsweetened soda water. We can also cut in half the amount of sugar we add to beverages such as coffee or tea or possibly eliminate it altogether.
- Mindful attention to snack foods in the home. We eat what is close, which could be a bag of chips, a handful of nuts, a piece of fruit, or carrot sticks.
- Portion control
- Creation of daily food habits that balance nutrition, caloric intake, ease, taste, and cost. If meals are planned in advance versus done on the fly or when the diner is famished, there can be greater control over their nutritional and caloric impact.

Hunger for Food and its Relationship to Drug Cravings

There are numerous similarities in the physiological pathways (dopamine/meso-limbic system) involved in hunger and cravings for food and those found with substances that provide pleasurable responses. The release of endogenous opioids and dopamine, which we experience as pleasure, serve important survival functions because they ensure that we eat and procreate. They also play a role in our need/hunger for social interaction. However, these same mechanisms also drive cravings for drugs and play a role in disordered and compulsive eating patterns.

Our experiences and memories of pleasure with sex, food, and drugs play important roles in the generation of future cravings. We want what feels good. However, we often find a decrease in the positive experience with repeated use. So, while the craving/hunger persists and returns, it does not get satisfied or fully satisfied. This is likely one mechanism that contributes to increased substance use with less effect (tolerance). Brain imaging studies in people with obesity and substance use disorders show similar patterns of decreased dopamine receptors in key portions of the brain.

Clinically, the connections between substances of misuse and hunger/craving can become a focus of treatment. A 12-step aphorism for things that can precipitate a lapse—HALT (hungry, angry, lonely, tired)—is supported by good experimental data. The reward system is also a target of certain medications used in the treatment of substance use disorders, most notably naltrexone and acamprosate. In cognitive behavioral models, the identification of cravings, coupled with targeted interventions and skills, can help a person acknowledge the hunger, learn how to lessen or appease it, and not act on it in a compulsive way. Strategies to manage cravings can include:

- Education about the relationship between the compulsive behavior or substance use and the brain's reward system
- Distraction techniques
    - Calling a friend, sober support, sponsor, or family member
    - Reading or watching a movie or TV show
    - Taking the dog for a walk
- Healthful snacks that will damp down hunger: "Eat a granola bar when you think about having a drink. See if that doesn't lessen the craving."
- Exercise

EXERCISE

The benefits of regular exercise (physical activity) have been found in many studies. While we associate exercise with weight loss, it appears to provide only a modest benefit of a few pounds unless it's of great intensity and duration (i.e., more than 225 minutes/week). The true payoffs lie in decreased heart disease, better respiratory function, improvements in depression and anxiety, better sleep, and overall better function and quality of life. Even in obese individuals, exercise appears to lower risks that come with the weight.

While physical activity has strong associations with better overall health but only minimal-to-moderate weight loss, it can diminish or prevent weight gain. This is an important point for people on medications that carry risks for weight gain and metabolic syndrome. Individuals who don't get enough physical activity increase their risks for obesity, sleep apnea, diabetes, coronary artery disease, and many other negative health outcomes.

So how much exercise do we need? While expert opinions vary, here are some guidelines:

- The American College of Sports Medicine recommends 150–250 minutes per week of moderate to vigorous physical activity.
- The American Heart Association recommends 150 minutes per week of moderate exercise or 75 minutes per week of vigorous exercise.
- The CDC recommends the following:
  o Children and adolescents should get 60 minutes/day of moderate to vigorous physical activity.
  o Adults should get 150–300 minutes/week of moderate-intensity physical activity or 75–150 minutes/week of vigorous-intensity aerobic activity.
  o There are specific recommendations regarding the type of physical activity a person gets, along with recommendations for older individuals and those with chronic health conditions. The guidelines are available online at: https://health.gov/paguidelines/second-edition/pdf/Physical_Activity_Guidelines_2nd_edition.pdf

---

What's the difference between moderate and vigorous exercise?

Moderate exercise increases heart and respiration rates, but you're still able to carry on a conversation and not become winded. Examples include brisk walks, bicycling or roller skating/blading on level ground, Vinyasa yoga, gardening, and mowing the lawn.

Vigorous exercise leads to greater elevations in pulse and respiration. While you can still carry on a conversation, you'll need to pause to catch your breath. Examples include running, jogging, biking uphill, basketball, swimming laps, and aerobics.

General recommendations for you and your clients:

- First, ensure that a person's health status is adequate for any recommended regimen. A general health assessment by the person's primary care medical provider—such as an MD/DO, APRN, or physician assistant—is a good idea.

- Pick activities that the person enjoys and will maintain. Make it fun.
  - What have they tried in the past and liked?
  - What have they wanted to try but haven't yet done?
  - Is this someone who will use a gym, or would they be better served setting up a home regimen or some combination of the two?

- Assess resources.
  - Are there low-cost or no-cost options in the community, such as yoga classes at a senior center or programs through a town's recreation department? Low-cost or even scholarship options through the local YMCA/YWCA?
  - What can they afford in terms of gym memberships, workout tapes, apps, equipment, and so forth?

- Increase how much you walk. Pedometers, which are devices that count our steps, can be a fun and useful way to increase activity. Less than 5,000 steps/day is associated with a sedentary lifestyle, and health benefits are found at 10,000 steps/day or more.

- Get a workout buddy. For some, combined physical activity and social interaction can provide a wellness twofer. Classes, scheduled jogs or walks with a friend, or the camaraderie that can be found in a supportive health club carry not only the expected health benefits from the physical activity but also from the positive interaction.

SOCIAL CONNECTIONS AND SUPPORTIVE RELATIONSHIPS

The quality and, to a lesser extent, quantity of key relationships in our lives have profound emotional and health implications. This starts in childhood with our coaches, teachers, parents, and other important family members, and it extends to our peer relations at school and play and onto our work relationships with colleagues and supervisors. During adolescence and through adulthood, the development of intimate connections and the establishment of marriage and marriage-type affiliations greatly impact all dimensions of our existence, happiness, and even life expectancy. Groups with whom we affiliate, co-workers, bosses, peers, faith-based groups, and others help us set behavioral norms that can promote or damage our emotional and physical well-being. The 12-step aphorism of "people, places, and things" is a reminder of the often insurmountable challenge to change drug behavior when surrounded by people who actively use and encourage others to do so: "You were more fun when you drank. You're not really an alcoholic."

There is an extensive and diverse literature on how we are shaped by our relationships and by the strength and nature of our attachment to important people in our lives. Key indicators often center around social isolation versus connection, support, and high strain/conflict. The links between our social relationships and various outcomes can then be divided into three broad and interconnected categories:

1. **How relationships impact behavior**

   From birth to death, we modify our behavior to coexist with those around us, from early parent-child training to peer affiliations to following the dress and conduct code at work. If we are surrounded by people who smoke, we're more likely to do so. If there's a push at work to reward everyone who gets in 10,000 steps a day and free pedometers are distributed, there's an increased likelihood that we'll join in. Intimate/marriage partners influence our every move, including what we eat, whether we get medical and dental follow up, how much exercise we get, and our drug-, alcohol-, and tobacco-related behaviors.

2. **How relationships impact emotional health**

   Throughout our lives, our emotional well-being is linked to our major relationships. Serious disruptions in the parent-child bond are associated with mental health problems throughout the life cycle—most notably anxiety and mood disorders—and influence our choices in future bonds.

   Intimate relationships can be sources of tremendous emotional support, joy, and nurturance, or they can spiral into discordant and damaging patterns of unresolved conflict, coercion, control, and domestic violence. Is the home a sanctuary or a fretful environment where one must walk on eggshells to maintain the peace? In addition, the loss of a spouse or partner through death or divorce is a major, and at times insurmountable, source of grief and depression.

   In multiple studies, American workers identify work as the major source of stress in their lives. It's no coincidence that the most important positive or negative factors that affect the workplace are how you get along with your boss and your colleagues. Positive and mutually supportive relationships make the workday fly by. But conflictual ones, which might include issues of bullying, coercion, sexual harassment, or discrimination, lead to sleepless nights and anxiety-riddled days. Our reliance on the day job for finances, health care, meaning, and personal growth often keeps people tied to positions where they become burned out, depressed, or even traumatized.

3. **How relationships impact physical health**

   The physiology and health consequences of our relationships have been studied for decades in both humans and animals. Perhaps the most important finding is the association between how long we live and the quality and duration of our significant relationships. In one meta-analysis, based on 148 studies and data from over 300,000 people, a 50 percent increased mortality risk was found for those with a combination of poor social relations and support, such as isolation and integration. When this data was broken down further, an even higher risk was assigned to those with low social support and poor social integration. To put this into context, this risk is similar to, and in the latter two instances greater than, the risk associated with cigarette smoking.

As in the two previous sections, this important thread carries across the lifecycle. Health indicators that correlate with the quality of our social relationships include blood pressure/hypertension, risk for obesity (BMI and waist circumference), and early death. Specific biomarkers include changes in the inflammatory process and elevations in markers and conditions associated with protracted stress, such as elevations in cortisol and epinephrine (stress hormones).

As you read through the previous paragraphs, it's easy to see how our relationships at work, home, and play impact everything: from what we have for supper to how long we live or whether or not we have that next drink, shot of fentanyl, or cigarette. Attention to healthy and supportive relationships, including the therapeutic one, can have a dramatic impact on your clients' progress in the direction of their goals. Specific interventions might include:

- Developing goals and priorities around important relationships or lack thereof in your client's life and developing ways to build and improve them

  Client: "I want to have friends who don't do drugs."

  Clinician: "Fabulous goal. Let's explore a couple of things you can do to make that happen."

- Early and ongoing identification of people in your client's life who support them in recovery
- Group or individual work that includes identified supports
  - "You mentioned your dad has been a big support. Would you be comfortable inviting him in for a session?"
  - "We do a Tuesday 'friends and family' group. There's pizza. What about coming with your friend Dennis?"
- Weaving in outside supports into structured daily interventions
  - Scheduled calls with sober supports, especially during high-risk times for use, such as evenings and weekends
  - Faith-based, community, or recreational activities
- Peer support groups, both in-person and online

A Sense of Purpose and Meaning

Over the years, my patients have helped me add to the 12-step aphorism about relapse—HALT (hungry, angry, lonely, tired). Two additions to keep in mind are pain (both physical and emotional) and boredom. The latter kicks off this discussion about a sense of meaning. What gives our days and lives purpose, importance, and direction?

While the term *meaning* can seem vague, it encompasses three broad and interdependent concepts:

1. **Purpose:** We establish goals and priorities and work toward and with them.
2. **Cognition:** We believe that our lives make sense.
3. **Significance:** What we do and how we do it matters.

Surveys indicate that there is a gender split between what women versus men identify as the major source of meaning in their lives. On average, more women report relationships and family as their greatest priority, while more men point to work and their careers. Keep in mind these are generalizations based on large surveys and there is variability.

Regardless of what someone identifies as their major source(s) of meaning and importance, it's easy to see how significant disruptions, disappointments, and failures in these areas come with a cost and how success, achievement, and acknowledgment of one's priorities bring a payoff. There is good evidence to show that people who maintain a sense of purpose and accomplishment are healthier, happier, and live longer. This literature has grown in the past decade and is supported by multiple studies that show improved psychological and physical health among those with a greater sense of meaning in their lives.

From a clinical stance, meaning, priorities, and a sense of purpose carry weight when helping someone move forward in recovery. Indeed, they provide the rudders for treatment: "What is it that matters to you?" and "What is it you'd like to achieve moving forward?"

For clinicians and other helpers, it's important to remember that these goals and priorities must be the client's. While you might believe that getting the heroin and fentanyl use under control is the most important thing, they may not. And for them, stable housing or a job is their top priority. It may be that having a job and a place to come home to will allow them to finally work on the heroin. After all, it's hard to work nine-to-five if you're nodding off at the computer. The "Your Goals and Priorities" handout in Chapter 5 can be used to help your clients articulate what most matters to them.

ATTENTION TO ACUTE AND CHRONIC MEDICAL PROBLEMS

Our emotional stability and resolve to resist urges to misuse substances can unravel when we are sick or in pain. Indeed, much of our current opioid epidemic stems from the over-prescription and overpromotion of opioid pain medications for myriad chronic conditions. For most of us, all we need to do is think about a time when we were sick or in pain to realize the truth in the aphorism "If you don't have your health, you don't have anything."

As we look at wellness and whole-person approaches to treatment, physical health cannot be ignored. Problems left unaddressed and unattended can quickly turn from a minor annoyance to the cause of disability and even death. While we'll cover specific serious health concerns related to intravenous drug use, certain medications, and other substances throughout this book, a few points to consider include:

- Once a health issue is identified, it must be addressed. Even though you or your agency might not provide medical or specialty health care, referral to an appropriate provider is essential. While this is just good care, it's also covered in regulatory standards, such as those seen with the Joint Commission and with State Departments of Public Health.

- All clients should have a primary care provider or identified clinic. Ideally, they will have a provider they trust and feel heard by.

- Up-to-date releases of information should be obtained and maintained for the person's health care provider(s) to allow for communication.

RESILIENCE

Clear connections between trauma, childhood trauma, and negative physical and psychological problems have been drawn. When faced with data related to high adverse childhood experiences, or ACEs, we see myriad negative outcomes that range from elevated levels of obesity, heart disease, hypertension, and even cancer to high levels of anxiety, depression, substance misuse, and suicidality. But as this information has rolled in, important questions have emerged. Why do two people go through the same experience, but one is destroyed by it, and the other recovers and may even thrive? What factors allow us to weather both the daily and extraordinary stressors that come with life? Just as important—are there skills, attitudes, circumstances, and other factors that promote recovery?

While there is variability in how it's defined, *resilience* refers to a person's ability to both make it through the daily grind and recover from adversity. The literature that has emerged provides a positive counterpoint to what we've learned about trauma. Studies into what promotes resilience have come up with the following factors:

- Positive outlook (optimism), including humor, even in the face of adversity
- Supportive relationships and positive role models
- Meaning and a sense of purpose
- Hope or an unswerving belief that things will improve
- Physical health, wellness, and strength
- Flexibility and adaptability (i.e., being able to let get go of one set of plans and shift to another)
- Spirituality (may or may not be based in a particular religion)

HYGIENE AND SANITATION

Human life expectancy has nearly doubled since the early nineteenth century. This has more to do with advances in sanitation and personal hygiene, less-crowded housing, improved prenatal and perinatal care, education, and personal hygiene—indoor plumbing in particular—than with any medical discoveries. In 1840, the average person lived to their mid-forties, and in 2020, the average lifespan is over age seventy—and depending on which country you live in, can be well into the eighties.

In 2020, the COVID-19 pandemic hit, and amid great uncertainty, the interventions that decreased the rate of transmission of the virus were those that focused on hygiene and physical distance. Hand washing for at least twenty seconds, using hand sanitizers, cleaning potentially contaminated surfaces, wearing masks, and keeping six feet apart when in public were commonsense and effective public health strategies to slow the spread of the disease.

COVID is a reminder that we live surrounded by microbes—bacteria, viruses, and fungi. For the most part, our relationships with these microscopic entities is benign and even symbiotic. For instance, without the billions of bacteria that live in our gastrointestinal systems, we'd be unable to digest much of our food.

What maintains this generally healthful relationship is our immune system. When this becomes weakened, our defenses against potential invaders is diminished. This underscores the importance of other wellness strategies mentioned in this chapter, such as sleep, exercise, and proper nutrition, all of which promote maximum immune function.

But even before we need to call on our immune system, we can do much more. For instance, the surface of our skin is covered with microbes. For the most part, these won't bother us, but when the surface of our skin is broken, whether from a cut, splinter, or the use of intravenous drugs, we risk the introduction of these potential pathogens into the skin/dermis, muscle, bone, and blood. The results can be mild, such as we see with acne caused by staphylococcus, to catastrophic, from abscesses, cellulitis, and bone and muscle infections to sepsis, heart failure, and death.

We know the hygiene basics, but the key is to double down and ensure that they're incorporated into our daily habits:

- Wash your hands frequently, especially after being out in public and after going to the bathroom.
- Keep hand sanitizer in your vehicle and purse/briefcase.
- Make hand sanitizer available in your office and other public places.
- Shower or bathe daily if possible.
- Brush your teeth at least twice/day, floss, and use an antimicrobial mouthwash.
- If you are ill, seek medical care as needed and stay home. This is to protect others and decrease transmission.

MENTAL DISORDERS, THEIR PRESENTATION(S), AND TREATMENT APPROACHES WITH CO-OCCURRING SUBSTANCE USE DISORDERS

CHAPTER 10

Co-Occurring Attention-Deficit/Hyperactivity Disorder and Related Disorders

OVERVIEW

Attention-deficit/hyperactivity disorder (ADHD), a persistent problem with attention and focus often accompanied by hyperactivity and impulsive behavior, is associated with significant impairment in a child's development and achievement in school, in social settings, and at home. Once thought to be rare in adults, multiple studies show that it persists from childhood in as many as 75 percent of adolescents and 50 percent of adults.

It is estimated that between 5 percent and 9 percent of children and 2.5 percent to 5 percent of adults meet criteria for ADHD (4.4 percent in the National Comorbidity Survey).

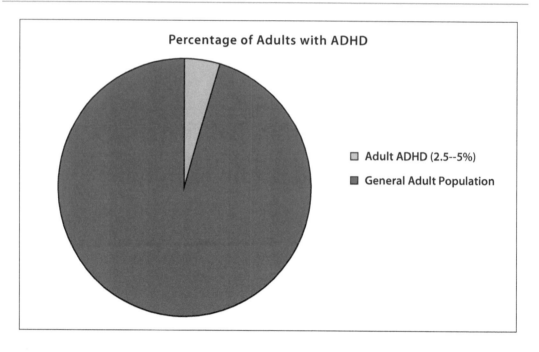

The relationship between ADHD and substance use disorders is well established. Studies that have looked at the overlap between these disorders have found that between 10 percent and 24 percent of adults with ADHD will also have at least one non-tobacco substance use disorder. And the overall risk for developing any substance use disorder is 2.5 times more than the general population.

In addition to the relationships between ADHD and substance use disorder are the findings that oppositional defiant disorder and conduct disorder are linked as well. The latter, which involves disregard for rules and the rights and feelings of others, is considered the child and adolescent precursor to adult antisocial personality disorder.

Conduct disorder carries a high lifetime co-occurrence with all substance use disorders. Studies that looked at individuals with conduct disorder, ADHD, and substance use disorder found the link between conduct disorder and substance use disorder to be greater than the link between ADHD and substance use disorder. Some researchers have proposed a model whereby ADHD leads to conduct disorder, which in turn greatly increases the risk of developing substance use disorders.

ADHD, frequently first diagnosed in childhood, is somewhat unique among co-occurring disorders. In many instances, the mental disorder preceded the substance use disorder. Therefore, a diagnosis of ADHD in a child or adolescent can be considered a significant risk factor for the development of one or more substance use disorders. In individuals who also meet criteria for conduct disorder, this risk increases as much as threefold.

For parents and those who work with children and adolescents, diagnoses of ADHD, oppositional defiant disorder, and conduct disorder should be warning flags to assess for the presence of substance use problems and to begin early interventions to prevent their development.

Children and adolescents with ADHD begin substance use at a younger age and progress more rapidly to misuse and dependence. Substance use findings among children, adolescents, and adults with ADHD include:

- As many as 50 percent of adolescents with substance use disorders will meet criteria for ADHD.
- Children with ADHD are three times more likely to have a nicotine use disorder in adolescence.
- Childhood ADHD is linked to alcohol and drug use disorders in adults. They are:
  - Twice as likely to develop a cocaine use disorder
  - 1.5 times more likely to develop a cannabis use disorder
  - Almost twice as likely to develop an alcohol use disorder
- Earlier onset and greater severity of substance use disorders are seen in adults with ADHD.
- Adults with ADHD are less likely to stop smoking.
- ADHD is associated with early onset of cigarette smoking (under age fifteen), which in turn is associated with other substance use disorders.

Because of the connections between ADHD and substance use disorders, and the persistence of symptoms into adulthood, it is important to screen for ADHD in people who seek treatment for substance problems. This is especially true for women, who more often have the inattentive symptoms as children and adolescents and are less frequently given the diagnosis.

Studies that have assessed the presence of co-occurring ADHD in adults with substance use disorders find consistently high rates that range between 15 percent and 35 percent. This contrasts sharply with the number of people in those same studies (less than 5 percent) who had been previously diagnosed with ADHD as children. This disparity underscores the importance of assessing ADHD symptoms in adults with substance use disorders.

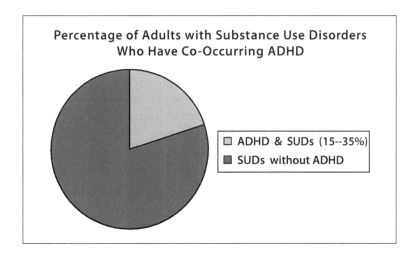

Among individuals with co-occurring substance use disorders and ADHD, preferred substances include cannabis, cocaine, stimulants, alcohol, opioids, and tobacco.

ADHD, Substance Use Disorders, and Co-Occurring Mental Disorders

While the overlap between ADHD, substance use disorders, and other "externalizing" disorders—such as oppositional defiant disorder and conduct disorder—is robust, it's important to note that other psychiatric disorders—such as depression, bipolar disorder, PTSD, personality disorders (antisocial and borderline, in particular), and anxiety disorders—commonly coexist in people who have both ADHD and substance use disorders.

There are significant implications for treatment and prognosis with people who have multiple psychiatric disorders. They are prone to greater disability and severity of substance use problems, and the complexity of their symptoms can complicate and confuse diagnoses.

- Is the hyperactivity and inability to sit still from their ADHD?
- Are they hypomanic or manic?
- Is the individual's current state a symptom of opioid withdrawal? Stimulant intoxication?

As with all co-occurring disorders, the presence of multiple psychiatric disorders needs to be addressed, and diagnostic confusion can be clarified over the course of treatment.

Assessment of ADHD

Children and Adolescents

The assessment and diagnosis of ADHD in children and adolescents includes multiple sources of information: parents, teachers, and possibly other clinicians, such as a school psychologist, social worker, or nurse. Where there is a strong hereditary or genetic component to ADHD, the presence of the disorder in other close family members (parents and siblings in particular) should be explored.

In the DSM-5, symptoms must have been present for at least six months and be accompanied by six or more inattentive and/or hyperactive/impulsive symptoms. Several of these symptoms must have been present before the age of twelve (in the earlier DSM-IV-TR, this was age seven), the symptoms must occur and cause impairment or disrupt multiple aspects of the individual's life (school, home, sports, recreation, friendships), and finally, the symptoms must not be the result of some other medical condition, mental disorder, medications, drugs, or alcohol.

Combined with direct observation and clinical assessment, standardized questionnaires and screening tools completed by parents, teachers, and possibly clinicians and the child are the mainstays of making the diagnosis of ADHD in children and adolescents. Commonly used screening tools and questionnaires for children and adolescents include:

- Attention Deficit Disorders Evaluation Scale (ADDES-3)
- ADHD Rating Scale-IV
- SNAP-IV Rating Scale (available in its entirety on the American Psychiatric Association's website: www.psychiatry.org/practice/dsm/dsm5/online-assessment-measures#Level2)
- Conners' Rating Scale

Adults

Assessing ADHD in adults with co-occurring substance use disorders, and possibly other mental disorders as well, presents challenges. It is important to differentiate signs and symptoms that might be associated with active drug use and/or withdrawal and intoxication syndromes from the inattention, impulsivity, and fidgeting seen with ADHD. Similarly, symptoms such as hyperactivity, easy distractibility, and inattention are found in other mental disorders, such as bipolar spectrum disorders. Certain medical conditions, such as hyperthyroidism, can also mimic ADHD. Keys to better assess ADHD in adults include the following:

- Ask questions regarding symptom history:
  - Does the person have a prior childhood diagnosis of ADHD? And what was this based on?
  - If there's not a prior diagnosis, is there evidence that symptoms of ADHD were present before age twelve? (DSM-5 criteria)
  - Is there a family history of ADHD?
  - Does the person display the requisite number (at least five for adults) of hyperactive/impulsive and/or inattentive symptoms as specified in the DSM-5? And have they persisted since childhood?
- Gather multiple sources of information. Just as multiple informants are helpful in the assessment of children and adolescents, a parent, significant other, and/or clinician who knows the individual can provide their observations and aid in the evaluation.
- Rule out potential medical causes for the observed symptoms.
- Use screening tools. As with children and adolescents, the use of screening tools in adults, while not diagnostic, adds important information. When used as part of an intake process, they can also help flag previously undiagnosed cases of ADHD. Screening tools for adults include:
  - Conners' Adult ADHD Rating Scales-LV (CAARS): A sixty-six-item self-report and observer scale that uses 0–4 Likert ratings. A score greater than 65 is suggestive of ADHD.

o Brown Attention Deficit Disorder Scale (BADDS): Developed by Dr. Thomas Brown, a variety of age-specific scales are available. A forty-item scale for adults and adolescents uses 0–4 Likert ratings. A score greater than 50 is suggestive of ADHD.

o Wender Utah Rating Scale for ADHD: This sixty-one-item Likert-based scale assesses ADHD symptoms in adults based on the individual's ability to recollect what symptoms were present during childhood.

o Adult ADHD Self-Report Scale (ASRS-v1.1): An eighteen-item questionnaire completed by the patient. It is copyrighted by the World Health Organization and is reprinted here in its entirety. It takes approximately five minutes to complete. The first six items (Part A) can be used as a brief screening tool. It is not meant to be diagnostic but can bring to attention the potential for ADHD. Any four of the six items marked off in the shaded boxes on the form are suggestive of ADHD. There are no scores assigned to part B, but items checked off in the shaded boxes should prompt further investigation for the presence of ADHD.

Adult ADHD Self-Report Scale (ASRS-v1.1) Symptom Checklist

Patient name	Today's date				
Please answer the questions below, rating yourself on each of the criteria shown using the scale on the right side of the page. As you answer each question, place an X in the box that best describes how you have felt and conducted yourself over the past 6 months. Please give this completed checklist to your health care professional to discuss during today's appointment.	Never	Rarely	Sometimes	Often	Very Often
1. How often do you have trouble wrapping up the final details of a project once the challenging parts have been done?					
2. How often do you have difficulty getting things in order when you have to do a task that requires organization?					
3. How often do you have problems remembering appointments or obligations?					
4. When you have a task that requires a lot of thought, how often do you avoid or delay getting started?					
5. How often do you fidget or squirm with your hands or feet when you have to sit down for a long time?					
6. How often do you feel overly active and compelled to do things, like you were driven by a motor?					
7. How often do you make careless mistakes when you have to work on a boring or difficult project?					
8. How often do you have difficulty keeping your attention when you are doing boring or repetitive work?					

9. How often do you have difficulty concentrating on what people say to you even when they are speaking to you directly?					
10. How often do you misplace or have difficulty finding things at home or at work?					
11. How often are you distracted by activity or noise around you?					
12. How often do you leave your seat in meetings or other situations in which you are expected to remain seated?					
13. How often do you feel restless or fidgety?					
14. How often do you have difficulty unwinding and relaxing when you have time to yourself?					
15. How often do you find yourself talking too much when you are in social situations?					
16. When you're in a conversation, how often do you find yourself finishing the sentences of the people you are talking to, before they can finish themselves?					
17. How often do you have difficulty waiting your turn in situations when turn taking is required?					
18. How often do you interrupt others when they are busy?					

©2003 World Health Organization (WHO)
Reference: Kessler, R. C., Adler, L., Ames, M., Demler, O., Faraone, S., Hiripi, E., Howes, M. J., Jin, R., Secnik, K., Spencer, T., Ustun, T. B., & Walters, E. E. (2005). The World Health Organization Adult ADHD Self-Report Scale (ASRS). *Psychological Medicine*, 35(2), 245–256.

TREATMENT OF CO-OCCURRING SUBSTANCE USE DISORDERS AND ADHD

Effective treatment-and-recovery plans for people with co-occurring substance use disorders and ADHD may require both sequential and integrated treatment. While there are limited studies that examine co-occurring treatment for substance use disorders and ADHD, research and clinical experience offer the following guidelines:

1. Acute and active substance use and/or withdrawal states will need to be addressed first. This makes sense both from a diagnostic and a treatment perspective because when a person is actively using or in a state of withdrawal, it is unclear what symptoms are caused by intoxication, withdrawal, or the ADHD.

2. Psychosocial treatments such as CBT have been shown to be of benefit for both ADHD and substance use disorders. Results are more uniformly positive in adults than in children.

3. Psychopharmacology might include medications to address ADHD, as well as medications to treat specific substance use disorders.

PSYCHOSOCIAL TREATMENTS FOR ADHD

There are no well-controlled studies that look at particular therapies in adolescents and adults with co-occurring substance use disorders and ADHD. Clinicians need to look at what has been found to be effective for ADHD and incorporate it into the person's overall treatment. The evidence supports the use of behavioral therapies and CBT in children, adolescents, and adults with ADHD. As with all CBT, success hinges on the client's willingness to participate, both in session and through homework completion and practice. This is how they will develop the skills and generalize them into their daily lives. Areas of focus will include:

- Skills training
  - o Time management
  - o Organization
  - o Prioritization
  - o Breaking down tasks into small, manageable components
  - o Identification of problems with task initiation and low motivation
  - o Interpersonal skills training and communication skills
- Cognitive training to address distorted patterns of thought, especially negative self-talk the individual has about their capabilities to stay on task and to be successful. Emphasis is put on identifying and working with impulsive urges and behaviors. This is to develop long-range goals versus immediate gratification, such as the misuse of drugs and alcohol.

Medications for ADHD

FDA-approved medications for the treatment of ADHD include the following:

1. **Psychostimulants:** These are the first-line treatment for ADHD. They are effective in managing symptoms in children, adolescents, and adults. However, these medications include risks for misuse, diversion, and dependence, and a black box warning was recently added to all stimulants regarding the risk of sudden cardiac death.

    All stimulants can cause insomnia, increase blood pressure and heart rate, and decrease appetite. Prior to starting one of these medications, a medical history and physical examination, likely including an ECG, should be conducted, especially if there is a history, or a family history, of heart disease.

    Other common side effects and adverse effects include increased energy and behavioral and emotional changes that can include anxiety, mania, depression, paranoia, and other psychotic symptoms. Available stimulants include the following:

    a. Methylphenidate hydrochloride

        i. Ritalin and Ritalin SR (sustained release tablets)

        ii. Concerta (extended/osmotic-release tablets)

        iii. Metadate CD (extended release capsules)

        iv. Daytrana (a patch)

        v. Methylin (liquid solution and chewable tablets)

    b. Mixed amphetamine salts

        i. Adderall, Adderall extended release

    c. Lisdexamfetamine dimesylate (Vyvanse)

    d. Methamphetamine hydrochloride

        i. Desoxyn

    e. Dexmethylphenidate

        i. Focalin, Focalin extended release

    f. Dextroamphetamine sulfate

        i. Dexedrine

2. **Nonstimulant medications for ADHD**

    a. Atomoxetine (Strattera): Similar in structure to some of the older antidepressants, which act on the neurotransmitters serotonin and norepinephrine, atomoxetine is an FDA-approved medication for the treatment of ADHD in children, adolescents, and adults. It is often tried as an alternative to stimulant medication and might be considered with someone who has a history of stimulant misuse.

    b. Bupropion (Wellbutrin): This antidepressant medication is used to treat ADHD but is contraindicated in individuals with a history of seizure disorder and those with significant eating disorders. It is not FDA-approved for ADHD, so it would be considered off-label.

   c. Guanfacine: Initially a medication for blood pressure (alpha-blocker), it is FDA-approved for the treatment of ADHD in children ages six to seventeen.

      i. Tenex

      ii. Intuniv (extended release form)

   d. Tricyclic antidepressants: Even though they do not carry the FDA indication for ADHD, there is a literature to support the off-label use of some of the older tricyclic antidepressants (desipramine and nortriptyline), which inhibit the reuptake of both serotonin and norepinephrine. These medications do not carry significant misuse potential, but they are associated with significant cardiac side effects and can be fatal in overdoses. An ECG should be obtained prior to starting one of these medications and again when the stable dose is achieved.

MISUSE AND DIVERSION OF STIMULANT MEDICATIONS

Stimulant medications, such as amphetamines (Adderall, Dexedrine) and methylphenidate (Ritalin), are often used for their euphoric effects and are a favorite among high school and college students when pulling "all-nighters." They can be misused by people who want to lose weight, as well as those with eating disorders who take them for their appetite-suppressant and weight-loss side effects. Others, such as long-distance truck drivers, have been known to use psychostimulants to ward off fatigue. Because of their euphoric properties, these medications have significant "street value" and can be sold or traded. Some will combine them with other substances, such as alcohol, opioids, or other sedatives, to achieve particular highs.

Concerns about misuse and diversion of stimulant medication, both in minors and adults, need to be addressed. The risk of misuse and diversion increases further if there is a history of oppositional defiant disorder, conduct disorder, and/or antisocial personality disorder.

Strategies to decrease misuse include the following:

1. Use long-acting versus immediate-release stimulants. These carry less of a euphoric effect and are less readily snorted or injected. Transdermal (via the skin) preparations of methylphenidate also carry a lower likelihood for misuse.

2. Drug screens can help verify that a person is in fact taking the medication.

3. When prescribing stimulants to children and/or adolescents, be aware of other family members who might divert the medication. Children and adolescents should have a responsible parent or guardian oversee their medication and keep it secure.

4. For children and adolescents who take medication at school, it should be overseen by the school nurse (which is the law in most states).

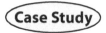

Jayna Carver

Jayna is a nineteen-year-old single woman and college sophomore who is self-referred to the university mental health center for long-standing problems with focus and attention. "As a kid, they just passed me through school, but most of the time I spaced out. It hasn't gotten better. I'm smart, but you'd never know it. I need to be on meds."

Jayna describes how, as a child in elementary school, she was often reprimanded for inattention. "But because my grades were okay, nothing happened. And in high school, if a course had homework, I'd drop down a level to where I didn't have to do any. A couple times, my parents got called in. I know the school counselors recommended I get evaluated for ADHD, but my dad was dead set against anything having to do with meds."

Things worsened her first year at college. "It's a miracle they didn't kick me out." Her first semester, she was enrolled for sixteen credits (full time) but only completed half her courses. "I was on academic probation for a semester and somehow managed to pull it off. But I have to do better if I'm going to make it into a nursing program. The financial aid office told me I need to get a 2.0 or better to keep my package." Her career goal is to become a nurse practitioner (APRN). "I'd like to work with kids."

When asked about her freshman-year performance, she admits it was a struggle to make it to her morning classes, "I'm not an early bird, and they were all nine o'clock classes." But she adds, "I also partied more than I should have. I've got to keep that to just the weekends. I will for a little bit, and then…" At present she states she'll go out with friends to dorm, house, and dance parties, or to bars off campus two to four times a week and "sometimes more." "I can't remember the last time I paid for a drink, and I don't really get wasted the way I used to. "Everybody knows which places card and which don't."

She quantifies her alcohol consumption as zero on nights she stays in and anywhere from between "a few beers and maybe a couple shots" to "a lot more on the weekends." She does not believe she is a problem drinker, but if she's not careful, it could become an issue. "I know when to cut myself off… usually, and I never drive if I'm drunk." She has tried marijuana. "I'm not a pothead or anything, but if someone has a joint, I'll take a few hits." She denies current or past use of opioids or anxiolytics. "I've tried Molly and Ecstasy—not for me. I can't stand being out of control." She has tried stimulant medication given to her by friends, both methylphenidate (Ritalin and other brands) and amphetamine salts (Adderall, Vyvanse, and other brands). "I think that's what I need. I can focus when I take that stuff." She frequently asks her friends for some of their ADHD medication on days she has tests or to help her study. On two occasions, she's purchased it illegally. "I'm scared to do that, because you never know what you're actually getting." She does not smoke cigarettes or vape.

Jayna is the oldest of two in an intact family. Her father works for the Department of Transportation as a road-crew supervisor, and her mother is an ICU nurse. Her younger brother is a high school junior who excels in athletics. She describes a mostly positive childhood. "My parents never fought around us, but there were times you could tell they had problems." She has never witnessed domestic violence or been sexually assaulted. "I had a bad experience with a boyfriend in high school who'd try to get me drunk and do stuff. Once I figured what he was up to, I ditched him." She is not currently in a significant relationship and identifies as heterosexual.

She has no prior history of mental health or substance use treatment and is unaware of any family history of emotional or substance problems. "My dad drinks too much, but it's not every night, and he's a happy drunk—falls asleep in front of the TV, snores like a log. It annoys the hell out of my mom, but mostly she doesn't say anything." She describes how, as a high school junior and senior, she'd go to parties where alcohol was served. "We all knew who the cool parents were." And on several occasions, she'd have an older cousin purchase alcohol for her and her friends. "You can't always be the moocher." She denies any history of blackouts.

On mental status, she is articulate, humorous, and poised. Her speech is fluent and not pressured. She admits to mild anxiety, largely related to school performance. She has no depressive symptoms and is future focused. She has no evidence of psychosis or imminent risks for self-harm or harm to others. A self-report screen for depression (the PHQ-9) is negative, as is one for trauma. She scores a 3 out of 4 on the CAGE-AID questionnaire.

She has no active medical problems and is on birth control. Her vital signs are within expected ranges, and there is no evidence of any active withdrawal or intoxication. A review of the prescription drug program reveals no prescribed controlled medications. A drug screen and breathalyzer were not obtained, per this clinic's practice.

Step One: Level of Care Determination and Discussion

Jayna presents with two clusters of concerns: her problems with attention and school performance combined with an escalating pattern of substance use (mostly alcohol). She has clear career goals, came self-referred to the evaluation, and is in a contemplation-to-action stage with regard to her attentional problems, but she does not currently believe her substance use is problematic (precontemplative). However, based on her current usage, she could meet criteria for an alcohol use disorder. Also, while she attributes her problems of poor academic performance to her long-standing issues with inattention and concentration, it's likely that her escalating use of alcohol, late nights, and partying contribute to her financial and academic jeopardy. She has no identified high-risk issues and would be appropriate for further outpatient evaluation and treatment.

Step Two: Construct the Problem/Need List

The significant information (data) from the case study can be divided into two broad categories: ADHD/mental health and substance use. Some information will apply to more than one category, and a medical column is included to ensure that no issues are left behind.

Substance Use	Mental Health	Medical
Goes out to drink with friends two to four times per week	Problems with focus and attention that date to childhood	No active medical problems
Underage drinking that started in high school	Dropped course levels in high school due to lack of attention	On birth control
Does not believe she has a problem with alcohol but thinks it could become an issue	Parents recommended to have ADHD evaluation, which did not happen	Normal vital signs
Binge drinks on weekends	Dropped half her courses first semester of college	
Used stimulants obtained from friends and purchased it illicitly	Financial aid package jeopardized due to poor school performance	
Has tried Molly, Ecstasy, and cannabis. Denies habitual use	On academic probation due to poor school performance	
Father drinks heavily	Has tried stimulant medication and found it helps her with studying	
Drinks more with less effect	Motivated to be on medication to improve her focus, concentration, and school performance	
Positive CAGE-AID questionnaire	Anxiety (mild) due to school stress	

With these three categories, an initial problem/need list can be constructed. As there are no reported active medical issues, this can be trimmed to two items:

1. Serious problems with attention and focus that impair school function and date back to childhood; Current academic and financial jeopardy due to poor school performance

2. Alcohol use with increased intake, weekend binge drinking, underage drinking, and a family history of problem alcohol use; Positive CAGE-AID

Step Three: Establish the Initial Goals/Objectives for Treatment

Using the previous list, the patient and clinician will develop measurable, realistic, behavioral, and desirable goals for treatment. Where Jayna does not believe she has a problem with alcohol, the approach will be to meet her where she is around her drinking (motivational enhancement):

1. Severe problems with attention and focus that impair school function and date back to childhood, as well as current academic and financial jeopardy due to poor school performance

    a. Short-term goal(s):

        i. Complete diagnostic evaluation of ADHD to include a standardized screen, input from client's parents (release in chart), and prior school records (release in chart/request for records sent)

        ii. Schedule psychiatric evaluation with an MD or APRN to review psychopharmacological and other treatment options

        iii. Engage in weekly CBT therapy with a focus on skills acquisition for concentration, attention, and improved academic performance

        iv. Achieve a grade point average for the current semester that will eliminate the risk of reduction/loss of either financial support or academic standing (3.0 or better)

    b. Long-term goal(s):

        i. Maintain a grade point average that will support admission to an advanced nursing program of Jayna's choice (3.0 or better)

        ii. Develop and maintain core skills related to focus and attention, which may include mindfulness practice, cognitive approaches, and the ongoing use of medication for ADHD

        iii. Decrease symptoms of ADHD to no more than a 2 using a 5-point scale

2. Alcohol use with increased intake, weekend binge drinking, underage drinking, and a family history of problem alcohol use; Positive CAGE-AID

    a. Short-term goal(s):

        i. Engage in a motivational dialogue around current use of alcohol

        ii. Complete a pros and cons assessment of alcohol consumption

b. Long-term goal(s):

 i. Prevent alcohol consumption from escalating beyond its current level

 ii. Prevent alcohol or other substance use from interfering with Jayna's goals

Step Four: Construct the Treatment-and-Recovery Plan

Once the problem/need list and the goals and objectives have been fleshed out, they are moved forward into the treatment-and-recovery plan where the specific interventions are identified, including information about frequency, duration, and who will be responsible for seeing that they happen.

Treatment-and-Recovery Plan

Patient's Name: Jayna Carver
Date of Birth: 6/12/2001
Medical Record #: XXX-XX-XXXX

Level of Care: Outpatient

ICD-10 Codes	DSM-5 Diagnoses
F90.0	ADHD, inattentive type
F10.10	Alcohol use disorder, mild

The individual's stated goal(s): "To get my grades together and get into a good advanced nursing program. To not have my drinking turn into an issue"

---

1. Problem/Need Statement: Severe problems with attention and focus that impair school function and date back to childhood, as well as current academic and financial jeopardy due to poor school performance.

Long-Term Goal(s):
1. Maintain a grade point average that will support admission to an advanced nursing program of Jayna's choice (3.0 or better)
2. Develop and maintain core skills related to focus and attention, which may include mindfulness practice, cognitive approaches, and the ongoing use of medication for ADHD
3. Decrease symptoms of ADHD to no more than a 2 using a 5-point scale

Short Term Goals/Objectives (with target date):
1. Complete diagnostic evaluation of ADHD to include a standardized screen, input from client's parents (release in chart), and prior school records (release in chart/request for records sent) (12/1/20)
2. Schedule psychiatric evaluation with an MD or APRN to review psychopharmacological and other treatment options (12/1/20)
3. Engage in weekly CBT therapy with a focus on skills acquisition for concentration, attention, and improved academic performance (12/8/20)
4. Achieve a grade point average for the current semester that will eliminate the risk of reduction/loss of either financial support or academic standing (3.0 or better) (5/1/21)

2. Problem/Need Statement: Alcohol use with increased intake, weekend binge drinking, underage drinking, and a family history of problem alcohol use; Positive CAGE-AID.

Long-Term Goal(s):
1. Prevent alcohol consumption from escalating beyond its current level
2. Prevent alcohol or other substance use from interfering with Jayna's goals

Short-Term Goals/Objectives (with target date):
1. Engage in a motivational dialogue around current use of alcohol (12/8/20)
2. Complete a pros and cons assessment of alcohol consumption (12/8/20)

Interventions					
Treatment Modality	**Specific Type**	**Frequency**	**Duration**	**Problem Number**	**Responsible Person(s)**
Psychological Assessment/ Medication Consultation	MD/APRN evaluation	Once (with ongoing follow-up)	1.5 hours	1, 2	Dr. Greene
Individual Therapy	Co-occurring focused CBT with motivational component	Weekly	1 hour	1, 2	G. Stango, LCSW
Lab Work	1. EKG 2. Drug screen 3. Blood work, as needed 4. Pregnancy test	1. Prior to initiation of medication 2. Random 3. As needed	N/A	1, 2	Dr. Greene
Peer Support	Online group of client's choice	At least 1/ week	Ongoing	2	Ms. Carver

Identification of strengths: Motivated to improve school performance. Willing to discuss alcohol and potential pros and cons related to her current consumption

Peer/family/community supports to assist: Views her parents as supports but does not want them involved at this time other than to provide past history

Barriers to treatment: None identified at this time

Staff/client-identified education/teaching needs: To learn treatment options for ADHD and to identify effective strategies to manage symptoms. To explore issues related to alcohol and options to prevent it from escalating and interfering with her life goals

Assessment of discharge needs/discharge planning: Achieve stated goals, at which time discharge to a less intense service level for maintenance

Completion of this treatment-and-recovery plan was a collaborative effort between the client and the following treatment team members:

SIGNATURES		Date/Time:
Client:	Jayna Carver	11/24/2020, 2:00 p.m.
Physician:	Peter Greene, MD	11/24/2020, 3:15 p.m.
Primary Clinician:	Gloria Stango, LCSW	11/24/2020, 2.00 p.m.

CHAPTER 11

Depressive Disorders and Co-Occurring Substance Use Disorders

OVERVIEW

Every year, nearly 7 percent of Americans will meet criteria for major depression, with women carrying a two- to threefold greater risk than men. A first episode of depression can occur at any age, with the greatest incidence in the late teens and twenties.

Based on two large surveys, the lifetime prevalence of depression in the United States ranges from 13 to 16 percent. Broken down, the lifetime prevalence of major depressive disorder as a standalone problem is 7.41 percent, and the lifetime rate of major depression with a co-occurring substance use disorder is 5.82 percent. Rates of all substance use disorders are significantly higher among people with major depression than the general population.

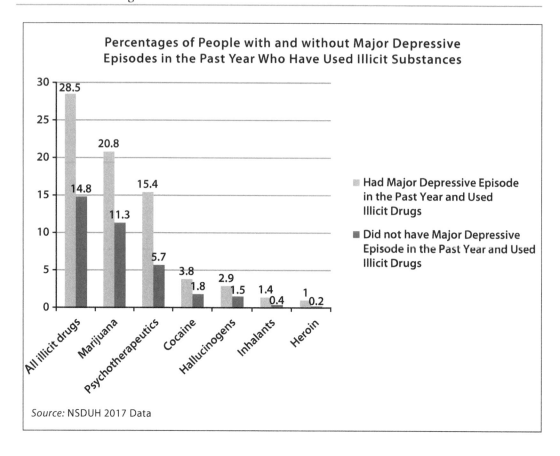

Percentages of People with and without Major Depressive Episodes in the Past Year Who Have Used Illicit Substances

Had Major Depressive Episode in the Past Year and Used Illicit Drugs

Did not have Major Depressive Episode in the Past Year and Used Illicit Drugs

Source: NSDUH 2017 Data

Co-occurring depressive disorders occur in more than 40 percent of people with alcohol use disorders and in more than 17 percent of people with all nontobacco substance use disorders. Depression with co-occurring substance use disorders is associated with more severe depression, multiple co-occurring mental disorders, and more suicide attempts.

The course of depression varies and can be a chronic problem similar to hypertension or diabetes. An untreated depressive episode can last from months to more than a year. The more episodes of depression a person has had increases the likelihood of future episodes.

Symptoms of Depression

In the current DSM, the key to the diagnosis of a depressive episode is that it is a sustained mood state of at least two weeks' duration, although people will typically report symptoms on the order of months or even years.

A diagnosis of a depressive episode is based on a constellation of symptoms, one of which must be a depressed/sad/unhappy mood and the other the loss of interest or pleasure (i.e., anhedonia). Other symptoms include:

- Changes in sleep (either too much or too little)
- Changes in appetite (either increased or decreased and may be accompanied by weight loss or gain)
- Changes in energy (typically loss of energy and chronic feelings of fatigue but may also be agitated, irritable, and anxious)
- Poor concentration (difficulty focusing and attending to activities that require sustained attention)
- Excessive and often inappropriate guilt
- Feeling of worthlessness and low self-esteem
- Hopelessness (feeling that it will never get better)
- Thoughts of death
- Thoughts of suicide, including plans and/or attempts

Key Issues in the Assessment of Co-Occurring Depressive and Substance Use Disorders

It is not always easy to tease apart a primary depressive disorder from other mental disorders, such as bipolar disorder, PTSD, and borderline personality disorder. And many substances and medications can cause depressive syndromes. For instance, alcohol-induced depression in individuals with alcohol use disorders can account for more than 30 percent of depressive episodes in that population. In the case of alcohol-induced depression, if lasting abstinence is achieved, the depressive symptoms may resolve without further treatment. Finally, many medical conditions can manifest with symptoms of depression. These range from depression following strokes or heart attacks to certain malignancies, such as pancreatic cancer and infectious diseases, such as mononucleosis.

For some with depressive episodes, there may be no identifiable psychosocial stress connected to the depression. For others, there will be a clear relationship between life events (e.g., breakups, financial stressors, loss of a job, housing problems, legal difficulties, etc.) that precipitate the mood episode.

In the assessment of a person with co-occurring depressive and substance use disorders, it is important to not jump to conclusions about the nature or cause of the depression but to keep an open mind and attitude of flexibility. Questions include the following:

- Has the person had other mood episodes, such as any prior periods of mania or hypomania? If yes, then the diagnosis will be in the bipolar spectrum.
- Does the person have a history of depressive episodes that predates the substance use problems?
- Is the person on medications that could cause the depressive symptoms?

- Is the person in a withdrawal or post-intoxication state (crash) that can cause symptoms of depression?
  - Opioid withdrawal
  - Acute post-intoxication state from cocaine, methamphetamine, or other stimulants
  - Alcohol or benzodiazepine withdrawal
- Is there a family history of depression and/or other mood or mental disorders?
- Is a medical condition present that might worsen or cause the symptoms of depression?
- What psychosocial stressors may be worsening or even causing the current depressive episode?

Assessment and Screening Tools

Screening tools can be valuable assets in both the initial assessment and ongoing treatment of depression. Certain instruments, such as the ones described here, can help clarify diagnosis and be followed over time to track changes over the course of treatment. Ones such as the PHQ-9 have become industry standards and are incorporated into many electronic health records.

- **Beck Depression Inventory-II:** This widely used twenty-one-item questionnaire is completed by the client. It takes approximately five minutes and utilizes Likert-style severity ratings. It is copyright protected and available for purchase through Pearson Education (www.pearsonassessments.com).

- **Hamilton Rating Scale for Depression:** This is another frequently used twenty-one-item assessment tool (versions with seventeen to twenty-seven items) that is completed by clinicians. It uses ratings of 0–2, to 0–4. Downloadable copies are available online.

- **Patient Health Questionnaire 9 (PHQ-9):** The PHQ-9 is a widely used instrument that is completed by the client. As with all screening tools, it should be used in conjunction with a thorough clinical assessment before making a diagnosis. An adapted version of the PHQ-9 is available from the American Psychiatric Association (www.psych.org). In that version, the client is asked to rate symptoms over the past one, not two, weeks. The PHQ-9 is in the public domain and can be freely copied.

Patient Health Questionnaire (PHQ-9)

Name:_____   Date:_____

Over the past two weeks, how often have you been bothered by any of the following problems? Circle the number that corresponds with your answer.

		Not at all	Several days	More than half the days	Nearly every day
1	Little interest or pleasure in doing things	0	1	2	3
2	Feeling down, depressed, or hopeless	0	1	2	3
3	Trouble falling or staying asleep, sleeping too much	0	1	2	3
4	Feeling tired or having little energy	0	1	2	3
5	Poor appetite or overeating	0	1	2	3
6	Feeling bad about yourself—or that you are a failure or have let yourself or your family down	0	1	2	3
7	Trouble concentrating on things, such as reading the newspaper or watching television	0	1	2	3
8	Moving or speaking so slowly that other people could have noticed. Or the opposite—being so fidgety or restless that you have been moving around a lot more than usual	0	1	2	3
9	Thoughts that you would be better off dead, or of hurting yourself	0	1	2	3
	Column totals				
	Add columns together				
	Total Score				

Scoring the PHQ-9:

Total Score	Depression Severity
1–4	Minimal depression
5–9	Mild depression
10–14	Moderate depression
15–19	Moderately severe depression
20–27	Severe depression

PSYCHOSOCIAL TREATMENTS

Several psychotherapies for depression have been shown to help reduce symptoms. These include CBT, interpersonal psychotherapy, and psychodynamic psychotherapy. However, little research has methodically assessed these same therapies in individuals who have both substance use disorders and depressive disorders. One study, using a small sample size and no control group, did find positive outcomes for both depression and alcohol-related issues with CBT.

The clinical consensus is that psychotherapy, whether in group or individual format, should be offered to patients with co-occurring depressive and substance use disorders. The selection of a therapy will be based on issues such as:

- Patient preference
- Availability
- Evidence to support particular approaches in individuals with co-occurring depressive and substance use disorders

From a pragmatic perspective, the inclusion of psychotherapy provides an ongoing relationship between the individual with depression and the therapist. Active stressors and problems are addressed, and connections and the interplay between negative mood states (depression, irritability, anxiety) and the problem substance use can be made. So too, whole-person approaches to wellness (Chapter 9) can be incorporated into treatment, with goal setting to help manage the depression, real-life stress, and problem substance use.

PHARMACOLOGY

Most practice guidelines recommend the use of antidepressants in individuals with moderate or severe depression. However, few studies have looked at specific medications in people who have both mental and substance use disorders. Studies that have been done tend to have small numbers and often lack control groups.

A further finding is that response to antidepressant medications in people who actively drink and use other substances is less strong than for people with depression alone. This is an important educational point to teach clients: Not only is depression worsened by substance use, but as someone continues to use, they are less likely to get the benefit, or the full benefit, of the medication.

In the past, it was thought that prescribing antidepressants while people still used drugs and alcohol was a bad idea. This approach may have been fueled both by earlier sequential paradigms for the treatment of co-occurring disorders (i.e., treat the drugs and alcohol first, and then address the mental illness) and by the risks involved with some of the older antidepressants, such as the tricyclic antidepressants, which can be fatal in overdose situations due to their effects on the heart. A third hypothesis as to why pharmacological treatment for depression is sometimes held back is articulated in these questions: Is this a substance-induced mood disorder? And if it is, will it resolve when the problem substance is stopped?

The current consensus is to proceed with caution and to offer medication when a diagnosis of a depressive disorder has been made and the person is not in an active withdrawal or intoxication state. In the absence of clear best choices of medications in clients with co-occurring depressive and substance use disorders, the prescriber needs to look at available medications for the treatment of depression and, based on an overall understanding of the client's specific situation, history, and symptoms, make recommendations. Issues that might sway the decision for one agent over another include:

- **Client preference and/or experience:** "That one worked for me before." "I tried that one, and it didn't do anything for me."

- **Side-effect profile:** Side effects can be both a positive and a negative. Certain drugs might be avoided because of concerns regarding weight gain and metabolic syndrome (central obesity, development of type 2 diabetes, elevated cholesterol, etc.). Others might be useful because the client has trouble falling asleep and the medication is sedating and could be given prior to bed.

- **Cost:** Will the person's insurance cover the medication, or will they have to pay out of pocket?

- **Potential interactions** with other medications the client is on

- **Safety of the medication**, especially in a person with a history of overdose or thoughts of overdosing, as well as if a person takes it with alcohol or illicit substances. For instance, sedating medications, when combined with opioids, increase the risk of respiratory depression, coma, and death.

- **Potential benefit/risk in other co-occurring conditions**, such as:
  - A patient who smokes might want to try bupropion, which also has the FDA indication for smoking cessation.
  - A person with a comorbid anxiety disorder might benefit from an antidepressant that can treat both anxiety and depression.
  - Someone with weight loss and poor sleep as symptoms of their depression might be a good candidate for an agent that helps with sleep, such as mirtazapine (Remeron), which can also increase appetite.
  - A person with certain pain conditions might be a candidate for duloxetine (Cymbalta), which carries the FDA indications for fibromyalgia and diabetic peripheral neuropathy.
  - Someone with liver disease should avoid medications that have been associated with liver failure.

Antidepressants

Among numerous FDA-approved antidepressants, little data demonstrates that any one is superior. The pills all take at least two to four weeks, at times longer, to show clinical benefits. Some of the older antidepressants—the monoamine oxidase inhibitors (MAOIs)—appear to have greater efficacy in the treatment of depression, but their side effects and potential for dangerous adverse reactions have relegated them to a rarely used status.

And newer treatments, such as infusions and intranasal administration of esketamine combined with an oral antidepressant for treatment-resistant depression, have widened the array of options. Choices of agents include:

- **Selective serotonin reuptake inhibitors (SSRIs):** fluoxetine (Prozac), sertraline (Zoloft), paroxetine (Paxil), citalopram (Celexa), escitalopram (Lexapro), vortioxetine (Brintellix), and fluvoxamine (Luvox—does not have the FDA indication for depression, but is an SSRI). Common side effects include sexual dysfunction in both men and women, weight gain (especially true for paroxetine), headache, discontinuation syndromes (which can be severe), and manic activation.

- **Serotonin norepinephrine reuptake inhibitors (SNRIs):** venlafaxine (Effexor), desvenlafaxine (Pristiq), duloxetine (Cymbalta), and levomilnacipran (Fetzima). Side effects are similar to the SSRIs and include sexual side effects, withdrawal syndromes, and manic activation. They can also be associated with elevations in blood pressure.

- **Bupropion (Wellbutrin):** Its mechanism of action is not well understood but involves dopamine and norepinephrine. It is associated with decreased nicotine cravings. It should be avoided in people with certain eating disorders (e.g., bulimia and anorexia) and in individuals with a history of seizures.

- **Trazodone (Desyrel):** Trazodone has its effect on the serotonin system but is not an SSRI or SNRI. It is infrequently used as an antidepressant due to sedation and is often used off-label to help with insomnia. It can rarely cause priapism—a sustained painful erection—which may require medical attention. In addition to sedation, common side effects include blurred vision, dry mouth, headache, and intense dreams.

- **Mirtazapine (Remeron):** Mirtazapine acts on both serotonin and norepinephrine. Its main side effects include sedation, increased appetite, and weight gain.

- **Tricyclic antidepressants:** Once popular, these medications, which include amitriptyline (Elavil), nortriptyline (Pamelor), and desipramine (Norpramin), are infrequently used as antidepressants in the United States due to their side effects and potential lethality in overdoses. Typical side effects include dry mouth, urinary retention, constipation, and increased appetite. Because of their cardiac effects, they should be avoided in people with a history of coronary artery disease. An ECG should be obtained prior to treatment and monitored once a therapeutic level has been achieved. They should also be avoided in people with certain types of glaucoma.

- **Monoamine oxidase inhibitors (MAOIs):** Rarely prescribed, these include isocarboxazid (Marplan) and phenelzine (Nardil). They are effective antidepressants that require adherence to a diet free from tyramine, a substance derived from the essential amino acid tyrosine. Tyramine is found in many foods, such as aged cheeses, Chianti wine, pickled and smoked meats and fish, chocolate, and soy sauce, to name a few. The potential interaction can lead to a hypertensive crisis, which can be life-threatening. This same interaction can occur when MAOIs are combined with many other medications, including over-the-counter cold preparations and other antidepressants. Prior to taking an MAOI, there should be at least a two-week washout period for any other antidepressant, and longer for those with longer half-lives, such as fluoxetine (Prozac). Common side effects of the MAOIs include headache, insomnia, and weight gain.

- **Esketamine:** At the time of this publication, this medication, which is available as an infusion or nasal spray, is reserved for people with treatment-resistant depression. This is defined as two or more failed trials with different oral antidepressants at an adequate dosage and duration. It is an analog of the anesthetic drug ketamine and does carry potential risks for misuse and physiologic dependence. Common side effects include sedation, dissociation, and elevations in blood pressure. For these reasons, clients need to be monitored for two hours after each administration and should not drive or operate heavy machinery for twenty-four hours. The patient self-administers the nasal preparation (Spravato) under medical supervision. Initially this is done weekly, and based on response, the doses become less frequent.

ELECTROCONVULSIVE THERAPY, TRANSCRANIAL MAGNETIC STIMULATION, AND VAGUS NERVE STIMULATION

Electroconvulsive Therapy

Electroconvulsive therapy (ECT) is a well-established treatment for severe depression. It is typically reserved for individuals who have not responded to multiple medication trials and is highly effective for individuals with psychotic depression. The treatment involves the creation of a seizure through the administration of a dosed electric current. Modern ECT includes the use of rapid-onset anesthesia and paralytic agents to prevent patients from having a physical seizure in which they could harm themselves. Side effects of ECT include memory loss, typically for the time around the procedures, but some individuals have reported more sustained problems with memory. Other side effects include headache, nausea, muscle aches, and side effects associated with the anesthetic agents used.

ECT requires a series of treatment, on average six to twelve sessions. When a response is achieved, the person may be offered a course of maintenance ECT (i.e., less frequent treatments) to help them sustain symptom remission. ECT can be offered on an inpatient or outpatient basis.

Transcranial Magnetic Stimulation

Transcranial magnetic stimulation (TMS) involves the noninvasive exposure of the brain to brief electromagnetic pulses. It requires multiple treatments, typically twenty to thirty treatments over the course of four to six weeks. Side effects are minimal and mild and include headache. There have been rare reports of seizure and manic activation with TMS. Overall, the results have not been strongly positive.

Vagus Nerve Stimulation

Vagus nerve stimulation received FDA approval for refractory depression (i.e., at least four failed trials of medication) in 2005. It involves the surgical implantation of a device that stimulates the left vagus nerve. Common side effects include vocal changes, hoarseness, and coughing. Adverse reactions include the development of obstructive sleep apnea, cough, and vocal changes.

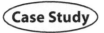

Jacqueline Ford

Jackie is a sixty-nine-year-old widowed mother of three and grandmother of four who works full time as a sales representative and cashier for a large chain store. She presents to a mental health clinic after her previous psychiatrist retired. "I'm just about out of my medication, but they don't do much." She adds, "I'm so used to being depressed, I've forgotten what it's like to feel normal. I have no energy, can't fall asleep. I have no appetite, I am constantly tired, and the panic has gotten to where I can barely function. It's every day and even worse when I run out of the pills. Will I be able to see the doctor today?"

She's struggled with her mood, anxiety, insomnia, and panic attacks since she was a teenager. "Maybe always. I was a nervous kid." Four years ago, things worsened when her husband, Frank, a self-employed plumber, died of heart disease. "Welcome to the golden years." She describes how their retirement savings were wiped out by his hospitalizations and medical costs and by drug treatment for her oldest child. "I've got two mortgages, and I'll work till I drop. Which, according to my primary care physician, could be any day. And to be honest, I'm so tired… all the time. I don't think death is such a bad thing… and no, I'm not suicidal. Not now, at least. I don't have time for it."

She reports multiple sources of active stress. "Where to start? My oldest lives in the basement and has been in and out of more detoxes and rehabs than I can count. He says he's not using and goes to a methadone clinic, but I don't believe him. I can't. I know it's the drugs talking, but he lies, and he's stolen from me. I've been to so many groups telling me I should tough love him and kick him out. But I can't. I won't. He's overdosed multiple times, and I know that one day I'll come home… and he'll be dead. My daughter—middle child—is with a man who treats her like crap. Doesn't hit her, at least that she's told me, but she only stays because of the kids." Her affect brightens as she describes her four grandchildren, ages seven to nineteen. "My youngest boy is career military—married, two kids. Knock on wood, other than having to move every two years and I never get to see him and the kids, he's okay."

Jackie was in her early thirties the first time she saw a mental health professional. She's had multiple courses of psychotherapy and been on at least eight different antidepressants. "I can't remember them all." Her current antidepressant regimen includes an SSRI and bupropion. She has been prescribed anxiolytics and benzodiazepines for at least twenty years. A review of the prescription drug monitoring database confirms this but shows she receives two monthly prescriptions: one for diazepam (Valium) 10 mg, three times a day, and one for alprazolam (Xanax) 2mg, four times a day, from two separate prescribers (her psychiatrist and her primary care physician). She is also on zolpidem (Ambien) 10 mg at bedtime. Her last month's refill of diazepam was two weeks prior to this appointment, and she states she has less than a week's worth left. "It's been a bad week, and I sometimes take an extra pill here and there when I get really shaky. My doctor said it's okay to do that. The alprazolam helps a little, but a couple hours later and the shakes are back. And some nights I'll wake up in a cold sweat, and if I don't take two, I won't be able to get back to sleep." She adds that she keeps her medications hidden because her son has stolen them in the past. She has never been psychiatrically hospitalized and denies any history of suicide attempts, though at times she has thought about ending her life. "I'm Catholic. It's not an option."

Jackie grew up in a working-class home outside of Cincinnati. She graduated high school and attended college for two years. "Never graduated. Got married and pregnant... and not in that order." She is the middle of three children. Her mother is ninety-five, has Alzheimer's, and is in an area nursing home. "The care in that place is awful, but I couldn't keep her with me anymore. She doesn't even know who I am now." Her father passed away over twenty years ago. She reports her parents fought when she was a child but that it never got violent. She believes her mother also suffered with depression, and in addition to her son, several relatives have problems with drugs and/or alcohol.

She denies active use of alcohol and does not believe it has ever been an issue for her. She tried marijuana in high school but never became a habitual user. She was a smoker for forty-five years (up to a pack and a half/day) but gave it up when her husband was told he had to quit for his health eight years ago. "I did it for him. Thought about starting up again after he died, but he'd have hated that."

Her medical history includes hypertension, controlled with two medications. She had three vaginal deliveries, has no allergies, and is scheduled to meet with a pain specialist for knee, hip, and chronic lower back pain that she scores as an 8/10 (10 being worst). "I don't know what they can do for me other than pills. I'm on my feet eight hours a day. What do you expect?" She has no history of seizures and denies having ever hallucinated.

On mental status, she is a thin, neatly dressed woman in a blouse and skirt. She appears older than her stated age and has deep circles under her eyes and a resting tremor that is visible in her hands and lips. Her mood is described as depressed and anxious, which is congruent with her affect. She is restless and frequently shifts in her seat. When you shake her hand, it is clammy and moist. Her short-term memory shows impairment, as she can only recall one out of three words after three minutes and twice loses track of the conversation. "What were we talking about?" But otherwise she is fully alert and oriented.

She does not think she'll ever feel better but consistently denies plans to harm herself, though she has contemplated suicide in the past. There is no evidence of psychosis. Her self-report screen for symptoms of mania via the Mood Disorder Questionnaire (MDQ) is negative. Her PHQ-9 screen for depression is strongly positive at 19. A screen for PTSD—the PCL-5—shows mild symptoms at 25, which mostly coincides with her depression and anxiety symptoms but is not specifically connected to identifiable trauma. Her blood pressure and pulse are both mildly elevated (pulse 104, BP 140/90). Her score on the Clinical Institute Withdrawal Assessment for Benzodiazepines (CIWA-B), which is a measure of withdrawal symptoms (see Chapter 17) is 40, indicating moderate to moderately severe withdrawal. Her insurance is unmanaged Medicare with no supplemental coverage.

Step One: Level of Care Determination and Discussion

Ms. Ford presents with a complex but common combination of severe and persistent stressors, treatment-resistant depression, anxiety, daily panic attacks, worrisome benzodiazepine use that involves high dosages and a pattern of escalation, cognitive problems (memory impairment), and active medical concerns. At first glance, this could seem overwhelming, but if you identify those items that are urgent versus ones that are important but need not be addressed today, you can develop an early plan.

The best place to start is what brought her in for today's visit. She's run out of her medications, and while she focuses on the antidepressants, the pressing concern is her benzodiazepine use. She is about to run out, might already have done so, and displays symptoms that likely represent intermittent withdrawal (e.g., tremor, elevated blood pressure and pulse, anxiety, and panic). Benzodiazepine withdrawal, like alcohol withdrawal, can be dangerous and even life-threatening. Her age, coexisting medical conditions, and extensive daily use of benzodiazepines at high doses increase her risk for serious withdrawal.

As can happen at an intake appointment, an element of urgency/crisis led to today's visit. A frank and nonjudgmental discussion should quantify the amount of benzodiazepine she takes each day and how much she has left in the bottles. This provides an opportunity to discuss and educate about the potential dangers of withdrawal, along with signs and symptoms. She needs to be evaluated by a prescriber, preferably today. Outcomes of that consultation could range from an urgent/same-day referral for inpatient stabilization and possibly detox to a less intensive level of care, such as a PHP or IOP, where some degree of medical monitoring can be provided.

As one can imagine, a person who presents for outpatient mental health treatment and is told she needs an inpatient detoxification might struggle with this recommendation. Her financial concerns (e.g., co-pays, deductibles, loss of income), worry for her son and what he might do if she's not home, inadequate understanding of the seriousness of withdrawal, level of depression and hopelessness, and other issues can all factor into her willingness to enter treatment.

Step Two: Construct the Problem/Need List

Substance Use	Mental Health	Medical
Running out of her benzodiazepines early	Struggled with depression and anxiety most of her life; "Anxious kid"	Poor sleep (chronic problem); On high-dose nightly zolpidem for sleep
Two separate prescribers for different benzodiazepines	No energy. Constantly tired	Elevated blood pressure and pulse; On two medications

• Lorazepam 10 mg three times/day • Clonazepam 2 mg three times/day • Running out one week early	Panic attacks (daily)	Resting tremor
Has been prescribed benzodiazepines for twenty plus years	Numerous trials of antidepressants (at least eight) without good response	Chronic lower back, knee, and hip pain
Son and multiple family members with substance use problems	Numerous courses of psychotherapy	Ex-smoker (forty-five years)
Ex-smoker (forty-five years)	Short-term memory impairment	Short-term memory impairment
Receives benzodiazepines from two separate prescribers	Active psychosocial stressors: • Mother with Alzheimer's • Son with opioid use disorder living at home • Financial stress • Daughter in abusive relationship • Husband's death	CIWA-B score of 40 (moderate/moderately severe withdrawal)
CIWA-B score of 40 (moderate/moderately severe withdrawal)	Hopeless	
	Contemplated suicide but states she won't act on these thoughts for religious reasons	
	PHQ-9 positive; MDQ negative; PCL-5 score 25	
	Mother had depression	

Step Three: Establish the Initial Goals/Objectives for Treatment

Using the previous list, the patient and clinician can now develop an initial problem/need list with measurable, realistic, behavioral, and desirable goals for treatment. In addition, the problem list must support the medical necessity for whatever level of care is recommended:

1. Dangerous benzodiazepine use, AEB increased use over time, high total dosage, and multiple prescribers; overuse, AEB prescriptions running out too soon, intermittent withdrawal (tremor, panic, worsened anxiety, restlessness, elevated pulse and blood pressure, sweating, sleep disturbance), probable cognitive side effects (memory loss), and CIWA-B of 40

    a. Short-term goal(s):

      i. Eliminate symptoms of withdrawal (CIWA-B < 5)

      ii. Quantify current use

      iii. Stabilize (minimize) daily dose and eliminate use of PRNs (i.e., use of medications as needed)

      iv. Provide education regarding risks/benefits of benzodiazepines and help client identify short- and longer-term goals around use

    b. Long-term goal(s):

      i. Decrease benzodiazepine use to no more than a 4 mg lorazepam equivalent daily dose and to consider eventual full taper

      ii. Be free from symptoms of benzodiazepine withdrawal and craving

2. Severe depression and anxiety, AEB a depressed mood, anhedonia, poor sleep, chronically low energy, hopelessness, suicidality without intent, multiple active stressors, panic attacks, and anxiety

    a. Short-term goal(s): Experience a 50 percent or greater decrease in depressive and anxious symptoms using 10-point self-rating scales and the PHQ-9

    b. Long-term goal(s):

      i. Experience symptoms of depression and anxiety no greater than a 2 out of a possible 10

      ii. Have a PHQ-9 score of < 10

      iii. Be free from panic attacks

3. Active medical issues: chronic insomnia, hypertension, chronic pain, tremor, short-term memory impairment

    a. Short-term goal(s): Complete assessments of sleep and pain problems

      i. Refer to a sleep clinic (probable sleep study)

      ii. Refer to a multidisciplinary pain specialist or clinic

      iii. Complete cognitive testing and diagnostic workup to assess memory loss and ascertain its cause (Long-term goal will be based on outcome(s) of this workup.)

    b. Long-term goal(s):

      i. Be able to manage pain and have it at to no more than a 4–5 on a 10-point scale

      ii. Get six and a half hours (at least) of restorative sleep/night

      iii. Be normotensive

Step Four: Construct the Treatment-and-Recovery Plan

Treatment-and-Recovery Plan

Patient's Name: Jacqueline Ford

Date of Birth: 12/2/1952

Medical Record #: XXX-XX-XXXX

Level of Care: Inpatient medically supervised benzodiazepine detoxification

ICD-10 Codes	DSM-5 Diagnoses
F13.239	Benzodiazepine withdrawal without perceptual disturbance with benzodiazepine use disorder, severe
F33.1	Major depressive disorder, recurrent episode with anxious distress and panic

The individual's stated goal(s): "To not feel so awful all the time. To stop these panic attacks"

1. **Problem/Need Statement:** Dangerous benzodiazepine use, AEB increased use over time, high total dosage, and multiple prescribers; overuse, AEB prescriptions running out too soon, intermittent withdrawal (tremor, panic, worsened anxiety, restlessness, elevated pulse and blood pressure, sweating, sleep disturbance), probable cognitive side-effects (memory loss), and CIWA-B of 40.

Long-Term Goal(s):

1. Decrease benzodiazepine use to no more than a 4 mg lorazepam equivalent daily dose and to consider eventual full taper
2. Be free from symptoms of benzodiazepine withdrawal and cravings (CIWA-B <5)

Short-Term Goals/Objectives (with target date):

1. Quantify current use (10/2/22)
2. Decrease symptoms of withdrawal, AEB a CIWA-B < 5 (10/4/22)
3. Stabilize (minimize) daily dose and eliminate use of PRNs (10/4/22)
4. Provide education regarding risks/benefits of benzodiazepines and help client identify short- and longer-term goals around use (10/2/22)

2. **Problem/Need Statement:** Severe depression and anxiety, AEB a depressed mood, anhedonia, poor sleep, chronically low energy, hopelessness, suicidality without intent, multiple active stressors, panic attacks, and anxiety.
Long-Term Goal(s):
1. Experience symptoms of depression and anxiety no greater than a 2 out of a possible 10.   2. Have a PHQ-9 score of < 10   3. Be free from panic attacks
Short-Term Goals/Objectives (with target date):
1. Experience a 50 percent or greater decrease in depressive and anxious symptoms using 10-point self-rating scales and the PHQ-9 (11/15/22)

3. **Problem/Need Statement:** Chronic insomnia, hypertension, chronic pain, tremor, short-term memory impairment.
Long-Term Goal(s):
1. Be pain free   2. Get six hours (at least) of restorative sleep/night   3. Be normotensive
Short-Term Goals/Objectives (with target date):
1. Complete an assessment of sleep and refer for a sleep study if necessary (10/5/22)   2. Complete an assessment of pain and address underlying causes (10/5/22)   3. Complete cognitive testing to clarify source of memory loss (10/5/22)

Interventions					
Treatment Modality	**Specific Type**	**Frequency**	**Duration**	**Problem Number**	**Responsible Person(s)**
Medical and Psychiatric Assessments	History and physical, complete biopsychosocial assessment	Upon admission, and follow-up as needed	45–60 minutes	1,2,3	Physician/ APRN
Nursing Assessment	Nursing assessment	Upon admission, and as per the CIWA-B protocol* for benzodiazepine withdrawal	1 hour on admission, and multiple times/day as per the CIWA-B protocol	1,2,3	RN

Withdrawal Protocol	CIWA-B*	Based on symptom severity	Until patient has safely tapered down to target dose with a CIWA-B score of less than 10	1	RN, treating physician
Individual Therapy	Co-occurring focus CBT	3x/week	50 minutes for duration of admission	1,2	Ms. Ford and primary therapist
Group Therapy	Substance abuse education	Daily	50 minutes for duration of admission	1,2	Ms. Ford and group leader
	Peer-led recovery groups	Daily	1 hour for duration of admission	1	Ms. Ford and group leader volunteer
	Relapse prevention	3x/week	1 hour for duration of admission	1	Ms. Ford and group leader
	Wellness and recovery group	Daily	1 hour for duration of admission	1,2,3	Ms. Ford and occupational therapist
	Mindfulness and skills training group	Daily	1 hour for duration of admission	1,2	Ms. Ford and group leader
	Multiple family support and education group	1x/week	90 minutes	1,2	Ms. Ford and group leader (any family members she wants invited)
Lab Work	Blood work/ ECG, other labs as indicated	Upon admission, and as needed	N/A	1,2,3	MD/APRN
Specimen Collection	Breath analysis/ urine drug screen	As ordered	For duration of admission	1,2	Clinician or designee

Identification of strengths: Has a strong work ethic and desire to feel and function better. Identifies herself as a loving mother and grandmother who wants to be healthy and available to her family

Peer/family/community supports to assist: Three children, whom she identifies as supportive but not available

Barriers to treatment: Concerns that her medical-leave benefit and health insurance will not adequately cover the cost of treatment. Fear that she might lose her job

Staff/client-identified education/teaching needs: To understand the nature of her benzodiazepine use and how it impacts her mood, panic, and quality of life. To develop healthier coping and wellness skills, including the use of psychosocial and possibly pharmacological treatments to manage her anxiety and depression

Assessment of discharge needs/discharge planning: Ms. Ford will be medically stable to where she can continue her treatment at a less restrictive setting, likely in a PHP or IOP with co-occurring capability.

Completion of this treatment-and-recovery plan was a collaborative effort between the client and the following treatment team members:

SIGNATURES		Date/Time
Client:	Jackie Ford	10/2/22, 3:00 p.m.
Physician:	Louella Grant, MD	10/2/22, 3:20 p.m.
Primary Clinician:	Gerald Singh, RN	10/2/22, 3:00 p.m.
Other Team Members:	Blanche Crane, AT/OTR	10/2/22, 4:15 p.m.
	George Pick, PCA	10/2/22, 4:15 p.m.
	Lydia Flores, recovery specialist	10/2/22, 4:30 p.m.

*The CIWA-B is similar to the CIWA scale used to assess signs and symptoms of alcohol withdrawal.

CHAPTER 12

....

Bipolar Disorder and Co-Occurring Substance Use Disorders

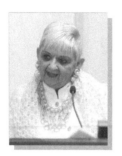

My Story

By Karen Kangas, EdD

Director of Recovery and Family Affairs, Behavioral Health Network of Hartford HealthCare, Leader in the National Client Advocacy Movement

> "I don't like the way we treat people with mental illness.
> We lock them up in cages."

The Patient with Keys

I grew up in Montana. My dad, Toby Kangas, was a famous high school basketball coach, and Mom was a housewife. She also suffered with what they called agitated depression and had problems with alcohol and prescription pills.

I was a hyper kid and the oldest of two. I didn't sleep much, stayed up all night and got stuff done. I was the head majorette, studied hard, and got A's I breezed through my undergraduate work, graduated with honors, and started to teach fourth grade at the age of twenty in Tacoma. With my first paycheck, I bought a pair of five-inch heels with rhinestones. I loved that job, and every summer I'd go home to Montana, where my dad would put up scaffolding and I'd paint the house.

During this time, my mother would go to the emergency room, but they wouldn't keep her long. Once they gave her a hundred Xanax, and I watched them disappear, along with alcohol. She'd end up in bed for days, and at some point, my dad decided she had to be in a hospital—but not in Montana, because of his reputation.

In my early twenties, my roommate—also a teacher—and I headed east. We got hired by the Hartford public school system. It was an inner-city school, unlike anything I'd ever known, with 2,000 kids, K through eight. I taught fourth grade and loved it. There I met and married another teacher. We honeymooned in Atlantic City, bought a nice house in the suburbs, and had two children. My parents would visit, my husband and dad would golf, and my mom sewed us curtains. I continued to be an unbridled ball of energy. When I got pregnant, I sewed all my maternity clothes, slept little, and showed up to work in a different outfit every day.

The marriage looked good, but there were problems. We moved down south and then back to Connecticut. I got my doctorate in education, started literacy programs, became a principal, took care of the house, didn't sleep, and was in nonstop motion.

The marriage worsened and ended. My daughter stayed with me, and my son went with his father. My mood crashed. I saw a lot of doctors, but no one told me what was wrong. One day I was having what I didn't know was a panic attack, and a doctor suggested a shot of whiskey and "Let's see what happens." It worked, and I discovered that alcohol slowed me down and decreased my unbearable anxiety. That doctor was the first who said, "Something is going on with you," though he didn't say what.

My father and had me see a psychoanalyst who put me on Elavil. It was awful. I became so high that I had to drink more to come down. I stopped the medication and stopped seeing him. I don't know if I became psychotic, but I imagined someone came in and molested me. I was coming apart.

That was the first time I got admitted to a psychiatric hospital. I signed out against medical advice the next day. It was horrible. No one paid attention or wanted to help me or tell me what was wrong. To date, I've been in psychiatric hospitals eighteen times. I don't like them. When you're in that much pain, you want to know that someone's going to help you, that there's hope, that you're going to get back to your career. But instead, they lock the door, restrict your visitors and your ability to use the phone, and you can't even go to the gift shop.

I finished the school year, called my parents, and said, "I can't do this. I need to come home." I was forty-three, and I believed I was going home to Montana to die. For months I'd paint the house and cry, listen to music and cry, and I didn't sleep. It's what they call a mixed episode, where you're both depressed and racy.

One night I took all my father's heart pills, all my mother's pills, and lithium, which I was now on, albeit at too high a dose. I wrote a note and thanked my parents. I got in bed and said, "Okay God, I'm ready to die." But my stomach curled from the pills, and I vomited. I told no one, and I threw out the note.

Finally, my dad brought me to a hospital and had me see his internist, who referred me to a psychiatrist, who asked some questions I'll never forget.

"Do you have clothes in your closet at home that still have tags on? Do you have many clothes?"

I said, "I do."

"Do people tell you that you need to slow down? That they can't quite understand you?"

"Yes."

"Well," he said, "I think what you have is cyclothymia. And we're going to start you on some medication." I agreed, and eventually that diagnosis turned to manic depression or bipolar. But at least now I *had* a diagnosis. This thing had a name. "I have manic depression."

I bounced back. I applied for a job as a principal in Montana, went for the interview wearing yellow shoes, and got the job. But by the end of the academic year, I was as high as can be. At one point, I drove to Denver and bought fifteen pairs of shoes I didn't need. I drank and went into school disheveled. One day the superintendent was waiting for me, and I ran out. I knew I needed help. I went home, saw a TV ad for a drug-and-alcohol rehab program that had a woman on a horse. That seemed to make sense—to be outdoors, to get exercise. I drank a beer on the way to make sure they'd take me. But while I was there, the superintendent visited and told me, "When you come out, we're going to fire you."

I was devastated. I got an attorney to try and fight for my job while doctors told me I'd never work again, which is the worst thing someone can do—take away hope. And I thought, *This is it for me, no job, no marriage, no life.*

What started to turn things for me was a support group for people with mental illness. Many were professionals like me, and their lives weren't over. There were two doctors—one had bipolar and the other had schizophrenia. We met every week, and it was wonderful. They were vibrant and funny and could talk and laugh about the stuff that no one else would. It saved me.

I lost my court case and my job, and with $100 in my pocket, I returned to Connecticut. I was forty-four, had no money, and stayed in a friend's living room. I tried real estate and then saw an ad for an advocate at Fairfield Hills State Hospital. It said, "A person with a history of mental illness is encouraged to apply." I did and got hired.

Fairfield Hills was a large state hospital where people would stay for years and decades. It was the first time I saw people with mental illness who were not well. There I met a woman named Gerta who become my mentor. She was a Holocaust survivor whose family had put her in the hospital for OCD symptoms when she was thirty-two. They were told, "It's best not to visit." She'd remain there for forty years. I first met her walking on the grounds. She said, "I like your necklace," to which I replied, "I like yours." That was our connection— jewelry.

I spent a lot of time with her. She called me her girlfriend, and the staff would let me take her places. Once, I asked her where she wanted to go.

She said, "McDonalds."

"Why there?"

"Because that's where the kids are." And she shared her regrets—how she'd never had children, never made love to a man, and "never even had a cat."

She taught me that she was a human being with desires and wants, and why did she have to live this way!

Around that time, I, along with others in recovery, began to meet and then set up consumer groups around the state. Many had been patients in the state hospitals. We talked about what was needed, what would help. But for any real change to occur, we needed a place at the table, to have someone in the Commissioner's office. In time, with perseverance and the threat of a media-covered strike in front of the commissioner's home in New Haven, I was hired into this new role. I became known as the patient with keys. And people called. They'd want to meet for lunch or coffee and share their histories of mental illness—things they were too frightened to divulge lest they jeopardize their jobs, their insurance, or their relationships. And almost always they'd ask, "Will this ever pass? Will I ever be well?"

To which I answer, "Yes. You must have hope. Believe that you're going to get well. Take the medications if they help. When you have a bad day, don't get into it. Get out of bed and call me."

So what is my role as an advocate? It's like being a coach, like my dad. I get to know people, listen to their stories, and share some of the struggles I've seen others and myself go through. The biggest thing is the connection and professional friendships within certain boundaries. The people I work with know they can trust me and tell me things they won't or can't share with their treatment team. Most important is to give hope, to let them know that, even though they're not the way they want to be, this will pass and they'll learn to have the life they want.

I now run the Recovery Leadership Academy at Hartford Health Care. It's an eighty-hour course that teaches people in recovery how to be advocates and recovery-support specialists. The curriculum is ambitious—how to write resumes, how to get jobs, how to testify at the legislature, and how to have choice and self-determination. We make sure that people know their rights, that they're heard, are treated with respect, are free from cruelty and from restraints—physical or chemical. We show people how to get the help they need and that they can and will have the lives they want.

OVERVIEW

Bipolar disorders, characterized by disabling and sustained mood swings (mania, hypomania, and depression), are among the most common psychiatric disorders in people with substance use problems. Per the National Comorbidity Replication Study, about 1 percent of the population meets criteria for bipolar I disorder, 1.1 percent for bipolar II disorder, and another 2.4 percent for subthreshold bipolar.

The lifetime prevalence of nontobacco substance use disorder in people with bipolar disorders ranges between 50–60 percent, with many having multiple substance use disorders. The three most common with bipolar disorder are alcohol, cannabis, and cocaine. This strong connection between substance use disorders and bipolar disorders is summed up well by Karen Kangas, EdD, a leader in the consumer advocacy movement, who observed, "I don't ask people with bipolar disorder if they have ever used substances. Instead I ask, 'What substances did you use?'"

Some of the reasons why people with bipolar disorder are drawn to substances can include the following:

- To decrease symptoms of bipolar disorder by self-medicating with alcohol, cannabis, and opioids. For example, drinking alcohol can combat the racing thoughts that make it impossible to sleep. The use of cannabis, alcohol, and other sedatives can provide short-term relief from anxiety and depression. Some with bipolar disorder report they experience a paradoxical effect with cocaine in that it helps them calm down. (This is also seen in some with ADHD.)

- To maintain or increase the pleasurable (euphoric) experience of mania or hypomania with substances, such as cocaine, amphetamines, bath salts and other synthetic stimulants, and alcohol. The substance use can be symptomatic of the impulsivity seen when people are manic or hypomanic.

- To get high

- To be social

The clinical course and prognosis for people with co-occurring bipolar and substance use disorders are poorer than for people with just bipolar disorder. Findings for people with co-occurring bipolar and substance use disorders include:

- Earlier onset of bipolar symptoms

- More frequent mood episodes

- Longer time to recover between mood episodes

- Higher rates of rapid cycling (four or more mood episodes per year)

- More episodes with mixed features (presence of both depressed and manic/hypomanic symptoms at the same time)

- More psychotic symptoms (especially true for cannabis use)

- Higher rates of unemployment

- Higher rates of hospitalization
- Poorer response to medications, including lithium
- Higher rates of incarceration
- Higher rates of violence
- Lower treatment adherence
- Lower quality of life
- Roughly twice the number of suicide attempts
- Increased mortality from completed suicide and medical causes

GENETICS OF BIPOLAR DISORDER AND THE DEVELOPMENT OF CO-OCCURRING SUBSTANCE USE DISORDERS

Bipolar disorder has a strong genetic component, and up to 80 percent of people with the disorder report a family history. This, combined with genetic aspects of substance use disorders, place children of people with co-occurring bipolar disorder at tremendous risk. Because of the strong genetic component to bipolar, it's important to get both a careful family psychiatric and substance use history. This should also include family members who might never have been diagnosed but who the patient feels have severe mood episodes with or without substance problems.

Substance use disorders develop early in the course of bipolar disorder and peak between the ages of fourteen and twenty. In some cases, individuals can identify mood episodes that preceded their substance use disorder. For others, it appears the substance use came first.

Early identification and intervention for children at risk for bipolar disorder, especially children of those with co-occurring bipolar and substance use disorder, may decrease the likelihood that they will develop substance use problems and the related worsened prognosis.

DIAGNOSTIC DILEMMAS WITH BIPOLAR DISORDER

Bipolar disorders are among the most missed and misdiagnosed disorders in psychiatry. On average, people do not receive an accurate diagnosis until they have had symptoms for a decade or more. Missed diagnoses and misdiagnoses are compounded when co-occurring substance use disorders cloud the diagnostic picture, as do other comorbid psychiatric disorders, which run high in people with bipolar (lifetime comorbidity rates of 42 percent). Common co-occurring mental disorders include anxiety disorders, such as generalized anxiety disorder (GAD), panic disorder, PTSD, and ADHD. There is also significant comorbidity with personality disorders.

People with bipolar disorder more commonly seek treatment when they are depressed, often with mixed features and intense anxiety and irritability. They may not consider their past episodes of mania or hypomania as unusual. Many with bipolar disorder view the increased energy, diminished need for sleep, and productivity that accompany hypomanic episodes as times they felt well.

When manic, people with bipolar disorder may have psychotic symptoms and often believe there is nothing wrong (i.e., anosognosia). They will not be interested in treatment and may only come to the attention of clinicians if their behavior is so extreme, risky, or dangerous that they are brought in by family, friends, or police for an emergency evaluation and possibly hospitalization or even arrest.

When people are intoxicated or in a withdrawal state, it's difficult to differentiate which symptoms are related to substances and which are due to mental illness:

- Is the irritability and aggressiveness part of hypomania with mixed features, or is it opioid withdrawal?
- Is the pressured speech and risk-taking behavior the result of mania or intoxication with cocaine, bath salts, methamphetamine, or other stimulants?

When multiple psychiatric disorders are present, accurately teasing them apart is a challenge:

- Is the hyperactivity from bipolar disorder, ADHD, or both?
- Are the frequent mood swings evidence of a rapid-cycling bipolar, or are they more consistent with borderline personality disorder, where a person's mood state can change rapidly and dramatically?

As a result of the at-times-confusing clinical picture, people with bipolar disorder are at high risk for inaccurate diagnoses, with unipolar depression (major depressive disorder) being the most frequent. The risk here is that certain treatments for unipolar depression, such as antidepressant medication, can worsen the symptoms of bipolar disorder through increased irritability and manic switching/activation, which can include psychotic symptoms and increased frequency of mood episodes.

MAKING THE DIAGNOSIS OF BIPOLAR DISORDER

In order to diagnose bipolar disorders, you need a careful history. You must find out if, over the course of this person's life, they have ever had a manic or hypomanic episode. Indeed, the diagnosis of bipolar I hinges on the singular criterion of a just one episode of mania, even one that might have been brought on by medication.

- **Manic episodes:** A period of sustained elevated or irritable mood that lasts at least one week or any length if the person is hospitalized. Untreated, manic episodes can last months or, in some cases, years. When manic, individuals may not realize anything is wrong, and in fact, euphoria (feeling wonderful) can be a symptom. Along with this elevation in mood, mania can include:
  o Seemingly boundless energy and enthusiasm
  o Rapid/pressured speech and thought. This can be so extreme that it's impossible to carry on a conversation.
  o Tangential and circumstantial speech (thought) patterns. Here it's hard to follow the person's train of thought as it jumps rapidly from topic to topic.

When asked to answer a question, they may start on topic but quickly wander off to where the original question is never answered.

o Decreased sleep without complaints of tiredness

o Inflated sense of importance or grandiosity. In mania, this can become delusional to where the person believes they are an important figure, such as Jesus, a prophet, a rock star, a business mogul, or the devil. They may believe they possess special powers and abilities (e.g., mind reading, being a wizard or prophet, etc.).

o Increased goal-directed activity, such as writing a novel in three days, painting nonstop, or doing some other activity in a driven and relentless fashion. This behavior is accompanied by intense enthusiasm: "This is going to set the world on fire and make me a billion dollars!"

o Shifting enthusiasms and distractibility

o Impaired concentration

o Risk taking and/or impulsive and unwise behaviors, including using drugs, engaging in random sex, gambling, excessive shopping, maxing out credit cards, high-risk online investing, and spending retirement accounts, to give a few examples.

o Irritability. When people are manic, they often don't respond well to being questioned or challenged.

- **Hypomanic episodes:** Hypomania is less intense than mania but includes similar symptoms (e.g., non-delusional grandiosity, rapid speech, racing thoughts, increased goal-directed activity, etc.). While mania can include psychotic symptoms, such as delusions and even hallucinations, they are not present in hypomania. In the DSM-5, the duration criterion for a hypomanic episode is at least four days. And where the intensity of a mania often necessitates intervention, such as a hospitalization, a person who is hypomanic continues to function at work and home—often at a high, driven, and intense level—but there is a noticeable change in their behavior.

- **Depressed episodes:** In the DSM-5, depressed episodes in bipolar disorder are of at least two weeks' duration and include at least five of nine symptoms. One of these must be either a sustained depressed mood and/or persistent loss of interest or pleasure (anhedonia). Other symptoms include disturbances in sleep and appetite, guilt and feelings of worthlessness, poor concentration, low energy, apparent agitation or diminished movement, and thoughts of death and suicidality (ranging from thoughts to actual attempts).

- **Mixed features:** A significant change between the DSM-IV-TR and the DSM-5 is the elimination of the mixed episode diagnosis. Instead, in the current diagnostic manual, both depressive disorders and bipolar disorders can have mixed features as a specifier. For instance, someone who is clinically depressed but also experiences racing thoughts, distractibility, and diminished sleep without complaints of tiredness could be classified as having a depressed episode with mixed features.

In assessing for the presence of a bipolar disorder in someone who is currently depressed, it is useful to focus on their specific symptoms of depression, as there can be differences between typical "unipolar" depression (i.e., people who have never had a manic or hypomanic episode) and what is called "atypical" depression, which is more associated with bipolar disorders. Symptoms of bipolar depression are more likely to include:

- Excessive sleepiness and time spent in bed (as opposed to insomnia and trouble sleeping)

- Constant feelings of tiredness, low energy, heaviness, or being weighed down

- Increased appetite (as opposed to the loss of appetite seen more in unipolar depressions)

- The presence of mixed features (e.g., racing thoughts, inability to concentrate, pressured speech, etc.)

- Anxiety

- Agitation

- Irritability

MOOD CHARTS

A mood chart, where a person recollects all significant mood episodes over the course of their lifetime, can aid in diagnosis. Even though it is common for a first major mood episode (depressed, manic, or hypomanic) to occur in the context of a significant life stress, such as military bootcamp, going off to school, pregnancy, and so on, future mood episodes in bipolar disorder may not correlate to an identifiable stress.

In women, it is crucial to ask about mood episodes related to pregnancy, especially in the third trimester and postpartum (peripartum). Women with bipolar disorder are at extremely high risk for severe mood episodes during these periods. Although not diagnostic on its own, the history of a peripartum depression or other mood episode should raise suspicion for the presence of a bipolar disorder.

MOOD CHART

Instructions: Please write down times in your life when you felt either moderately or severely depressed, as well as any periods where you had tremendous energy (i.e., were hyper). Include any significant events or stressors that were going on at that time and whether you were using any substances, including alcohol. Use a 10-point scale for both periods of depressed mood and hyper mood, with 10 being the most depressed or most hyper and 0 being not at all depressed or hyper. Write in your age on the bottom line (see sample), starting at the point you believe you first had a serious problem with your mood.

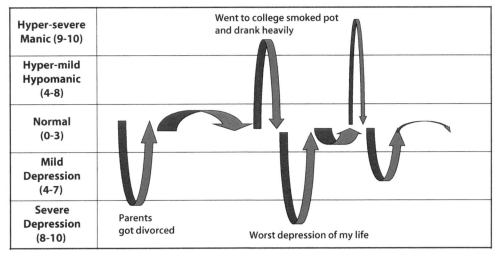

Hyper-severe Manic (9-10)	
Hyper-mild Hypomanic (4-8)	
Normal (0-3)	
Mild Depression (4-7)	
Severe Depression (8-10)	

Age (years)

SCREENING AND ASSESSMENT TOOLS FOR BIPOLAR DISORDER

Screening tools and instruments that help quantify the severity of mood and behavioral symptoms in bipolar disorder provide useful adjuncts to clinical assessment and to measuring treatment progress. In particular, instruments that flesh out prior episodes of mania or hypomania can aid in arriving at an accurate diagnosis. Frequently used tools for depressed episodes include:

- **The Beck Depression Inventory-II:** This twenty-one-item patient-completed questionnaire uses severity ratings for symptoms of depression. It is useful for putting a number on the patient's current level of depression and can be administered throughout treatment to chart progress.

- **The Hamilton Depression Scale (HAM-D):** Clinicians complete this twenty-one-item tool (longer and shorter versions are available) that is widely used in studies of depression and can help track response to treatment. It takes approximately twenty minutes to complete.

- **The Patient Health Questionnaire-9 (PHQ-9):** This easily completed self-report screening tool corresponds to the symptoms of depression in the DSM. A copy is included in this manual.

Tools to assess mania and hypomania include:

- **The Young Mania Rating Scale:** This eleven-item clinician-administered tool is used to evaluate the presence of current symptoms of mania or hypomania. It can be repeated to show changes in symptoms.

- **The Mood Disorder Questionnaire (MDQ):** The MDQ is the most widely used screening tool to assess for the presence of prior mania or hypomania. It is completed by the client and when combined with a careful history and clinical assessment, can aid in making an accurate diagnosis of bipolar disorder. When using the MDQ, it is important to spend time with clients to review their responses and to clarify the following:

  o How long did their symptoms last? Do their endorsed symptoms meet the DSM-5 duration for a manic episode (at least one week or any length of time if the symptoms are so severe the person requires hospitalization) or hypomanic episode (at least four consecutive days)?

  o Did these symptoms only occur in the context of drug or alcohol use, or did they occur even when drugs and/or alcohol weren't involved?

  o Are the symptoms of hyperactivity, high energy, and poor concentration due to bipolar disorder, or are they more chronic and in keeping with possible ADHD? Conversely, do the shifting moods last on the order of hours, which might be more consistent with a personality disorder or an impulse-control problem, such as borderline personality disorder or intermittent explosive disorder?

Remember, a positive screening test is not diagnostic but it should alert the clinician to take a thorough history and fully assess for the presence of a bipolar disorder.

The Mood Disorder Questionnaire (MDQ)

Instructions: Please answer each question as best you can.

1. **Has there ever been a period of time when you were not your usual self and...**

Place a check in each appropriate box	Yes	No
... you felt so good or so hyper that other people thought you were not your normal self, or you were so hyper that you got Into trouble?		
... you were so irritable that you shouted at people or started fights or arguments?		
... you felt much more self-confident than usual?		
... you got much less sleep than usual and found you didn't really miss it?		
... you were much more talkative or spoke much faster than usual?		
... thoughts raced through your head or you couldn't slow your mind down?		
... you were so easily distracted by things around you that you had trouble concentrating or staying on track?		
... you had more energy than usual?		
... you were much more active or did many more things than usual?		
... you were much more social or outgoing than usual, for example, you telephoned friends in the middle of the night?		
... you were much more interested in sex than usual?		
... you did things that were unusual for you or that other people might have thought excessive, foolish, or risky?		
... spending money got you or your family into trouble?		

2. If you checked "yes" to more than one of the above, have several of these ever happened during the same period of time? (circle one) Yes   No

3. How much of a problem did any of these cause you—like being unable to work; having family, money, or legal troubles; or getting into arguments or fights? (circle one response)

   No Problem   Minor Problem   Moderate Problem   Serious Problem

4. Have any of your blood relatives (i.e., children, siblings, parents, grandparents, aunts, or uncles) had manic-depressive illness or bipolar disorder? (circle one) Yes   No

5. Has a health professional ever told you that you have manic-depressive illness or bipolar disorder? (circle one) Yes   No

Scoring the MDQ

The screen is considered "positive" if the client:

1. Endorses seven or more "yes" items in question number 1

And

2. Answers "yes" to question number 2

And

3. Indicates "moderate" or "serious" to question number 3

Psychosocial Treatment of Co-Occurring Bipolar Disorder and Substance Use Disorders

Limited studies look specifically at the treatment of co-occurring substance use and bipolar disorder. However, those studies that have been done, combined with common sense and clinical experience, show that combined/integrated treatments have better clinical outcomes than treatments that attempt to address and treat one issue until it's resolved and then move on to the next (i.e., sequential treatment).

That said, in the face of multiple issues, the clinician will have to prioritize treatment needs based on a thorough clinical assessment, along with the patient's specific needs, goals, and priorities. Where acute safety issues are present (e.g., withdrawal states, suicidality, and out-of-control behaviors that can be associated with manic and depressed states), they will need immediate attention. Similarly, major social concerns that interfere with treatment (e.g., homelessness, unsafe housing, legal difficulties, custody disputes, severe financial problems, lack of transportation, etc.) will need to be addressed early in treatment.

An integrated clinical approach for bipolar disorder and substance use disorders includes the following:

1. **A thorough clinical assessment**, as outlined in Chapters 2–4 and expanded in this chapter (e.g., use of screening tools, careful history of mood episodes, and possibly the completion of a mood chart)

2. **Patient education** about both the substance use and bipolar disorder: This can be incorporated into both individual sessions and group therapies. Specific topics for bipolar that need to be covered include:

   a. Education about bipolar disorder, geared to the cognitive level and interest of the specific person: A diagnosis of bipolar disorder can be scary. Helping someone demystify the illness gives them a greater sense of control and of being able to manage their symptoms. Steering clients to useful websites, pamphlets, and books is a good way to start. (See Resources and References for this chapter, which are provided at the end of this book).

   b. Medication education: As medications are a common component of treatment, it is critical that the person understands what each drug does, as well as its risks, potential side effects, adverse reactions, and hoped-for benefits.

c. The beneficial use of peer supports: These can be local groups or peer-run programs where they get a firsthand look at other people with bipolar disorder who successfully manage their illness and their lives. Having peers with bipolar disorder and often a history of co-occurring substance use problems, who can share their experiences, can be powerful and inspiring.

d. Education around the importance of adequate restorative sleep: For many with bipolar disorder, changes in sleep patterns may be the first—and possibly only—warning sign of an impending mood episode. When individuals are manic or hypomanic, sleep is diminished. When individuals are depressed, sleep and time spent in bed increase. Learning to regulate sleep can be an effective strategy to prevent or decrease mood episodes. For some individuals, it can be effective to have discretion over whether or not to take a sedative if they are having difficulty sleeping. Good sleep habits and sleep hygiene (see Chapter 9) should be taught and reinforced.

e. Helping clients identify their specific warning signs of an impending mood episode: In the early or prodromal stages of a mood episode, it is often possible to take action that can lessen the overall severity of the mood episode or head it off entirely. In addition to changes in sleep patterns, other warning signs can include:

  i. Noticeable changes in mood: Feeling "too happy," depressed, anxious, or irritable

  ii. Changes in thought and speech patterns: Becoming wired or racy

  iii. Behavioral changes: This is often unique to the individual and can include shopping sprees they can't afford, impulsive decision making at home or work, and preoccupation with specific activities.

  iv. Return of delusional thoughts

f. The importance of daily routines to help regulate mood: Evidence indicates that sticking to a regular routine can decrease the frequency of mood episodes. On the flip side, frequent changes in schedules, such as rotating shift work, can contribute to mood destabilization. It is most important to establish a regular sleep and wake times.

g. Education around the positive benefits of healthy habits (wellness) as part of a person's daily routine:

  i. Teaching clients about nutrition and exercise (especially important when people are on medications that can cause weight gain and metabolic syndrome)

  ii. Emphasizing the importance of clean and sober supports in a person's life, which may will involve changes in who they associate with

h. Education around specific linkages between substance use and bipolar disorder: Although clients may perceive real benefits from the use of cannabis, alcohol, and other substances, these effects are short term. The evidence is clear that people with bipolar disorder who use substances have worse outcomes (e.g., less response to medication, more frequent hospitalizations, more mood episodes, and greater incidence of suicide attempts and unintended overdoses).

3. **Inclusion of supports**, such as family or close friends, in treatment: This is to both provide education and to help increase the level of support for the person with bipolar disorder. These educational efforts could include directing family and friends to organizations, such as NAMI (www.nami.org), which offer both support groups, as well as thoughtful and up-to-date trainings for family and peers.

4. **Evidence-based psychotherapies** for bipolar disorder

   a. Integrated group therapy: Developed by Roger Weiss, MD, integrated group therapy is a cognitive behavioral group therapy designed for people with co-occurring substance use and bipolar disorders. It is a manualized, twelve-session therapy (also studied in a longer twenty-session format) used in conjunction with medication. It addresses both disorders simultaneously (i.e., "bipolar substance abuse"). Common features of both disorders are stressed. Thoughts and behaviors that aid recovery are encouraged, and conversely, those that increase the risk of relapse with substance use or into a mood episode are discouraged. Connections between the two disorders are highlighted, and clients learn how substance use worsens their bipolar symptoms and how going off their medication can lead to relapse of both a mood episode and substance use.

   b. Family-focused treatment: Developed by David J. Miklowitz and Michael J. Goldstein, this is a manual-driven, twenty-one-session therapy that brings together both the person with bipolar and that person's family. The emphasis is on education about bipolar disorder and on how to resolve family conflict. Family members are taught how to recognize symptoms of impending mood episodes, and problem-solving techniques are stressed. Family-focused treatment is associated with a decreased relapse rate of mood episodes and improved family communication and problem solving.

   c. Interpersonal and social rhythm therapy: Developed by Ellen Frank, PhD, this psychotherapy helps people with bipolar disorder stabilize their mood by establishing healthy and regular routines and by actively decreasing interpersonal conflict. It incorporates education around bipolar and helps the individual learn techniques to decrease conflict.

5. **Other psychotherapies** can be adapted to incorporate issues relevant to both substance use and bipolar disorder. They include CBT, REBT, DBT, and others. Motivational interviewing techniques can be incorporated to help people change problem behaviors related to the substance use and the bipolar disorder, such as poor adherence to a medication regimen and continued problem substance use.

PHARMACOTHERAPY

People with bipolar disorder should be offered initial and ongoing assessment for medication. This regimen will likely include the use of mood stabilizers, as well as medications to assist with cravings and other comorbid psychiatric disorders and symptoms.

Few studies look at specific medications in individuals who have both bipolar disorder and substance use disorders. Most drug studies exclude subjects with co-occurring disorders to decrease confounding variables. In general, those studies that have looked at specific mood stabilizers in people with co-occurring substance use disorders and bipolar disorder show a positive effect in both directions. That is, if you treat the bipolar disorder, the substance use disorder improves, and when people are abstinent from substances, their bipolar symptoms improve.

The primary goal for medication in bipolar disorder is to achieve mood stabilization, which means the person does not experience episodes of depression, mania, and/or hypomania. Common secondary targets for medication include improving sleep disturbances (e.g., insomnia, hypersomnia, sleep apnea), anxiety, and irritability.

Many effective pharmacological treatments are available for the symptoms of mania and hypomania. When people are manic, tranquilizers, often combined with mood stabilizers, are used to decrease the symptoms of excitement, agitation, and psychosis. However, far fewer medication options are available for the treatment of the depression associated with bipolar disorder. Antidepressants, which are used in unipolar depression and many of the anxiety disorders, are not first- or second-line treatments for bipolar depression because they can trigger mania and hypomania and may worsen the frequency and severity of mood episodes (i.e., rapid cycling).

Prescribers need to factor in many variables in order to select appropriate medication. If someone has a history of overusing or abusing anxiolytic medications, such as the benzodiazepines—clonazepam (Klonopin), diazepam (Valium), alprazolam (Xanax), etc.—or they are on opioid replacement therapy (buprenorphine or methadone), these medications can present challenges and an increased risk for overdose. Benzodiazepines should be avoided if someone actively misuses alcohol because the synergistic effects can lead to increased impulsivity, oversedation, and in extreme instances, respiratory depression and death. If someone is overweight or is concerned about medications that can cause significant weight gain and metabolic syndrome, that will limit available options.

Medications for bipolar disorder include mood stabilizers—lithium, lamotrigine (Lamictal), and valproate (Depakote)—which are often augmented with tranquilizers/neuroleptics. Some of the atypical neuroleptics—such as quetiapine (Seroquel), aripiprazole (Abilify), and ziprasidone (Geodon)—have also received FDA approval as mood stabilizers, both to augment lithium and valproate but also as monotherapy.

Patient education should be provided for all medications, both in verbal and written form (e.g., patient-information sheets specific to the medication). Special attention should be paid when using lithium so that the patient is aware of expected side effects, as well as more dire—and potentially life-threatening—signs of lithium toxicity (e.g., worsening tremor, slurred speech, unsteady gate, nausea, vomiting, confusion).

When using lamotrigine (Lamictal), which involves a slow titration (up to a couple of months), clients need to be alert to the signs of a serious and potentially fatal allergic reaction that takes the form of a severe rash and sores: Stevens-Johnson syndrome. If patients complain, notice sores in their nose or mouth, or develop a significant rash on the trunk, thighs, and extremities, this warrants an emergency evaluation, and if the rash is thought to be caused by the medication, it should be discontinued.

Most of the atypical antipsychotics carry significant risk for the development of metabolic syndrome, which includes weight gain, elevations in lipids (cholesterol, triglycerides), and the development of type 2 diabetes, as well as hypertension and coronary artery disease. Some of these agents, such as olanzapine (Zyprexa), can be associated with weight gain on the order of one pound per week. Others, such as risperidone (Risperdal) and quetiapine (Seroquel), have weight gain averaging half a pound per week. To date, the only atypical that does not appear associated with significant weight gain is ziprasidone (Geodon).

It is important to pay attention to a person's baseline health status and to changes in weight and laboratory values during treatment. Medication education should include discussion about the risk for metabolic syndrome, as well as pragmatic nutritional counseling about portion control, food choices, and daily exercise. Patients should be weighed at regular intervals and their BMI monitored. (There are a number of free smartphone and computer applications for BMI calculation, including ones through the National Institutes of Health and the CDC.)

The older antipsychotic medications, such as haloperidol (Haldol) and others, are often used in emergency -room and inpatient settings when rapid tranquilization of an agitated mania is required and are often administered in combination with a benzodiazepine, such as lorazepam (Ativan). The long-term use of this older group of antipsychotics has become less common in maintenance therapy due to concerns of a potentially irreversible movement disorder called tardive dyskinesia.

Mood-Stabilizing Medications			
Name	**FDA-Approved Indications**	**Major Side Effects and Adverse Reactions**	**Monitoring**
Lithium	• Mania and maintenance treatment of bipolar disorder	• Weight gain, increased thirst, diarrhea, tremor, psoriasis • Dangerous/life-threatening toxicity if levels are too high • Can damage the thyroid gland and kidneys • Associated with increased rates of cardiac birth defects	• Lithium level • Renal function • Thyroid function tests • Weight/BMI • Pregnancy

Lamotrigine/ Lamictal	• Bipolar I disorder in patients over age eighteen • Maintenance treatment.	• Risk of a dangerous allergic reaction (Stevens-Johnson Syndrome) • Some concern about subtle birth defects	• Liver function • Pregnancy
Valproic acid (Depakote)	• Treatment of acute mania • Not FDA-approved as a mood stabilizer in the United States	• Weight gain, metabolic syndrome, sedation, mental sluggishness, hair loss, tremor • Birth defects (should be avoided in pregnant women or women likely to become pregnant)	• Liver function • Weight/BMI • Lipids • Blood sugar • HgA1C • Pregnancy
Carbamazepine (Tegretol)	• Not FDA-approved in the United States as a mood stabilizer	• Agranulocytosis (i.e., loss of white blood cell production)	• CBC • Liver function • Pregnancy

Second-Generation Tranquilizers/Neuroleptics/Antipsychotic Medications			
Name	**FDA-Approved Indications**	**Major Side Effects and Adverse Reactions**	**Monitoring**
Aripiprazole/ Abilify	• Schizophrenia (adults and adolescents) • Acute mania and mixed episodes in bipolar I (ages ten and up)* • Maintenance treatment in bipolar I, both as monotherapy and as an adjunct to lithium or valproic acid (adults) • Adjunctive treatment in major depressive disorder	• Weight gain, metabolic syndrome	• Weight/BMI • Lipids • Blood sugar • HgA1C • Pregnancy
Asenapine (Saphris)	• Schizophrenia (adults) • Acute mania or mixed episodes in bipolar I (adults)*	• Weight gain, metabolic syndrome	• Weight/BMI • Lipids • Blood Sugar • HgA1C • Pregnancy

Clozapine (Clozaril)**	• Treatment-resistant schizophrenia • Reducing the risk of suicide in people with schizophrenia or schizoaffective disorder	• Agranulocytosis • Weight gain, metabolic syndrome • Hypotension	• CBC (weekly, then biweekly, and then monthly) • Weight/BMI • Lipids • Blood sugar • HgA1C • Pregnancy
Iloperidone (Fanapt)	• Schizophrenia (adults)	• Weight gain, metabolic syndrome	• Weight/BMI • Lipids • Blood Sugar • HgA1C • Pregnancy
Lurasidone (Latuda)	• Schizophrenia • Depression associated with bipolar I	• Weight gain, metabolic syndrome • Sedation • Restlessness	• Weight/BMI • Lipids • Blood Sugar • HgA1C • Pregnancy
Olanzapine (Zyprexa)	• Schizophrenia (ages thirteen and up) • Bipolar I (both as monotherapy and as an adjunct to lithium or valproic acid) • Combined with fluoxetine (Prozac) for the treatment of depression associated with bipolar I (branded as Symbyax)	• Weight gain, metabolic syndrome • Sedation	• Weight/BMI • Lipids • Blood Sugar • HgA1C • Pregnancy
Paliperidone (Invega)	• Schizophrenia (adult) • Schizoaffective disorder (ages twelve to seventeen) as monotherapy and as an adjunct to mood stabilizers and/or antidepressants	• Weight gain, metabolic syndrome	• Weight/BMI • Lipids • Blood Sugar • HgA1C • Pregnancy
Quetiapine (Seroquel)	• Schizophrenia • Bipolar I disorder, mania and mixed* • Bipolar disorder depressive episodes • Adjunctive therapy in major depressive disorder	• Weight gain, metabolic syndrome • Sedation	• Weight/BMI • Lipids • Blood Sugar • HgA1C • Pregnancy

Risperidone (Risperdal)	• Schizophrenia • Bipolar mania • Irritability associated with autism spectrum disorder (Pediatric indication)	• Weight gain, metabolic syndrome	• Weight/BMI • Lipids • Blood Sugar • HgA1C • Pregnancy
Ziprasidone (Geodon)	• Schizophrenia (adults) • Bipolar I disorder, acute mania or mixed, as monotherapy (adults)* • Adjunctive maintenance treatment with lithium or valproate (adults)	• Cardiac conduction problems, especially when combined with other medications	• Weight/BMI • Lipids • Blood Sugar • HgA1C • EKG • Pregnancy

*Mixed episodes are not included in the DMS-5. Now noted with the specifier "mixed features."

**Clozapine is infrequently used in bipolar disorder due to the risks associated with this medication.

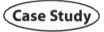

Chad Jenkins

Chad is a twenty-eight-year-old freelance graphic designer, photographer, and vlogger with a successful YouTube channel where he posts instructional tech videos. He is self-referred to a mental health clinic with a chief complaint of "crushing depression and wicked-bad anxiety." He adds that his "sleep sucks, but it always has. Either I get none, or I stay in bed all day… and I'm not kidding—all day." He has no children and is in a committed same-sex relationship of two years. "We're not married, but I wouldn't mind, and I know that my mood swings bother Jim, especially when I crash. He also thinks I drink too much… which I do." He adds, "There's a seasonal pattern to things. I have tons of energy in the spring, feel amazing, don't need much sleep, get a ton of stuff done, but toward the end of fall, like now, when the days get short, the depression hits, and it's worse every year. I'm like a bear. I just want to crawl into bed and stay there… for months. I also pack on pounds, which I can't stand, when I get like this."

Chad reports his mood problems go back to early childhood. "It was a typical suburban upbringing… which means screwed up." He's the youngest of four and the only boy. "I hated school and made up all sorts of excuses not to go. It's amazing I graduated. Junior high was the worst. I was the awkward kid who didn't play sports and got picked on. Coming home from school on the bus was a nightmare. I'd sometimes get followed home by some moron who thought it was fun to beat me up and throw my books into poison ivy. To avoid the hassle, I'd walk home, which was a couple of miles." His parents are still together and, while concerned about his freelance career, are supportive. He came out gay to his family in his late teens. "I could tell my parents—especially Dad—had issues, but they're on board now. I had a good friend, at least I thought he was a good friend, stop talking to me, and one of my sisters won't let me near her kids. That sucks, and she and I don't talk." He attended college and has a Bachelor of Fine Arts and significant school debt. In addition to his freelance work, he teaches computer graphics at a state college. "It forces me to keep my skills on point."

His psychiatric history is significant for having seen three therapists, and when he was nineteen, he saw a psychiatrist for a medication evaluation. "He put me on Prozac, and it made me crazy, like literally. I got paranoid, stopped sleeping altogether, and hallucinated… and not in a fun way. He wanted to put me in a hospital. I freaked out, stopped the medication, and never saw him again. It took over a month for me to feel even close to normal." He's never been hospitalized but admits to two suicide attempts, both by overdose: one with oven cleaner when he was thirteen and the other with over-the-counter medications when he was a teenager. Neither of these did he report. When asked about the precipitants, he states, "The first was because of the bullying, and the second was getting my heart broken. Apparently, I can't handle rejection."

He smokes cannabis daily, which he does not view as a problem. "It keeps me calm." He first smoked at fourteen, but now prefers to vape, uses THC tincture, and makes edibles. He admits to alcohol consumption at least four times per week. "It's crept up, and there are weeks, months if I'm honest, where I drink every night. Not so much to get drunk, but when I can't sleep, which is a lot, it knocks me out. I've gone weeks or even a month or two without a drop, but then something happens, and suddenly it's every night again." He tried hallucinogens in college, as well as cocaine and heroin, but has never injected drugs. "Back when I partied more, I'd take Ecstasy, Molly, and whatever else was around. Now it's weed and booze." He does not use tobacco.

His family history is significant for a maternal uncle who committed suicide. "I didn't really know him. He had schizophrenia and lived in group homes. He'd show up at family events and always seemed sad and out of place." He reports a sister with anxiety problems and panic attacks and believes his mother has similar problems with her mood, though she's never been treated or diagnosed. "As a kid, she always seemed mad and you knew to stay out of her way. But she never hit us, and I think maybe I got spanked twice for doing something really awful."

His medical history is significant for an appendectomy as a child. He's allergic to bee stings but is otherwise in good health, except for migraines (one to four/month). He does not currently have a medical provider and uses pharmacy instant clinics for annual flu shots and when his headaches are bad.

His mental status exam is of an articulate, at times humorous, man. He is dressed in cargo pants and a graphic T-shirt, which he designed. He is fully oriented and makes good eye contact. His speech is rapid, at times pressured, though he can be interrupted. His mood is described as anxious and depressed. His affect is full range and appropriate to content. Thought processes are logical, at times mildly tangential, but organized. He denies any psychotic symptoms and has no current thoughts of self-harm or harm to others.

His PHQ-9 is positive at 15 (moderate depression). He describes his current level of anxiety as between a 7–9 on a 10-point scale. His MDQ is positive with affirmative answers to all but one question. A screen for PTSD using the PCL-5 is positive at 45. A quick-read urine is positive for cannabis/THC only. His breathalyzer is negative. A review of the prescription drug monitoring database shows no prescriptions for controlled substances. His vital signs are normal, and his BMI is 24 (normal). He is insured through the exchange at the lowest level and asks about sliding-scale fees.

Step One: Level of Care Determination and Discussion

Mr. Jenkins presents with chief complaints of anxiety, depression, and mood swings and also acknowledges that he drinks most nights and smokes cannabis. He relates both alcohol and cannabis use to managing symptoms of anxiety and insomnia.

His history, which includes an episode of antidepressant-precipitated mania with psychosis, multiple sustained depressive and hypomanic episodes, and a strong family history of bipolar disorder, will meet criteria for bipolar I disorder. As there are no current emergent or high-risk issues, outpatient services that are tailored to his needs, priorities, and budget should be pursued. Options could include a private multispecialty behavioral health and co-occurring practice; an integrated co-occurring mental health and substance use clinic, such as a local mental health authority, hospital-based outpatient or not-for-profit clinic; or a federally qualified health care center (FQHC) with strong integrated behavioral health and primary care medical services.

Step Two: Construct the Problem/Need List

Substance Use	Mental Health	Medical
Drinks most nights	"Crushing depression and wicked-bad anxiety"	Appendectomy as a child
Daily cannabis use; Began smoking at age fourteen; Now vapes and uses/ makes edibles	Poor sleep; Too much or too little	Allergy to bee stings
Believes he might drink too much (contemplative)	Mood swings characterized by sustained depression and hypomania	No current medical provider
Alcohol use has increased in both quantity and frequency	Seasonal pattern (high in the spring, depressed in the fall and winter)	Migraines
Multiple attempts to decrease alcohol intake and frequency	Bullied as a child	
No reported symptoms of alcohol withdrawal	Has experienced negative consequences and loss of relationships due to being gay	
Does not believe his cannabis use is problematic	In a supportive long-term relationship	
	Supportive parents	
	Uncle with schizophrenia and completed suicide	
	PHQ-9 score of 15 PCL-5 score of 45	

(Continued)

(Continued)

Substance Use	Mental Health	Medical
	Strongly positive MDQ screen for bipolar disorder	
	History of fluoxetine-precipitated mania with psychosis	
	Rapid speech	
	History of two unreported suicide attempts, last at age nineteen	
	Never hospitalized; Has been in therapy three times	

Within these categories, an initial problem/need list can be constructed that contains three primary issues:

1. **Recurrent and severe mood episodes**, with recurrent depression, hypomania, and anxiety; Current episode depressed with increased sleep and appetite; Current PHQ-9 score of 15, strongly positive MDQ; Two unreported suicide attempts by overdose and poisoning; Significant early trauma (bullying)

2. **Problematic alcohol consumption and daily cannabis use.** Increased frequency and quantity of alcohol consumption with unsuccessful attempts to decrease use and related relational conflict; Not interested in addressing cannabis use as client finds it helps with his anxiety and sleep

3. **No current primary care provider.** Has not been assessed and treated for recurrent migraines

Step Three: Establish the Initial Goals/Objectives for Treatment

1. Recurrent and severe mood episodes

   a. Short-term goal(s):

   i. Decrease depressive symptoms to < 10 on the PHQ-9

   ii. Stabilize sleep to between six and a half to eight hours/night

   iii. Decrease anxiety to no more than a 4 on a 10-point scale

   iv. Provide education on bipolar disorder and treatment options, including medication, psychotherapy, and wellness regimens

   v. Address symptoms of trauma and decrease severity by 20 percent or more as measured by self-report and with the PCL-5

   b. Long-term goal(s):

   i. Prevent annual recurrence of mood episodes

   ii. Decrease trauma symptoms by 50 percent or more

2. Problematic alcohol use and daily cannabis use
   a. Short-term goal(s):
      i. Clarify current consumption of alcohol and cannabis to include patterns, frequency, and quantity of use
      ii. Decrease alcohol consumption by 50 percent or more
      iii. Complete pros and cons assessment of both alcohol and cannabis
   b. Long-term goal(s):
      i. Maintain alcohol use within established guidelines for nonproblem drinking. If unable to do so, pursue abstinence
3. No current primary care provider
   a. Short-term goal(s):
      i. Obtain a primary care provider and have an initial evaluation to include assessment of migraines
   b. Long-term goal(s):
      i. Ongoing access to primary care and specialty care if needed

Treatment-and-Recovery Plan

Patient's Name: Chad Jenkins	
Date of Birth: 8/12/1994	
Medical Record #: XXX-XX-XXXX	

Level of Care: Outpatient

ICD-10 Codes	DSM-5 Diagnoses
F31.32	Bipolar type I, moderate, current episode depressed, with anxiety and sleep disturbance
F10.20	Alcohol use disorder, moderate
F12.10	Cannabis use disorder, mild

The individual's stated goal(s): "To stop this roller coaster of my mood swings and to not have my drinking ruin my relationship"

1. **Problem/Need Statement:** Recurrent and severe mood episodes, with recurrent depression, hypomania, and anxiety; Current episode depressed with increased sleep and appetite; Current PHQ-9 score of 15, strongly positive MDQ; Two unreported suicide attempts by overdose and poisoning; Significant history of trauma.
Long-Term Goal: Prevent annual recurrence of mood episodes.
Short-Term Goals/Objectives (with target date):
1. Decrease depressive symptoms to < 10 on the PHQ-9 (11/30/22)
2. Stabilize sleep to between 6.5–8 hours/night (11/15/22)
3. Decrease anxiety to no more than a 4 on a 10-point scale (11/30/22)
4. Provide education on bipolar disorder and treatment options, including medication, psychotherapy, and wellness regimens (10/31/22)
5. Address symptoms of trauma and decrease severity by 20 percent or more as measured by self-report and with the PCL-5 (11/30/22)

2. **Problem/Need Statement:** Problematic alcohol consumption and daily cannabis use; Increased frequency and quantity of alcohol consumption with unsuccessful attempts to decrease use and related relational conflict; Not interested in addressing cannabis use as client finds it helps with his anxiety and sleep.
Long-Term Goal: Maintain alcohol use within established guidelines for nonproblem drinking. If unable to do so, pursue abstinence.

Short-Term Goals/Objectives (with target date):

1. Clarify current consumption of alcohol and cannabis to include patterns, frequency, and quantity of use (10/20/22)
2. Decrease alcohol consumption by 50 percent or more (10/30/22)
3. Complete pros and cons assessment of both alcohol and cannabis (10/27/22)

---

3. **Problem/Need Statement:** No current primary care provider

Long-Term Goal: Maintain a primary care provider

Short-Term Goals/Objectives with target dates:

1. Obtain a primary care provider (10/31/22) and have migraines assessed

Interventions					
Treatment Modality	**Specific Type**	**Frequency**	**Duration**	**Problem Number**	**Responsible Person(s)**
Psychiatric Evaluation	Full MD or APRN diagnostic evaluation	Once	1.5 hours	1, 2, 3	MD/nurse practitioner and RN
Individual Psychotherapy	CBT and motivational approach with integrated co-occurring focus. Address trauma.	Weekly	50 minutes	1, 2	Social worker
Ongoing Pharmacological Management	Medication management	Initially weekly, then as needed	For the duration of treatment	1, 2, 3	MD/nurse practitioner
Family/Couples Counseling	Family and/ or couples sessions	Once, and then as needed	1 hour	1, 2	Social worker or marriage/ family counselor
Lab Work	Labs/blood work, urine toxicology, breathalyzer, other studies	As ordered	As needed	1, 2, 3	MD/nurse practitioner
Additional	Referrals to primary care, provide information on peer-led supports	Once, and then follow up in individual and medication-management sessions	30 minutes	1, 2, 3	Social worker, MD/nurse practitioner/ recovery specialist

Identification of strengths: Supportive family and partner. Motivated to address mood problems and alcohol use. Creative and intelligent

Barriers to treatment: Financial concerns regarding the expense of treatment and medication

Staff/client-identified education/teaching needs: To understand the nature of bipolar disorder and learn strategies to best manage his mood. To learn about possible medications for mood stabilization. To learn about the relationships between his alcohol and cannabis use and mood symptoms and trauma

Assessment of discharge needs/discharge planning: To have achieved his above-stated goals and require less intense treatment, such as ongoing medication management and some form of relapse prevention work

Completion of this treatment-and-recovery plan was a collaborative effort between the client and the following treatment team members:

SIGNATURES		Date/Time:
Client:	Chad Jenkins	10/13/2022, 11:00 a.m.
Physician:	Artem Baranski, MD	10/20/2022, 2:00 p.m.
Primary Clinician:	Louise Jefferson, LPC	10/13/2022 , 11:00 a.m.

....

CHAPTER 13

Anxiety Disorders and Co-Occurring Substance Use Disorders

OVERVIEW

All anxiety disorders carry high rates of co-occurrence with substance use disorders (more than threefold over the general population). In a large study of people who sought treatment for alcohol use disorders, more than 30 percent met criteria for an anxiety disorder. This makes sense when you consider the nature of sedative medications—such as alcohol, certain sleeping medications, opioids, and the benzodiazepines, including lorazepam (Ativan) and diazepam (Valium)—and the short-term relief they can provide from worry and anxiety. Through a behavioral lens, these drugs, when taken to reduce anxiety, produce an immediate reward (positive reinforcement), and their continued use may provide some relief from symptom recurrence (negative reinforcement).

225

However, as tolerance and physical dependence take hold—which can happen quickly with opioids and over a longer timeframe with alcohol and other sedatives—the need to maintain the substance carries the added imperative of preventing withdrawal symptoms.

Research shows that anxiety disorders, with the notable exception of PTSD, develop years before the substance use disorder. And there can be significant symptom and syndrome overlap among anxiety disorders. Most adults with anxiety disorders can trace their origins back to childhood, with symptoms of separation anxiety, school avoidance, specific phobias, and generalized anxiety. For many, anxious symptoms seem to "morph" over time, with periods of increased stress generating exacerbations that might include altogether new symptoms, such as panic attacks or agoraphobia.

The connections between substances and anxiety disorders make tremendous sense. Someone with OCD might experience panic attacks and periods of agoraphobia (fear of leaving the house) and use alcohol to muster up the courage to go to the grocery store. And many with opioid use disorders and PTSD will describe a profound sense of relief and well-being when they took that first hit of oxycodone, heroin, or fentanyl.

The fluid nature of anxiety disorders becomes more complex when substance use co-occurs. Not only can substances provide temporary relief from symptoms of anxiety, they can also cause anxiety syndromes, at times severe, especially when people go in and out of withdrawal states from alcohol, opioids, or other sedating medications. What the person identifies as an anxiety disorder may in fact be alprazolam (Xanax) withdrawal that has worsened and/or mimics the underlying condition.

An interesting relationship between substance use and anxiety disorders is that having one increases the probability of having the other, as well as hastens its development. The age of onset of anxiety disorders is up to seven years earlier in people with substance use disorders than those without. Children and adolescents with anxiety disorders have an increased risk for substance misuse as adolescents and adults. From a public health perspective, they present an opportunity for early intervention.

Compared to individuals who have either co-occurring anxiety or substance use disorders, people who have both have poorer outcomes that include higher rates of other psychiatric disorders (mood disorders in particular), increased rates of hospitalization, higher rates of disability, increased medical comorbidity, and increased suicide risk. Patterns of alcohol and substance use in people with anxiety disorders also tend to be more severe.

It's important to carefully assess each person's specific symptoms and syndromes, as clarification of anxiety diagnoses, substance use diagnoses, and other co-occurring medical and psychiatric disorders will guide treatment. A few points to remember in the assessment process include:

- If someone is in a withdrawal state (e.g., from alcohol, opioids, or benzodiazepines), this may worsen symptoms of anxiety, irritability, and depression. In the absence of a clear history, definitive diagnosis of a nonsubstance-induced anxiety disorder may need to be deferred until after the withdrawal has resolved.

- Intoxication with some substances (e.g., stimulants, bath salts, cannabis, hallucinogens, inhalants) can bring on anxiety symptoms or worsen underlying ones.

- After a binge with certain substances (e.g., cocaine, PCP, other stimulants), anxiety symptoms may be exacerbated and confuse the diagnostic picture.

- In taking the history, it is important, although not always possible, to identify which came first: the problems with anxiety, even if never formally diagnosed, or the substance use.

ASSESSMENT TOOLS AND RATING SCALES

It helps to create a common language between the client and the therapist for symptoms of anxiety. This can involve the use of screening and evaluation tools, as well as numeric scales, such as:

- **The Yale-Brown Obsessive-Compulsive Scale (Y-BOCS):** This scale helps to put a number and severity on current symptoms of OCD based on the amount of time an individual spends involved in OCD thoughts and actions daily.

- **Subjective Units of Distress (SUDs):** This is a useful scale, where the client rates their overall level of distress from 0 (no distress) to 100 (the most distress imaginable). Not only does this aid in quantifying distress at the time of evaluation, but it can be used to assess clinical interventions moving forward.

  o "Before you gave the talk, what was your SUDs? What was it during the talk? And what was it after?"

  o "What was your SUDs before you saw the picture of the spider? What was it during? Did it change as you sat with the anxiety and practiced mindful breathing? What was it after?"

- **Likert scales:** Likert scales are a common method to put a number on a symptom. These involve the use of 5-point scales, typically 0–4 or 1–5. The highest number will represent the most severe or extreme symptoms (or symptoms that are all of the time/constant), and the lowest number stands for none of that symptom or never.

0	1	2	3	4
(None)	(Mild)	(Moderate)	(Severe)	(Extreme)
1	2	3	4	5
(Never)	(Rarely)	(Often)	(Most of the time)	(Constant)

Likert scales comprise the bulk of many other assessment tools and can be applied to most symptoms.

- **10-point scales:** Ten-point scales can quantify the severity of a problem or symptom and track progress over time. When using a 10-point scale, define the parameters for your client. "Using a 10-point scale, where 0 is none and 10 is the worst anxiety anyone could ever have, what is your current level of anxiety?"

- **The Patient-Reported Outcomes Measurement Information System (PROMIS) Emotional Distress Short Form for Anxiety:** The PROMIS is a seven-item screening instrument/assessment tool completed by the client. It utilizes 5-point Likert scales. The copyright is held by the PROMIS Health Organization but can be reproduced without permission by clinicians for use with their patients. Copies, along with scoring guidelines, are available from the American Psychiatric Association at www.psychiatry.org/practice/dsm/dsm5/online-assessment-measures #Disorder, along with many other recommended assessment tools.

- **The Generalized Anxiety Disorder 7-Item Scale (GAD-7):** This is a widely used and efficient self-report tool that helps quantify the severity of anxiety symptoms and is a validated screening tool for GAD. It can also help identify symptoms associated with other anxiety disorders, such as social anxiety disorder, PTSD, panic disorder, and others. It is in the public domain, is available in over eighty translations, and can be accessed free online at www.phqscreeners.com.

Generalized Anxiety Disorder
7-Item Scale (GAD-7)

Over the last two weeks, how often have you been bothered by the following problems?	Not at all	Several days	Over half the days	Nearly every day
1. Feeling nervous, anxious, or on edge	0	1	2	3
2. Not being able to stop or control worrying	0	1	2	3
3. Worrying too much about different things	0	1	2	3
4. Trouble relaxing	0	1	2	3
5. Being so restless that it's hard to sit still	0	1	2	3
6. Becoming easily annoyed or irritable	0	1	2	3
7. Feeling afraid as if something awful might happen	0	1	2	3
Add the score for each column	+	+	+	
Total Score *(add your column scores)* =				

If you checked off any problems, how difficult have these made it for you to do your work, take care of things at home, or get along with other people?

Not difficult at all _____
Somewhat difficult _____
Very difficult _____
Extremely difficult _____

Scoring the GAD-7: Cut-off points of 5, 10, and 15 correspond with mild, moderate, and severe anxiety symptoms, respectively.

Source: Spitzer R. L., Kroenke, K., Williams, J. B., & Löwe, B. (2006). A brief measure for assessing generalized anxiety disorder. *Archives of Internal Medicine, 166*(10), 1092–1097.

ANXIETY DISORDERS WITH CO-OCCURRING SUBSTANCE USE DISORDERS

What follows are brief descriptions of the anxiety disorders and their associations with substance use disorders and other common comorbid disorders. PTSD and trauma, which frequently include anxious symptoms, will be addressed in the next chapter. The specifier "with anxious distress" can be applied to numerous nonanxiety disorders, such as the psychotic and mood (i.e., depressive and bipolar) disorders.

Generalized Anxiety Disorder

GAD includes protracted (i.e., more than six months) and excessive anxiety that is directed toward various situations and settings in a person's life (e.g., school, work, family, finance, health, etc.). In addition to anxiety, GAD can include irritability, poor concentration, muscle tension, and general and pervasive feelings of being "keyed up" and "on edge." The nervousness and worry often lead to significant problems with sleep.

GAD carries more than a twofold lifetime risk for developing a substance use disorder and nearly a sixfold risk for mood disorders. Alcohol use disorders, followed by other sedatives and anxiolytics, are the most common substance problems with GAD. People with co-occurring substance use and GAD have worse treatment outcomes, with increased levels of disability, more suicide attempts, and more frequent hospitalization.

Most people with GAD report the anxiety predated the substance use. As teens, people with GAD often discover that alcohol and other drugs provide temporary relief from their excessive worry and anxiety. On average, people with GAD develop problem substance use earlier than those who just have substance use disorders.

Heavy drinking and misuse of anxiolytic medication often complicate the diagnostic picture in GAD, especially if the substance use is unreported, unidentified, or minimized. When under the influence of alcohol and certain drugs, anxiety symptoms will diminish, and there can be tremendous symptom overlap between alcohol or benzodiazepine withdrawal and GAD, as well as other anxiety disorders.

Studies that have looked at the treatment of substance use and GAD show superior outcomes when both are adequately assessed and addressed in treatment.

Social Anxiety Disorder (Social Phobia)

Social anxiety disorder is characterized by intense, at times incapacitating, fear and dread of social situations. People with social anxiety disorder are often profoundly worried and ruminate about how others negatively perceive and judge them. They view themselves as defective, ineffective, and even unlovable. Social anxiety disorder carries high rates for comorbid and severe alcohol and drug use disorders. Individuals are also at a higher risk for both unipolar and bipolar depressive disorders.

Much substance use treatment involves group modalities, and these may present both a barrier to treatment—"I can't stand groups"—as well as have the potential for some exposure-based work to confront the anxiety.

Social anxiety disorder typically develops before the substance problem(s). Studies show that substance use problems develop somewhat later for social anxiety disorder than other anxiety disorders. One explanation is that people with social anxiety disorder avoid peer situations where drugs and/or alcohol will be available. However, as with the other anxiety disorders, patterns of substance use can be severe, especially alcohol, sedatives, painkillers, and anxiolytic medications, such as the benzodiazepines and opioids.

Panic Disorder

While all anxiety disorders can include panic attacks, panic disorder is characterized by recurrent panic attacks and intense fear or worry that the attacks will recur and/or efforts to avoid situations and settings that might precipitate an attack. In many instances, this fear of having a panic attack or of losing control can lead to agoraphobia, where the individual becomes frightened to leave their home. In the DSM-5, agoraphobia has been separated out from panic disorder, and where people meet criteria for panic disorder and agoraphobia, both diagnoses can be given.

Panic disorder is associated with a fourfold increase in rates of alcohol dependence, and the twelve-month comorbidity rates for mood disorders is over eightfold.

Panic attacks come on fast and can be triggered by specific situations or have no identifiable precipitant. Symptoms can be divided into three categories:

1. **Cognitive:** Intense anxiety that comes on fast and may be accompanied by thoughts of dread, a loss of control, or the belief that something horrible is about to happen

2. **Physiological:** Rapid pulse, sweating, heart palpitations, numbness or tingling in the extremities, lump in the throat, a sensation of light-headedness, or a sense of faintness/being about to pass out

3. **Behavioral:** Avoidance of situations and places that the person thinks can trigger an attack, which can progress to severe and disabling agoraphobia

Agoraphobia

Agoraphobia is the intense and disproportionate fear of specific situations, typically of being in public or even just being out of the home or going to a store. The fear and anxiety lead to avoidance, where people refuse to leave the home or do so only in the company of someone else. As with all anxiety disorders, it carries increased rates of co-occurring substance use problems.

Obsessive-Compulsive Disorder

OCD involves obsessive and intrusive thoughts, typically accompanied by intense urges to perform specific actions or think certain thoughts (i.e., compulsive behaviors or thoughts) to alleviate the anxiety associated with the obsession. Severity is based on the degree of resultant impairment and distress. In the DSM-5, modifiers are added to the diagnosis based on the person's level of awareness about their symptoms. This can range from a complete understanding that the thoughts and resultant behavior are not rational to a delusional belief that the thoughts and compulsive behaviors are founded in reality: "If I don't check the stove forty times the house will burn down." "If I don't wash my hands each time I touch a surface, I'll get the flesh-eating bacteria and die."

In both the initial assessment of OCD and in treatment, it's helpful to quantify how many hours a day a person engages in OCD thoughts and behavior. One useful instrument for this is the Yale-Brown Obsessive-Compulsive Scale, or Y-BOC. This, along with other assessment tools for OCD, are available online at the International OCD Foundation website: https://iocdf.org/wp-content/uploads/2014/08/Assessment-Tools.pdf.

Substance/Medication-Induced Anxiety Disorder

While many people with anxiety disorders turn to substances to relieve symptoms, there are also people who develop severe anxiety as a result of substances. This can include the presence of panic attacks and generalized anxiety. There are a broad range of substances that can cause anxiety disorders to develop, including caffeine, cocaine, opioids, other stimulants (e.g., bath salts, methamphetamine, and medications used to treat ADHD), alcohol, over-the-counter cold medications, steroids, and benzodiazepines.

Treatment of Co-Occurring Anxiety and Substance Use Disorders

Psychotherapies

Many studies validate psychosocial and pharmacological treatments for anxiety disorders, but few have systematically studied anxiety disorders that coexist with substance use disorders. In recent years, however, studies that looked at CBT and motivational interviewing, both separate and combined, have observed positive benefits for both the anxiety and substance use disorders. So too mindfulness, which is based in Zen meditation, and other contemplative practices have proved beneficial.

Other forms of therapy, such as psychodynamic and eclectic, while not well studied in these populations, may also help, but the practitioner and client must address both problems. A tremendous amount remains to be studied on the efficacy of particular therapies and approaches for the treatment of co-occurring anxiety and substance use disorders, but the following interrelated points offer guidance:

- Abstinence from the problem substance(s) is associated with improvement in the anxiety disorder.
- Decreased symptoms of the anxiety disorder(s) increase the likelihood of abstinence from the problem substance(s). The anxiety symptoms are often triggers for drug cravings and for use.

Cognitive Behavioral Therapy. CBT has a long and established track record for treating the entire range of anxiety disorders and symptoms, from panic attacks and specific phobias (e.g., fear of spiders, snakes, small spaces, heights, etc.) to OCD. Based on the individual's symptoms, specific techniques are employed. These include graded exposure to a feared event, situation, or thing, combined with response prevention, such as not letting a person with OCD and germ-contamination fears wash their hands after touching a feared object. CBT is often a time-limited therapy with ten to twelve sessions, though booster sessions can be an option on an as needed basis.

Motivational Interviewing Techniques. Motivational interviewing techniques have shown effectiveness in helping people change problem behaviors and can be delivered alone or in combination with CBT techniques. Motivational interviewing can also be used in a "step-wise" fashion where one or two motivational interviewing sessions might then be followed by a longer ten- to twelve-week course of CBT.

Wellness

While easily incorporated into specific psychotherapies such as CBT, attention to an individual's overall wellness regimens can have a dramatic positive effect on both the anxiety and substance use problems. The trick is to create workable strategies with the client that build existing strengths, resources, and preferences. Key components to a wellness routine include:

- Adequate restorative sleep (at least six and a half to eight hours per night)
- Daily exercise: Studies have been generally positive in demonstrating that exercise improves both mood and anxiety symptoms. The type of exercise appears less important, but at least forty-five minutes daily is desirable. This can be anything from going to the gym to walking the dog.
- Healthful eating
- Treatment of active medical issues
- Caffeine restriction
- Attention to important social relations, such as spending time with sober family and friends
- Employment and/or other meaningful pursuits
- Contemplative practices, such as mindfulness meditation, yoga, prayer, and tai chi
- Hobbies, especially those where people get the experience of being completely involved. This may be experienced as "losing track of time," and the list is extensive and includes gardening, painting, playing and/or listening to music, writing/journaling, puzzling, playing games, and all forms of handicraft, such as knitting, sewing, and so forth.

Pharmacology

Few well-controlled studies directly assess individual medications for people with co-occurring substance use and anxiety disorders. Prescribing clinicians must combine information from available studies with standard-of-care practice for each disorder. In addition, the prescriber needs to ask whether this medication, intended for the one disorder, will potentially make the other worse or more problematic. A few points to keep in mind include the following:

- If benzodiazepines are to be used, they must be carefully prescribed and monitored. If possible, their use should be avoided in this population, and when used, avoid short-acting agents, such as alprazolam (Xanax). This becomes an even greater challenge with people on opioid replacement therapy (e.g., buprenorphine and methadone), as the combination of benzodiazepines with any opioid increases the risks for respiratory depression, overdose, coma, and death.

- Antidepressant medications typically take two to four weeks to elicit a response, possibly two to three times as long when used to treat anxiety disorders. Effectiveness of antidepressant medications is hindered by active substance use. For people with bipolar disorders with anxious and/or mixed features, antidepressants may worsen irritability and precipitate mania or hypomania.

Antidepressants. The mainstay of treatment for anxiety disorders are the antidepressants. Studies that look at the antidepressants in people with substance use problems are few and show mixed results. Older medications, such as the tricyclic antidepressants, may be more effective to treat both depression and anxiety in people with co-occurring substance use disorders. However, their toxicity, risk in overdose (e.g., cardiac conduction delays, heart block, and death), need for blood monitoring, and side-effect profile make them less attractive to both clients and prescribers.

The current standard of care is to use SSRIs and SNRIs first. For individuals with both depressive and anxious symptoms, this strategy makes tremendous sense, but if some improvement is not seen after four to six weeks of an adequate trial of a medication at an adequate dose, the clinician needs to consider dose adjustment, augmentation with another medication, or switching to another agent.

Selective Serotonin Reuptake Inhibitors (SSRIs)

Compound	Trade Name	Dose Range (mg/day)
Citalopram	Celexa	10–40
Escitalopram	Lexapro	10–20
Fluoxetine	Prozac	10–60
Fluvoxamine	Luvox	50–200
Paroxetine	Paxil	10–60
Sertraline	Zoloft	50–200
Vilazodone	Viibryd	20-40

Serotonin Norepinephrine Reuptake Inhibitors (SNRIs)

Compound	Trade Name	Dose Range (mg/day)
Duloxetine	Cymbalta	40–60
Desvenlafaxine	Pristiq	50
Levomilnacipran	Fetzima	40–120
Venlafaxine	Effexor, Effexor XR	75–375

Tricyclic Antidepressants

Compound Name	Trade Name	Dose Range (mg/day)
Amitriptyline	Elavil	50–300
Amoxapine	Ascendin	200–400
Clomipramine	Anafranil	150–250
Desipramine	Norpramin	100–300
Doxepin	Sinequan	150–300
Imipramine	Tofranil	150–300
Maprotiline	Ludiomil	75–150
Nortriptyline	Pamelor	50–150
Protriptyline	Vivactil	30–60

Benzodiazepines. All benzodiazepines can be habit forming and misused for their sedating, disinhibiting, and euphoric properties. For people with anxiety disorders, the benzodiazepines can provide prompt relief from symptoms of anxiety, as opposed to the SSRIs and SNRIs that will take weeks or months to achieve their maximum benefit.

Once someone is physiologically dependent on a benzodiazepine, they may be at risk for significant withdrawal syndromes, similar to those seen in alcohol. People who take these medications consistently for more than a couple of weeks should be tapered off with careful follow-up to assess for withdrawal. In this class, medications with shorter half-lives, such as alprazolam (Xanax) and lorazepam (Ativan), are associated with more severe and rapid onset of withdrawal symptoms and syndromes.

Benzodiazepines

Compound	Trade Name	Half-Life (hours)	FDA Indications
Alprazolam	Xanax	6.3–14	• GAD • Panic disorder
Chlordiazepoxide	Librium	5–30	• Anxiety and anxiety disorders • Preoperative anxiety • Alcohol withdrawal
Clonazepam	Klonopin	18–30	• Panic disorder • Some forms of seizure disorders
Clorazepate	Tranxene	40–50	• Anxiety • Alcohol withdrawal
Diazepam	Valium	20–80	• Anxiety and anxiety disorders • Alcohol withdrawal • Muscle spasm • Protracted seizures (status epilepticus)

(Continued)

(Continued)

Compound	Trade Name	Half-Life (hours)	FDA Indications
Flurazepam	Dalmane	50–90+	• Insomnia
Lorazepam	Ativan	10–20	• Anxiety and anxiety associated with depressive symptoms • Protracted seizures
Oxazepam	Serax	5–20	• Anxiety and anxiety associated with depression • Alcohol withdrawal
Temazepam	Restoril	5–17	• Short-term treatment of insomnia
Triazolam	Halcion	2–4	• Short-term treatment of insomnia

Other Medications with FDA Indications for Anxiety Disorders. Hydroxyzine (Vistaril, Atarax) is an antihistamine that can be used in an as-needed manner (PRN) for the treatment of anxiety and, per the package insert, "tension associated with psychoneurosis." It is sedating and is often prescribed off-label as a nonaddictive sleep aid. Typical doses range from 50–100 mg, up to four times per day as needed for anxiety. Some patients report significant relief with this medication and use it daily.

Buspirone (Buspar) is a medication that binds to serotonin receptors in the brain. It has FDA indication for GAD. Typical dose range begins at 7.5 mg twice per day and can be titrated up to 60 mg per day. Benefits from buspirone may take two to four weeks or longer to be felt.

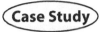

Janelle Compton

Janelle Compton is a married forty-five-year-old, self-employed certified public accountant and mother of two. She is self-referred to a mental health practice with a chief complaint of "My GYN has prescribed my alprazolam for years, but she retired, and I need someone to prescribe it for me." She is currently on 2 mg, three times a day. "I'm just about out, and I'm aware it's not something to just quit cold turkey. I wish I could be off this stuff, but that seems less and less possible."

She's struggled with anxiety her entire life. "My mother says I had separation anxiety, and I stayed home sick a lot. I'd get so worked up in elementary school that I'd throw up just thinking about getting on the bus. By junior high, I was good at hiding it, but I'd stay home sick or hide out in the bathroom when I'd get a panic attack." She reports her panic attacks are mostly controlled with alprazolam, but she still has one or two a month. She describes these as being proceeded by a sense of impending doom, "like something horrible is about to happen, or that I'm going to be in a situation and lose control or do something that will embarrass me." She identifies certain situations as triggers, such as supermarket checkout lines, evening-school activities where she feels judged by other parents, and increasingly, meetings with her clients at tax season. "I spin horrible scenarios, like they'll all find out what a terrible accountant I am. I'll lose all my clients, we won't be able to make the mortgage payments, or we'll lose the house. I know it's crazy, but it gets so bad my hands start to shake, and I think I'm going to black out." Additional symptoms include hyperventilating, rapid pulse, tingling in her extremities, and a choking sensation. She has also had panic attacks with no obvious precipitants. "Without the alprazolam, I can't function. Even with it, I wake up in the middle of the night, and I obsess about my kids, work, my husband… and I can't get back to sleep. It's worse during tax season."

Her social history is that she is the middle of three children to an intact suburban Italian American family. Despite problems with attendance, she excelled in school and is an accomplished violinist. "It's one of the few things I can do and feel calm." Her parents, both retired and in good health, are a retired teacher and an electrical engineer. She lived at home during her undergraduate years and attended business school out of state, where she met and eventually married her husband, Eric, an administrator for a state agency. They have two children—a daughter, twelve, and a son, nine. She describes her husband as generally supportive. "I don't let him know how bad my anxiety gets. He knows I have panic attacks, but I'm good at hiding them. My son, on the other hand, always knows, and I can see he struggles with what I had as a kid. He doesn't want to go to school and won't tell me why. If I can't fix myself, how am I going to help him?"

Past behavioral health services have been mostly focused on medication. She was first prescribed alprazolam by her pediatrician when she was fourteen. She has been on multiple antidepressants, believes they were helpful, but discontinued all of them due to a variety of side effects (e.g., sexual dysfunction, loss of dream sleep, headaches). In addition to alprazolam, she has been prescribed other benzodiazepines but reports the best results with her current regimen. But she adds, "I think I should go up a little." She has never been hospitalized and has no current or history of suicidal behavior. She has never been in psychotherapy. "I know I should, but who's got time for it? Between the kids, work, Eric, the house… give me the pills, and I'm good to go."

She reports no history of mental health problems in her family. However, she adds that her father is likely an alcoholic. "Growing up, you knew to stay out of his way when he'd had a few. He could be a happy drunk or a mean one. I get my nerves from my mother, who's been on Valium or Klonopin as long as I can remember."

She denies any active medical problems. She is a nonsmoker and consumes "an occasional glass of wine on the weekend."

Her mental status exam is that of an intelligent, accomplished, and well-dressed woman who makes good eye contact. Her mood is described as anxious 8/10, though she does not appear markedly nervous. Her speech is fluent and at times slightly pressured. Her thought processes are logical, and there is no evidence of disorganization. While she reports ruminative and anxious thinking, she denies any compulsive or ritualized behavior. She reports no psychotic symptoms or thoughts of harm to self or others. She scores a 12 on the PHQ-9 (mild depression) and a 15 on the GAD-7 (high anxiety). On a 10-point scale, she rates her current level of anxiety as a 9 out of 10.

She is reluctant to provide a urine drug screen and becomes anxious when asked to do so. When reassured that the results will not be shared and that it is essential, she agrees. The point-of-care results are positive for alprazolam, clonazepam, and oxycodone. A review of the state's prescription monitoring database shows that only the alprazolam was prescribed and that she should still have a two weeks' supply left from her thirty-day refill. She becomes tearful and says, "I sometimes borrow some of my mom's Klonopin, and I took half an Oxy (30 mg) that was left from my husband's knee surgery because I was so stressed by coming here. But I don't have a problem with opioids, I swear it."

Her vital signs are within normal limits, and there are no appreciable physical symptoms of any withdrawal.

Step One: Level of Care Determination and Discussion

While there are worrisome and urgent issues with Janelle Compton, such as her escalating benzodiazepine use, the presence of an opioid on her drug screen, and severe anxiety, there appear to be no emergent medical or behavioral health concerns. Outpatient care may be appropriate.

She will need a psychiatric assessment to clarify and better regiment her benzodiazepine consumption, as well as to provide options for other medications that could help diminish her symptoms. There is some urgency with this, as she is correct that she should not quit "cold turkey," and it will be important to decrease her current and potentially dangerous pattern of self-medication with substances she obtains from others. Further exploration of a potential opioid use disorder, along with education regarding the dangers of mixing opioids and benzodiazepines, should be provided.

Psychotherapy, possibly CBT, along with education regarding core wellness strategies and reinforcement of healthy habits, will offer her effective approaches to manage and decrease her anxiety and related symptoms.

Step Two: Construct the Problem/Need List

Mrs. Compton's data can be grouped into two large categories: one related to her symptoms of anxiety and the other related to her substance use.

Substance Use	Mental Health
Prescribed alprazolam 2 mg, three times/day; Running out two weeks early in a month's prescription	Anxiety her entire life
On benzodiazepines since age fourteen	Separation anxiety as a child
Has found antidepressants helpful but has not continued on any due to side effects	Panic attacks mostly controlled with alprazolam; Still gets 1–2/month
Father with alcohol problems	Sleep often broken by intense anxiety and panic
Will use mother's clonazepam	Ruminative thinking
Obtained oxycodone from another family member	Has never been in therapy but thinks it might help
	Mother with anxiety problems, also on benzodiazepines
	Feels calm when playing violin
	Unclear trauma history
	PHQ-9 score of 12, GAD-7 score of 15
	Current anxiety a 9 out of 10

This information can be constructed into the following problem/need list:

1. **Severe and persistent anxiety and panic**, AEB panic attacks and severe anxiety with a GAD-7 score of 15; Lifelong problems with anxiety that predate the use of drugs and/or alcohol

2. **Problematic substance use**, AEB exceeding prescribed dosage of benzodiazepine combined with additional benzodiazepine and opioids obtained from family

Step Three: Establish the Initial Goals/Objectives for Treatment

1. Severe and persistent anxiety and panic
    a. Short-term goals/objectives:
        i. Have symptoms of anxiety be no greater than 5 on a 10-point scale
        ii. Take only the prescribed amount of medications
        iii. Start weekly therapy that specifically addresses symptoms of anxiety and panic
    b. Long-term goal(s):
        i. Be free from panic attacks and have overall anxiety decreased by 50 percent or more (measured by self-report and with GAD-7 score no greater than 7)
2. Problematic substance use
    a. Short-term goals/objectives:
        i. Take medications as prescribed with no additional doses
        ii. Clarify and eliminate any nonprescribed use of opioids and benzodiazepines
    b. Long-term goal(s):
        i. Be on the lowest effective dose of benzodiazepines and, if possible, be off them altogether

Treatment-and-Recovery Plan

Patient's Name: Janelle Compton

Date of Birth: 9/14/1977

Medical Record #: XXX-XX-XXXX

Level of Care: Outpatient

ICD-10 Codes	DSM-5 Diagnoses
F41.1	Generalized anxiety disorder with panic attacks
F13.10	Anxiolytic use disorder, mild (benzodiazepine)

The individual's stated goal(s): "To be able to manage my anxiety and not be so dependent on these pills. Maybe to not need them at some point"

1. Problem/Need Statement: Severe and persistent anxiety and panic
Long-Term Goal: Be free from panic attacks and have overall anxiety decreased by 50 percent or more (measured by self-report and with a GAD-7 score less than 7)
Short-Term Goals/Objectives (with target date):
1. Have symptoms of anxiety be no greater than 5 on a 10-point scale (10/1/2022)
2. Take only the prescribed amount of medications (10/1/22)
3. Start weekly therapy that specifically addresses symptoms of anxiety and panic (10/7/22)

2. Problem/Need Statement: Problematic substance use
Long-Term Goals: Be on the lowest effective dose of benzodiazepines and, if possible, be off them altogether
Short Term Goals/Objectives (with target date):
1. Take medications as prescribed with no additional doses (10/8/22)
2. Clarify and address any nonprescribed use of opioids and benzodiazepines (10/8/22)

Interventions					
Treatment Modality	**Specific Type**	**Frequency**	**Duration**	**Problem Number**	**Responsible Person(s)**
Psychiatric Assessment	Complete diagnostic assessment	Upon admission	1–2 hours	1, 2	MD/nurse practitioner and RN
Individual Therapy	Integrated CBT	Weekly	12 weeks (50-minute sessions)	1, 2	Primary therapist
Ongoing Pharmacological Management	Medication evaluation and management	Initially weekly, then monthly or as needed	For as long as the client is in treatment	1, 2	MD/nurse practitioner
Lab Work	Urine toxicology, other labs as needed	As ordered	As needed	1, 2	MD/nurse practitioner
Peer Support	Online or in-person mutual self-help	At least weekly	Ongoing	1, 2	Mrs. Compton
Wellness	Exercise, get adequate sleep, play violin, spend time with children and husband	Daily	Ongoing	1, 2	Mrs. Compton

Identification of strengths: High level of motivation to address both anxiety and substance use problems. Identifies being a good mother and carrying at least half the family's financial needs as important and meaningful

Peer/family/community supports to assist: Husband, mother, children, few close friends

Barriers to treatment: Time constraints, especially around tax season

Staff/client-identified education/teaching needs: To understand the relationships between her anxiety problems and increased reliance on medication. To learn new ways to manage anxiety and negative emotions. To develop a support system

Assessment of discharge needs/discharge planning: When stated goals have been achieved, decrease frequency and intensity of service to maintain qains and promote ongoing recovery

Completion of this treatment-and-recovery plan was a collaborative effort between the client and the following treatment team members:

SIGNATURES		Date/Time:
Client:	Janelle Compton	9/24/2022, 2:00 p.m.
Treatment Plan Completed By:	Margaret Able, LCSW	9/24/2022, 2:00 p.m.
Medical Provider (Psychiatrist or APRN):	Virginia Able, APRN	10/01/2022, 10:00 a.m.

CHAPTER 14

....

Posttraumatic Stress Disorder and Co-Occurring Substance Use Disorders

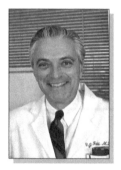

My Story

By Vincent J. Felitti, MD, FACP

my story

Origins of The Adverse Childhood Experiences (ACE) Study: Addiction as a Symptom of Trauma

The ACE Study began in the middle eighties because of counterintuitive findings from an obesity program that we ran at Kaiser Permanente's San Diego service network. We used the then-new technology of supplemented absolute fasting (no food whatever, but a supplement to maintain health and prevent death: 420 calories/day). This was with a Sandoz product, Optifast 70, now owned by Nestlé, and with it we could take a person's weight down 300 pounds in one year. It was enormously successful, and we have treated over 30,000 obese adults without one death.

About two years in, we noticed a high dropout rate that was limited to those who succeeded with their weight loss. I wondered, what's going on? They dropped the pounds but then regained all of it. A couple of women told us they left the study because of male sexual attention that came as they lost the weight. One shared her story of repeated molestation by multiple perpetrators as a child. It left her with profound anxiety, which she treated with three packs of cigarettes per day. Nicotine is an appetite suppressant, and it kept her weight down, as well as provided psychoactive anti-anxiety benefits. But at age thirty-five, her husband convinced her to quit smoking. Suddenly, she was flooded with unwanted male attention. Smoking three packs a day had kept people at a distance. She had no positive experience to deal with this attention, and she ate to reduce the anxiety, her weight going from 130 to 310 pounds. At that point, she developed both acute and chronic respiratory failure and had to go on twenty-four-hour oxygen. She came to our obesity program, and we took her from 310 to 150 pounds. We patted ourselves on the back and thought we'd done a terrific job. But as the weight came down, the sexual attention returned, and she made a conscious decision to go back to 320 pounds and oxygen.

What she shared stuck with me: "It's important to understand that weighing 300 pounds and smoking three packs per day are not my problem. They're *symptoms* of a deeper problem that goes back to my childhood." Indeed, they were the once-unconscious solutions she used to keep sexual attention away. I use the analogy of a house burning down. You see the smoke. It's a symptom, and it can kill you, but it's the fire, the cause, that needs treatment. Otherwise we'd fight fires with large fans.

I began to look at obesity and then at smoking, alcohol, drugs, promiscuity, and other potentially addictive behaviors that provide immediate relief from anxiety and depression, which are the *symptoms* of unrecognized causal issues that are often lost in time and that are further protected by shame and secrecy but are not the root problem. This raised a central question: If the addiction is a symptom, what's the cause? What our patients told us as they fled treatment was that early traumatic experiences from childhood were connected to the morbid obesity that had brought them to the clinic. Another observation was that it's rare to be born overweight. Most of our patients had gained the weight precipitously, often after a traumatic experience(s). One example was a woman who told me that at twenty-three, she was raped and gained a hundred and five pounds in the subsequent year. She then muttered, "Overweight is overlooked, and that's the way I need to be."

We used a group model in our obesity clinic, where patients could offer one another support and develop a deeper understanding about the conditions that had led to and perpetuated the obesity. We'd start with the following three questions:

- ***Why* do you think people get fat, not *how*?** What we heard back was "People will leave you alone," "Men won't bother you," "People expect less from you," and "Folks stay out of your way."
- **Sometimes people who've lost a great deal of weight regain it all and do so quickly. Why does that happen?** The repeated response was "Because if you don't deal with the underlying issues, it will come back."
- **What are the benefits of obesity?** And what they told us was, it's sexually and physically protective; people expect less of you.

In 1990, I presented our findings at a national obesity conference in

Atlanta. I shared what we'd learned that included these connections between obesity and early adverse experiences. In the question period at the end of my presentation, one physician got up and commented, "You really need to understand, Dr. Felitti, those statements by patients are fabrications put forward to provide a cover explanation for failed lives."

At the time, I didn't challenge him, but that night at a speaker's dinner, an epidemiologist from the CDC, Dr. David Williamson, commented that the information I'd shared was incredibly important but that it needed to be validated with an epidemiologically sound study based on thousands of patients. He invited me to speak at the CDC, where my information was well received. This eventually led to a long-standing collaboration with Rob Anda, an internist and epidemiologist at the CDC. Over the course of two years, we designed what would be known as the Adverse Childhood Experiences Study (ACE Study), where we would ask all new adult patients about childhood trauma (before age eighteen).

In 1994, we submitted the ACE Study proposal to the Kaiser Permanent Institutional Review Board (IRB). They turned it down flat, telling us, "You'll make patients decompensate, perhaps become suicidal, if you do this." We finally got approval, but under the condition that I would carry a cell phone 24/7 for three years to handle all the suicidal patients. It never rang, and we received completed responses from over 17,000 individuals about eight and then ten categories of adverse experience before age eighteen.

The results were unexpected and shocking to some. In this middle-class population (average age fifty-seven, 80 percent white, 10 percent Black, 74 percent college educated, all insured):

- 28 percent of the women admitted to contact childhood sexual abuse, as did 16 percent of the men.
- 28 percent reported physical abuse by their parents.
- 27 percent reported alcoholism or substance use in the household.
- 5 percent reported a household member had been incarcerated.
- 13 percent reported domestic violence.
- 23 percent reported divorce or loss of a biological parent.
- 17 percent reported depression or mental illness in the household.
- 10 percent reported physical neglect.

Since then, we have integrated what have come to be called the ACE questions into my department's ten-page health screening form that we have used with 440,000 adults coming in for comprehensive medical evaluation. There have been no patient complaints. Instead, I've gotten letters of thanks from people grateful that we asked these difficult questions. I remember one written on lined paper where an elderly woman wrote, "I feared I would die, and no one would ever know what had happened." Complaints, if we get them, come from colleagues who don't know what to do with the information. Indeed, it's the medical community where we've seen the greatest pushback to the data. There seems to be a deep-rooted belief that nice people don't talk about this stuff.

Our approach with the questionnaire information was to review it with the patients at their first visit. "You said on your questionnaire _____ happened to you as child. Can you tell me how that has that affected you later in your life?" We listened. And we accepted.

As we have then followed those 17,000+ ACE Study patients for over twenty years, we have generated robust and strong evidence to support dose-response connections between childhood adverse experiences and negative biopsychosocial outcomes, including depression, suicide, obesity, hypertension, cancer, smoking, alcoholism, drug misuse, teen pregnancy, multiple marriages, and sixteen autoimmune diseases. That is, risk increases with the number of ACE *categories* a person endorses and not the number of times the thing happened. As one CDC epidemiologist commented, "These are numbers you see once in a career." A few instances include:

- An ACE score of 6 or higher correlates with 19.7 years of lost life.
- Intravenous drug use carries a 4600 percent increased risk for a person with an ACE score of 6 or higher than it does for an ACE score of 0.
- There is a thirty-one-fold increased risk of a suicide attempt with an ACE score of 7 and above.
- There is a fivefold risk for an alcohol use disorder with a score of 4 or more.
- There is a sevenfold increased risk of having three or more marriages with a score of 5 or greater.

What to do with this information? First, we need to get it into routine medical practice. What we see by asking the questions—first via a questionnaire filled out at home and then with empathic and accepting face-to-face follow-up—are positive changes. These include reductions in both emergency room visits (-11 percent) and doctors office visits (-35 percent) in the subsequent year compared to their prior year. In large health care systems, these numbers correlate with billions of dollars in savings.

But the biggest public health advance I can conceive would be to get to the root causes and to improve parenting across this country. If we could decrease the incidence of these adverse childhood events, we would improve the nation's health, as well as people's lives. I think mass media may be a way to do this because it would involve teaching about thirty million young adults what supportive versus destructive parenting looks like and why this is important for their children's health and overall success in life. This might best be accomplished by storytelling and depiction—a serial TV show that provided illustrations of supportive and destructive parenting, with commentary about how these play out decades later. Some of our readers may know people in theater, psychology, public health, and broadcast TV who might be good participants in such a project. Opportunity awaits!

Links to learn more about ACES:

- The ACES site through the CDC: https://www.cdc.gov/violence prevention/childabuseandneglect/acestudy/index.html
- AcesTooHigh.com
- ACESConnection.com
- General internet and YouTube searches of "ACE Study" and "ACE Study—specific point of interest"

my story

Overview

PTSD affects more than five million Americans in any twelve-month period and has a lifetime prevalence of over 7 percent. It is somewhat unique among mental disorders, as its presence is predicated on a person having experienced or witnessed a traumatic event or series of events. It is common among victims of child abuse/neglect, sexual assault survivors, war veterans, prisoners, ex-convicts, and people who've survived man-made and natural disasters.

Rates of PTSD in people who seek treatment for substance use disorders are five times higher than those found in the general population. On the flip side, more than one third of people with PTSD have had at least one nontobacco substance use disorder. Histories of exposure to trauma (not necessarily with the development of PTSD) are found in most people with substance use disorders (90 percent). And 80 percent of women in treatment for substance problems report histories of physical or sexual assault.

The clinical course for people with co-occurring PTSD and substance use disorders is poorer than for either condition alone. PTSD is associated with increased drug/alcohol craving, poor adherence to treatment, decreased time to relapse, and higher relapse rates. People with both PTSD and substance use disorders often have multiple psychiatric diagnoses, more severe symptoms, poorer physical health, and diminished social functioning. Some people, such as those with histories of childhood sexual abuse and/or neglect, may present with complex symptoms that include recurrent suicidality, profound emotional vulnerability, and self-injurious behaviors (e.g., cutting, burning).

The good news is that symptoms of PTSD respond positively to treatment when substance use problems are in remission. Conversely, when PTSD symptoms are well controlled, people are less likely to engage in substance use. One study that looked at the correlation between abstinence from cocaine and/or alcohol showed a modest but significant reduction in PTSD symptoms, anxiety, and depression, especially during the first two weeks of abstinence. Also encouraging are clinical trials that have looked at treatment for both PTSD and substance use. Some studies have used sequential treatment and addressed the substance disorder first. Others have used parallel treatment, where one provider helps with the substance use problem and another with the PTSD, and some have used integrated models. Overall, the results for both the substance use and PTSD have been positive.

PTSD often precedes the substance use problem. This relationship lends credence to the self-medication hypothesis, where people turn to substances, hoping to relieve painful and negative emotions and thoughts. Certain symptoms of PTSD, such as flashbacks and cues to past traumas, can increase cravings for alcohol and other substances. From a behavioral perspective, this makes sense because the substance becomes associated with rapid relief from negative emotions (i.e., a reinforcer). Studies show that when PTSD symptoms are high, so too are cravings, relapse rates, and substance use.

For many, this tight relationship between drug use and PTSD goes unrecognized and untreated or under treated. To stop using drugs and alcohol only to become overwhelmed with anxiety, depression, nightmares, flashbacks, panic attacks, and suicidal impulses is not a good treatment outcome and is a setup for relapse.

SYMPTOMS OF PTSD

The symptoms of PTSD can be broken into the following clusters, and in the diagnostic DSM-5, a critical number, combined with clinical judgment, need to have been present for at least one month to make a PTSD diagnosis. The related diagnosis of acute stress disorder is applied for people whose symptoms last from three days to one month. Symptoms may manifest immediately after exposure to trauma or may be delayed for weeks, months, and even years:

1. Intrusive thoughts
   a. Intense and unwanted remembering of the traumatic experience
   b. Nightmares
   c. Flashbacks, where the person relives the event as though it is currently happening
2. Avoidant behaviors
   a. Deliberately avoiding situations and places that trigger memories of the traumatic event(s). For example:
      i. A rape victim who was attacked in a park now avoids all parks.
      ii. A resident of Manhattan who experienced 9/11 moves away and refuses to visit.
3. Arousal
   a. Hypervigilance—the feeling of always needing to be watchful and alert to the presence of danger
   b. Easily startled. For example:
      i. A combat veteran hears a loud noise, her pulse shoots up, and she reflexively dives for cover.
      ii. A victim of a home invasion hears a knock on the door and has a panic attack.
   c. Easily angered/hair-trigger temper
4. Negative emotional (mood) states
   a. Depression
   b. Irritability
   c. Anger
   d. Guilt and shame
   e. Helplessness
   f. Feeling numb

5. Disturbances in thought (cognition)

   a. Feelings of derealization and/or depersonalization; feeling disconnected from the world, oneself, and from others

   b. Amnesia related to the traumatic event(s)

   c. Unrealistic and/or exaggerated beliefs about the traumatic event, in which the person blames themself and/or others. For example:

   i. "I shouldn't have been walking alone."

   ii. "Why didn't I get an electrician in to check the wiring?"

   iii. "If I'd gotten home ten minutes earlier, this would never have happened."

   iv. "Someone should have known what he was up to."

Assessment and Screening Tools for PTSD

In addition to completing a comprehensive assessment (see Chapters 2–4) that includes a screening module for trauma, as well as assessments of dangerousness to self or others, specialized screening tools can be helpful in clarifying a PTSD or other trauma-related diagnosis. Tools that capture a timeframe, such as symptoms experienced over the last month, can be used to document response to treatment and be incorporated into treatment-and-recovery plans.

Recommended screening tools include:

- **Clinician-Administered PTSD Scale for the DSM-5 (CAPS-5):** This thirty-item structured interview has been widely used in research and has been revised to incorporate the changes to the PTSD criteria in the DSM-5. It utilizes a Likert scale rating (0–4) for symptom severity. It takes forty-five to sixty minutes to complete and assesses PTSD symptoms for the prior month. While primarily used in research, it can be used clinically by appropriately trained clinicians. A separate version is available for children and adolescents.

- **The Short Screening Scale for PTSD:** Designed for trauma survivors, this is a brief seven-item, yes-or-no questionnaire that includes items related to hyperarousal and avoidance. A score of 4 or more is considered positive and should warrant further clinical evaluation.

- **Trauma Screening Questionnaire:** This ten-item screen is used with trauma survivors. It includes five items related to reexperiencing and five related to arousal. A score of 6 or more is considered positive and should lead to a more detailed assessment of symptoms.

- **PTSD Symptom Checklist for DSM-5 (PCL-5):** This twenty-item self-report checklist can be used as a screening tool to aid in the diagnosis of PTSD and to follow up on response to treatment. It takes five to ten minutes to complete and utilizes a 5-point rating scale.

Copies of the PCL-5, as well as other screening tools for PTSD, can be obtained free of charge through the VA: www.ptsd.va.gov/professional/pages/assessments/ncptsd-instrument-request-form.asp.

TREATMENT OF CO-OCCURRING PTSD AND SUBSTANCE USE DISORDERS

Among the well-validated psychotherapies for PTSD, few have been systematically studied in people with co-occurring substance use disorders. To date, reviews that look at studies of specific psychotherapies for people with co-occurring PTSD and substance disorders have shown that many do indeed reduce symptoms of both, even months after the completion of treatment. What is not clear is whether these treatments are superior or greatly superior to treatment for substance use alone. While this finding may appear discouraging, it needs to be taken in the context of multivariable research that is difficult and expensive to conduct and control. Beyond that, when selecting the group to be studied, do you include all substances, or just alcohol or cocaine or opioids or...?

On the pharmacological side of treatment, few studies have examined specific drugs for PTSD and fewer still for the treatment of co-occurring PTSD and substance use disorders. At the time of this book's publication, only two agents have an FDA indication for PTSD—sertraline (Zoloft) and paroxetine (Paxil)—and their effectiveness for those conditions is at best, modest.

Psychotherapies

The therapies selected for inclusion in this book are those that have either been widely disseminated and/or have been studied in people with co-occurring disorders.

Non-Exposure-Based Treatments

- **Seeking Safety:** Developed by Lisa Najavits, PhD, this non-exposure, cognitive behavioral treatment is the most extensively studied of the non-exposure/present-based therapies for co-occurring PTSD and substance use disorders. Seeking Safety has five central principles:

  1. Safety: An overall focus on increasing safe behaviors and decreasing and eliminating unhealthy ones, such as the use of drugs and alcohol and being in abusive relationships

  2. Integrated treatment of PTSD and substance use problems: In all modules, both the PTSD and substance(s) are addressed (i.e., the treatment is fully integrated)

  3. Focus on ideals: Enhance the establishment/reestablishment of positive ideals, which include self-worth, integrity, honesty, and responsibility

  4. Four content areas:

     i. Cognitive: Use of cognitive restructuring and challenging beliefs, especially as they relate to the PTSD and the substance use, such as "I need to drink so I don't feel so much pain."

ii. Behavioral: Learn and implement coping skills along with a commitment to positive action.

iii. Interpersonal: Attention to better relationships and positive supports. This includes the option to invite significant people in to attend a session to help support the person in recovery.

iv. Case management

5. Therapist process: There is an emphasis on enhancing the therapist's skills, supporting them in the work, and respecting their individual styles.

Seeking Safety is both flexible and structured. It consists of twenty-five modules that can be provided in any order, based on need and preference. It can be provided in a group or individual format, and the actual number of sessions can vary. It can be used as a standalone therapy or with other treatment modalities, such as mutual self-help, pharmacotherapy, case management, relapse prevention, and exposure therapy. It has been studied in rape victims, incarcerated women, veterans, adolescent girls, and other populations. Seeking Safety has been shown to decrease both symptoms of PTSD and substance misuse. It can be combined with exposure-based treatment, such as eye movement desensitization and reprocessing (EMDR), discussed later in this chapter.

- **Target:** This gender-specific, group-based therapy is eight to nine sessions long and can be offered within substance use treatment. It utilizes psychoeducation and cognitive restructuring techniques (e.g., from CBT) and teaches emotion regulation skills.

- **Transcend:** This twelve-week partial hospital–based program includes ten hours of group therapy per week. It was studied in war veterans with PTSD and substance use disorders. It uses a manual, which includes a workbook for participants and guidelines for therapists. It is provided after the completion of a substance abuse program and includes concepts from a variety of therapeutic disciplines (e.g., CBT, psychodynamic, 12-step, relaxation training, and structured exercise). It does involve some in-group sharing of traumatic experiences. Groups are cohort based (i.e., the same participants start and finish together).

- **Trauma Recovery and Empowerment Model (TREM):** A thirty-three-session group-based treatment for women that is offered within substance use treatment, TREM teaches emotion regulation skills and includes psychoeducation and cognitive restructuring (e.g., from CBT). The manual includes brief trauma exposure. There is also an adapted gender-specific version for men, M-TREM.

- **Integrated CBT**: This has been studied as an eight-to-twelve-session protocol that includes psychoeducation and CBT skills, such as cognitive restructuring, breathing retraining, coping strategies, and relapse prevention. It is provided within substance treatment.

- **DART** for co-occurring disorders: DART includes psychoeducation and skills training for nine hours per week for twelve weeks. It is provided within substance use treatment.

- **Substance Dependency PTSD Therapy (SDPT):** This is an individual, cognitive-based therapy that focuses on coping skills and relapse prevention.

Exposure-Based Treatments. In all exposure-based therapies, by definition, the individual will explore some degree of their trauma. All these therapies prepare the client with a variety of grounding and/or cognitive behavioral training prior to the exposure components. This is to minimize traumatization. Proper training and supervision in these therapies is highly recommended prior to attempting their use.

- **Prolonged Exposure:** Developed by Edna Foa, PhD, prolonged exposure is an effective individual CBT-based treatment for PTSD. There have been multiple positive studies using prolonged exposure with people who have co-occurring PTSD and substance use disorders. Its efficacy as a treatment for PTSD is endorsed by the Institute of Medicine. In 2013, results of a large study of prolonged exposure in male and female veterans with PTSD (substance disorders were not specifically addressed) showed significant improvement in reducing symptoms of PTSD and depression.

    Prolonged exposure includes CBT elements, education about PTSD, and exposure to the trauma, which includes both imaginal remembering of the event and repeated in vivo (real life) exposure to feared situations and other cues the person has avoided since the trauma.

- **Cognitive Processing Therapy:** Developed by Patricia Resick, PhD, cognitive processing therapy is an eleven- or twelve-session manual-based treatment that has been used with sexual assault survivors and refugees, and the VA has adopted it for use with veterans. It has been used in both group and individual therapy formats. It includes education about trauma and how it changes a person's thoughts and beliefs. Cognitive processing therapy utilizes cognitive behavioral principles of identifying thoughts and feelings (and how they are connected) and then has the client challenge distorted beliefs. The exposure portions of this therapy involve written exercises (given as homework assignments) where the traumatic event(s) are recalled and written down in as much detail as possible and then reviewed with the therapist. Erroneous beliefs are challenged using CBT/Socratic-style reasoning. Specific issues of safety, trust, power, and intimacy are addressed.

- **Eye Movement Desensitization and Reprocessing (EMDR):** Developed by Francine Shapiro, EMDR utilizes exposure-based recollections of traumatic events in conjunction with deliberate and repetitive lateral eye movements. Its efficacy has been demonstrated in multiple clinical trials, and it is included in several practice guidelines as an evidence-based therapy. Its popularity and availability has grown. There is a certification program for practitioners that involves a standardized amount of training, with subsequent supervision.

- **Concurrent Treatment of PTSD and Cocaine Dependence (CTPCD)/ Concurrent Treatment of PTSD and Substance Use with Prolonged Exposure (COPE):** This individual therapy includes sixteen hour-and-a-half sessions. The therapy uses CBT, coping skills, psychoeducation, relapse prevention, and imaginal and in vivo exposure to past trauma (an adaptation of prolonged exposure). It is provided as a standalone therapy. Study results have been positive for both PTSD and substance use outcome measures.

Enhancing Resiliency, Safety, and Wellness

A growing body of research underscores the importance of resilience to counter the effects of trauma and stress. These are the factors that make people more able to handle the stress that life throws their way. It is what allows one person to endure and survive a horrific experience that leaves someone else destroyed. From clinical and wellness perspectives, the resilience literature provides a wealth of strategies that can be applied in work with people who have PTSD and related disorders.

But first, it is important to address issues of safety. Is your client currently in a situation that is stressful or traumatic?

- Is the home safe?
- Do people use drugs and alcohol in the home?
- Is the person in a significant relationship where they are physically, emotionally, or sexually abused?
- Are they in a domestic-violence relationship? Can and should they leave? This can involve financial, custodial, and personal safety concerns. People in abusive relationships are at the greatest risk for harm when they attempt to leave their abuser.
- Is someone's job, such as being a combat veteran deployed in the military, an ongoing source of stress and recurrent traumatization?
- Does this person have legal difficulties that include the threat of incarceration?
- Are they incarcerated?

For clinicians, understanding a client's active sources of distress and helping that person diminish, manage, and/or possibly eliminate them will be an important focus of treatment. There are many strategies to help foster resilience and wellness, many of which are incorporated into the therapies just reviewed. These include:

- Establish, reestablish, and strengthen positive supports and role models.
  - o Positive family relations
  - o Sober mentors, such as peer supports and 12-step mentors
  - o Attendance and participation in mutual self-help groups

- Address basic wellness needs.
  - Healthful and adequate nutrition
  - Physical activity and exercise
  - Attention to medical problems
  - Restorative sleep and good sleep habits
  - Pleasurable activities and hobbies
- Address issues of religion and spirituality. People are often able to draw strength from their faith, which includes finding meaning in the adversity they have had to endure.
- Promote cognitive flexibility and growth.
  - The importance of acceptance (This does not imply that one approves or endorses the experiences they have been through but that they acknowledge they occurred. Acceptance becomes an important step in allowing forward movement and growth.)
  - The use of humor to gain a sense of control over negative experiences
  - Finding meaning, and possibly purpose, in having survived the experience
  - Enhanced optimism (When life hands you lemons, make lemonade.)
- Enhance meaningful activities.
  - Work
  - Volunteerism/giving back to others
  - Attention to important relationships, such as caring for an elder parent or childcare

Pharmacological Treatments

As with all co-occurring disorders, few studies have adequately evaluated specific agents with people who have both substance use disorders and PTSD. Therefore, prescribers need to evaluate both halves of the equation—the PTSD and the substance problem(s)—and weigh the relative pros and cons of both on-label (FDA-indicated) and off-label (has not received FDA indication for a particular use) medications.

Pharmacological Treatment of PTSD

- **Selective serotonin reuptake inhibitors (SSRIs):** The only two medications (at the time of this publication) that have an FDA indication for PTSD are the SSRIs sertraline (Zoloft) and paroxetine (Paxil). Even though these agents have shown themselves to be superior to placebo, their overall effect on decreasing symptoms is modest.
- **Other antidepressants:** Other antidepressant medications that may be of benefit in PTSD include:
  - Other SSRIs
  - SNRIs, such as venlafaxine (Effexor) and duloxetine (Cymbalta)
  - Other antidepressants, such as the more sedating mirtazapine (Remeron)

- **Alpha-adrenergic antagonists:** These older blood pressure medications have been studied in PTSD. They may decrease symptoms of hyperarousal and distressing dreams. Frequently used agents include prazosin (Minipress) and clonidine (Catapres).

- **Atypical antipsychotics:** These agents are sometimes used off-label to target specific symptoms, such as hyperarousal. However, their potential benefit must be weighed against significant risks for adverse events, including weight gain and the development of metabolic syndrome.

- **Anticonvulsants:** There have been numerous studies looking at the potential benefits of agents like valproic acid (Depakote) and carbamazepine (Tegretol) in PTSD. The overall results have been mixed.

- **Benzodiazepines:** While these are often prescribed for their short-term relief of anxiety, studies in PTSD have not shown them to be of benefit. Because of their risk for abuse and dependence—especially in a person with co-occurring substance problems—they should be avoided. In practice, they are widely used.

Pharmacological Treatment of Substance Use Disorders in People with PTSD

In looking at the use of potential medications for substance use disorder in a person with PTSD, there are a few considerations: What is the substance being targeted? Are there specific agents that have been shown to be effective for that substance? Are those agents FDA-approved? Have they been studied in people with co-occurring PTSD?

Once we get beyond alcohol, opioids, and tobacco, there are no FDA-approved medications that target specific substance use disorders.

For people who have co-occurring opioid dependence and PTSD, replacement therapy is a likely option, such as buprenorphine and methadone. Similarly, if someone has an alcohol use disorder, medications such as the opioid antagonist naltrexone or acamprosate (Campral) could be considered.

Off-label studies of SSRIs, atypical antipsychotics, and anticonvulsants—like valproic acid (Depakote) and topiramate (Topamax)—may have some benefit.

What about cannabis for PTSD? Numerous states have legalized cannabis for medical use. Some have also approved it for recreational use. Among the states where it is legal for specific medical conditions, PTSD is often listed as an indication for marijuana. The challenge here is that there is little data to support the effectiveness of cannabis for symptoms of PTSD. The absence of evidence for or against cannabis has been fueled by federal regulations that still place it as a Schedule I substance along with heroin and cocaine (i.e., no legitimate medical use).

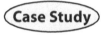

Jim Lathrop

Jim is a thirty-year-old, recently divorced father of one and a state trooper. He presents for treatment with a two-year history of severe mood swings, explosive rage, insomnia, and nightmares. He's dressed neatly in jeans and a flannel shirt, is clean shaven, and carries a faint odor of alcohol.

When asked about the symptoms that bring him in for his first encounter with a mental health professional, he is wary and wants reassurance that whatever he says will not get back to his place of work. "They wanted me to see the state shrink after it happened. No way in hell am I going to do that."

After the rules and potential exceptions to confidentiality are explained, he seems poised to leave but then says, "What the hell… I've got to do something. I need you to fix me because I can't go on like this. It's like living in hell. I can tell you exactly when it started." He describes a horrific and well-publicized multiple homicide/suicide, where he was a first responder and was present when a man who was recently laid off killed his three young children, his wife, and then himself. "I've been a trooper for nine years, and I've seen bad stuff." He chokes up. "It was seeing the kids. At first, I was just kind of numb, like there was a fog in my head, like things weren't real, like it was a movie or something. I figured it was normal and it would go away. It got worse. It's like my brain wouldn't shut up, and I kept seeing them and couldn't stop thinking about what they must have felt, how terrified they had to be."

As he speaks, Jim is distraught, and his mood shifts rapidly from profound sadness to anger. "You go through life thinking you're normal, and suddenly something happens, and it's like my brain won't shut up. When I try to relax, it gets worse—like there's something waiting for me to let down my guard, and there they are. I should have gotten there faster. I heard the shots. I should have broken in. We should have saved them, at least the baby." At times, he sobs when he describes how he unsuccessfully attempted to resuscitate the youngest child.

"It all went to shit after that. It's all I can do to show up to work, and being a trooper is all I ever wanted to do. Anything can set me off. It destroyed my marriage. I don't blame Kaitlin for leaving, and if something doesn't happen… I just can't go on feeling like this. Becky—she's three—she deserves a dad, and if I don't get fixed, it's not going to be me. I can't focus. I can't do anything right."

When asked specifically about suicidal thoughts or plans, he says, "Yeah, I think about it. But I'd make it look like an accident. That's the weird thing. Before this happened, I'd never thought about offing myself. Now a day doesn't go by where I don't at least wonder if I wouldn't be better off dead. Just turn the wheel hard to the right on the highway and go off a cliff. Get it over with." Upon further questioning, he admits that he doesn't want to end his life. "I couldn't do that to my little girl." As a state trooper, he does own and carry a firearm. He states that he has had no changes in his behavior toward his weapon and that after every shift, he removes the bullets and places the gun in a safe. He has no history of past suicidal thoughts or behaviors. He has no thoughts of harming anyone else. He denies any history of early childhood trauma. "I think my Dad spanked me twice, and both times I had it coming." His PCL-5 is strongly positive at 58.

As the interview shifts to the substance abuse history, Jim is frank about the increase in his alcohol consumption. "It used to be a couple beers after work, go out with the guys, nothing hard-core. Now I don't go out with anyone, and beer is too slow." He quantifies his daily consumption as at least a fifth, and sometimes a quart or more, of whiskey. In the past few months, it's progressed from drinks after work to a "slug or two in my morning coffee" to steady the shakes. He admits he had "a couple hits before coming here." He is a nonsmoker and denies any other drug use. He has never been in treatment for an alcohol use disorder. He has no history of seizures or delirium tremens.

He denies any known family history of mental illness but thinks his father and grandfather, both deceased, had problems with alcohol. He describes his suburban childhood as a happy one. He had friends, graduated high school, and received a bachelor's degree in criminal science. Prior to two years ago, he was active in his church, played league baseball, considered himself to be in a happy marriage, and had been overjoyed at the birth of his daughter. He and his ex-wife had planned to have three children. "That won't be happening now." He still talks with his ex-wife and has feelings for her. He is close with his mother and visits at least weekly. He views them as supports.

He has no active medical problems and is on no medications. His tonsils were removed. His breathalyzer shows a level of .08 (the legal limit to drive in his state), his pulse is mildly elevated at 102 beats per minute, and his blood pressure is 120/90. He does have a slight tremor when he holds his hands out. His CIWA score (Chapter 17) is 4, mostly based on his level of anxiety. He has no symptoms of a withdrawal hallucinosis.

Step One: Level of Care Determination and Discussion

The client in this case study displays a typical interplay between trauma and substance abuse. Because it has progressed to include signs and symptoms of physiological alcohol dependence, as seen by the mild withdrawal symptoms even while still under the influence, this individual will require a medically supervised detoxification. Additionally, his reports of daily thoughts of ending his life, accompanied by a plan, will need to be explored. He has multiple risks for making a suicide attempt, which include access to firearms, active and heavy drinking, depressive and PTSD symptoms, and recent major losses.

Options for the initial level of care will include an inpatient detoxification unit or psychiatric unit that is equipped to manage an alcohol detoxification, followed by a less restrictive treatment program, based on Mr. Lathrop's preferences, resources, availability, and clinical appropriateness. Or if Mr. Lathrop can put together a solid safety plan, a PHP that can provide a medically supervised detoxification, substance abuse treatment, and treatment to address his suicidality and PTSD might also be a more acceptable option to him.

In this instance, Mr. Lathrop expresses a strong desire to pursue outpatient treatment, at least initially. He is fearful that being on a locked inpatient unit will worsen his PTSD. Also, he has genuine and legitimate concerns that an inpatient admission could jeopardize his ability to carry a firearm, which is a requisite for his job. He is, however, willing to take a leave from his job and involve family (his mother and ex-wife) in the construction of a safety plan, which will include immediate removal of firearms from the home.

Step Two: Construct the Problem/Need List

Substance Use	Mental Health	Medical
Alcohol use has escalated since the trauma	Severe mood swings	Shaky hands when he doesn't have a drink
Daily drinking (one fifth to a quart of whiskey)	Rage attacks	Mildly elevated pulse and blood pressure
Morning drinking	Insomnia	CIWA score of 4
Shakiness in the morning	Nightmares	Positive breathalyzer
Has had alcohol prior to coming in for the evaluation	Symptoms started after direct involvement with a horrific tragedy	
No prior treatment for drugs or alcohol	Daily thoughts of suicide, thoughts of vehicular suicide to make it look like an accident	
Nonsmoker	Sadness and depression	
Does not use other drugs	Relates the loss of his marriage to his drinking and mood swings	
Family history of alcohol use disorders	Hyper startle response	

	Feelings of depersonalization and derealization	
	Flashbacks to the traumatic event	
	Guilt over not having been able to get there earlier and do more	
	No known family history of mental illness	
	Owns and carries a firearm	
	PCL-5 score of 58 (strongly positive)	

In this instance, where there is significant suicidal thinking, it is reasonable—and in many organizations expected—to address this as a separate problem/need. Where the medical issues appear to be related to the alcohol, those could be included in that problem/need statement:

1. **Active suicidality with daily thoughts of ending his life**, AEB thoughts of vehicular suicide. Other major risk factors include access to firearms, severe PTSD symptoms, and active alcohol use. Protective factors include his desire to be part of his daughter's life, supportive relationships with his ex-wife and mother, and the desire to return to a job that he loves. No history of prior attempts

2. **Active and severe alcohol use** with increased daily consumption and signs of early withdrawal

3. **Severe posttraumatic symptoms** with daily flashbacks, nightmares, hyper-startle response, mood swings, depression, anxiety, and rage attacks; PCL-5 score of 58

Step Three: Establish the Initial Goals/Objectives for Treatment

1. Active suicidality with daily thoughts of ending his life
   a. Short-term goals/objectives:
      i. Craft a safety plan, with specific contingencies, that includes his mother's involvement
      ii. Assess for the presence of any suicidal thoughts or behaviors
      iii. Remove all firearms and ammunition from the home
   b. Long-term goals: Have no suicidal thoughts

2. Active and severe alcohol use with daily drinking and signs of early withdrawal
   a. Short-term goals/objectives:
      i. Safely complete a detoxification from alcohol
      ii. Achieve early abstinence from alcohol

b. Long-term goals: Achieve sustained abstinence from alcohol

3. Severe PTSD symptoms

   a. Short-term goals/objective: Experience a 50 percent or greater reduction in PTSD symptoms by six weeks from today, AEB self-report and the PCL-5

   b. Long-term goals:

      i. Be as free from symptoms of PTSD as possible

      ii. Have no more than 30 percent of current levels as measured on the PCL-5

Step Four: Construct the Treatment-and-Recovery Plan
Treatment-and-Recovery Plan

Patient's Name: James Lathrop
Date of Birth: 6/2/1989
Medical Record #: XXX-XX-XXXX

Level of Care: Partial hospital program (PHP)

ICD-10 Codes	DSM-5 Diagnoses
F10.239	Alcohol withdrawal without perceptual disturbances with alcohol use disorder, severe
F43.10	Posttraumatic stress disorder with dissociative symptoms (derealization)
Z63.5	Disruption of family by separation
Z56.9	Other problems related to employment

The individual's stated goal(s): "To feel better. To not be so on edge and jumpy. To be able to control my anger. To not feel like my thoughts are so out of my control. To like my job again. To reconcile with my wife and to be a part of my daughter's life again. To not have so many nightmares and flashbacks. To stop drinking"

1. Problem/Need Statement: Active suicidality with daily thoughts of ending his life, including thoughts of vehicular suicide
Long-Term Goal: Have no thoughts of suicide
Short-Term Goals/Objectives (with target date):
1. Craft a safety plan, with specific contingencies, that will include involving the patient's mother in his treatment (by the end of today)
2. Assess for the presence of any suicidal thoughts or behaviors (daily)
3. Remove all firearms and ammunition from the home (by the end of today)

2. Problem/Need Statement: Active and severe alcohol use with increased daily drinking and signs of early withdrawal
Long-Term Goal: Achieve sustained abstinence from alcohol
Short-Term Goals/Objectives (with target date):
1. Safely complete a detoxification from alcohol (by one week to ten days from today)
2. Achieve early abstinence from alcohol (starting today)

265

3. Problem/Need Statement: Severe PTSD symptoms with daily flashbacks, nightmares, hyper-startle response, mood swings, depression, anxiety, and rage attacks; PCL-5 score of 58
Long-Term Goal: Be as free from symptoms of PTSD as possible; Have no more than 30 percent of current levels as measured on the PCL-5
Short-Term Goals/Objectives (with target date):
1. Experience a 50 percent or greater decrease in symptoms of PTSD by self-report and the PCL-5 (six weeks from today)

Interventions					
Treatment Modality	**Specific Type**	**Frequency**	**Duration**	**Problem Number**	**Responsible Person(s)**
Pharmacological Management of Alcohol Withdrawal	CIWA protocol for withdrawal	Daily	3–14 days	2	MD/APRN, RN, Mr. Lathrop, Mr. Lathrop's mother
Nursing Assessment	Comprehensive nursing assessment	Upon admission	1–2 hours	1, 2, 3	RN
Psychiatric Assessment	Complete psychiatric assessment	Upon admission	1–2 hours over the course of the first two weeks	1, 2, 3	MD/APRN, Mr. Lathrop
Ongoing Pharmacological Management	Medication management	Weekly for the first two weeks, then as needed	Over the duration of the admission	1, 2, 3	MD/APRN Mr. Lathrop
Lab Work	Complete metabolic profile, CBC, urine drug analysis, breathalyzer, and alcohol metabolites	Upon admission, urine screens ongoing	Over the course of the admission	1, 2, 3	MD/APRN
Safety Assessment	Suicide assessment	Daily	As long as the patient continues to experience suicidal thoughts or behaviors	1	Primary clinician or designee, Mr. Lathrop

PHP Group Therapy	Relapse prevention	Daily	50 minutes	2	Group leader, Mr. Lathrop
	Seeking Safety— integrated CBT for PTSD and substance use disorders	Daily	50 minutes	1, 2, 3	Group leader, Mr. Lathrop
	Psychoeducation	2x/week	50 minutes	1, 2, 3	Group leader, Mr. Lathrop
	Mindfulness	2x/week	50 minutes	1, 2, 3	Group leader, Mr. Lathrop
Individual Counseling	Integrated CBT with exposure	2x/week	50 minutes	1, 2, 3	Primary therapist, Mr. Lathrop
Peer Support	Online self-help group for law enforcement professionals or other in-person or online group	On all days client is not in program	1–2 hours	2	Mr. Lathrop

Identification of strengths: Wants to feel better and be able to participate more fully at work. Has a strong sense of morality. Has a strong work ethic and sense of duty to his family and his job

Peer/family/community supports to assist: Client's mother will drive patient to and from program while he undergoes the detoxification component and will stay with him until he feels well enough and safe enough to return to his own home. She will keep his firearms securely locked in a gun safe at her home

Barriers to treatment: The client is not sure how long he can remain out of work without a formal leave of absence. He is worried how being in treatment might hurt his ability to return to work

Staff/client-identified education/teaching needs: To understand the relationship between his PTSD symptoms and his drinking and how they influence each other in both positive and negative ways

Assessment of discharge needs/discharge planning: To be substance free and free from thoughts of self-harm

Completion of this treatment-and-recovery plan was a collaborative effort between the client and the following members of the treatment team:

SIGNATURES		Date/Time:
Client:	James Lathrop	6/12/22, 2:00 p.m.
Physician or APRN:	Carlton Blaise, MD	6/12/22, 4:15 p.m.
Treatment Plan Completed By:	James Lathrop & Debra Hayes, LCSW	6/12/22, 2:00 p.m.
Primary Clinician:	Debra Hayes, LCSW	6/12/22, 2:00 p.m.
Other Team Members	Mary Lathrop, (Jim's Mom)	6/12/22, 4:00 p.m.

CHAPTER 15

Schizophrenia, Other Psychotic Disorders, and Co-Occurring Substance Use Disorders

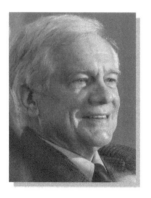

My Story

By Bob Drake, MD, PhD

"By and large you learn about what's helpful from the people who are having these experiences rather than from the experts."

Integrated Treatment for People with Psychotic Disorders and Substance Use Problems

In the late seventies, I was a psychiatric resident at Cambridge Hospital. One of my first inpatient rotations was on the dual-diagnosis unit at Westborough State Hospital, and this was a new thing. The literature was just emerging that with deinstitutionalization, people who had been in state hospitals, often for decades, now lived relatively independent lives in the community, but many had become involved with drugs, alcohol, and the legal system and were homeless.

From there, I began to work with the assertive community treatment teams (ACTT) at Cambridge Hospital, first as a resident and then as faculty. Our job was to help people who were incarcerated, homeless, or hospitalized get stable housing and do better in the community. At that time, we knew about providing assertive community treatment to people with serious mental illness but didn't know how to deal with the co-occurring substance use. So we tried different things.

My mentor and friend, George Valiant, was a real expert and a relative free thinker about alcohol and drug abuse. I'd meet with him weekly to think through what we were doing and debate about habit versus disease. We talked about the long-term course of substance use and that we tend to see people in crisis. But that's a tiny fraction of their lives and who they are. The second thing is that the longitudinal course is much different from the short-term course. And the third thing George always said—and it's proven true—is that the positive things in people's lives are much more important than the negative things.

As someone who has coached baseball for years, I like the ACTT model. It's all about building a team and getting eight to ten people to work together, to trust each other, and to be positive about what they're doing. It's exciting work. We get to help the most marginalized people in society, treat them with dignity and respect, and pay attention to what they tell us.

We had three teams—Cambridge, Somerville, and the dual-diagnosis team—that provided services across those areas. Most of the clients were people with schizophrenia and substance use problems. It was true ambulatory work, with a primary mission to help people become successful in the community when they had recently been in state hospitals, incarcerated, or homeless. We'd hold medication clinics in church basements that were used as drop-in centers. I attended a lot of AA meetings, and all the case managers knew that they could just bring a client in to see the doctor. It was all about outreach and engagement, often trying to connect with people who were homeless, had no medical record, and had been seriously mistreated and beaten down by having at least two serious illnesses.

It became clear that those who struggled the most had co-occurring substance use. We collected data and tried different things. We learned that the standard treatment of getting people admitted to a thirty-day substance abuse program just didn't work. They were a real disaster, run according to strict AA philosophies that you had to be off all medications. So they'd take our clients off their psychiatric medications, and they'd become psychotic.

When I moved to New Hampshire in 1984, I started a team like this at West Central, a Dartmouth-affiliated mental health center. We did a pretty good job, and the director of the state's mental health department asked if we would help with research, planning, and development for the state. He, as well as several leaders of mental health centers, recognized that co-occurring disorders would become more of a problem as time went on. These were the clients who didn't come in for appointments, ended up homeless, got arrested, were abused in the streets, and so on.

Our project, which received grant funding, put co-occurring teams into each of the state's mental health centers. For the next six to eight years, we had teams statewide. I met with each of them once a month. We'd go over the research and clinical issues, and we'd interview clients. We wanted to know what worked, and we tried new types of supported housing, group homes, scattered-site housing, specialty co-occurring groups within the mental health centers, different approaches to medications, and new family interventions. It was the early days of harm reduction work and meeting people where they were at.

We assessed and followed over 200 people for sixteen years. We learned how they adjusted to life in the community, what their service use was like, and how they did. We developed measures that showed us that people with psychotic disorders were negatively affected by small amounts of substance use compared to others. Someone with schizophrenia could smoke pot a couple of times and have it precipitate a major psychotic episode. We found that almost no one in our sample could sustain what we'd consider mild drinking and that our clients got into lots of trouble—like getting arrested or kicked out of their home—with small amounts of alcohol. They could not maintain social drinking. And this was all new information.

And we were lucky because we received grant support that let us explore, ask questions, and test hypotheses. We even had an anthropologist who spent hours a day with the clients to better understand their lives. And we did a lot of hard-nosed research to make sure we had valid data. We learned that people with co-occurring disorders often had serious trauma histories that had gone unidentified and that those individuals were much less able to sustain abstinence. The reason seemed to be that, when they did not use alcohol and drugs, they became overwhelmed with nightmares, flashbacks, and symptoms of PTSD. It was during that time that Kim Mueser, PhD, joined our team at Dartmouth and developed and studied PTSD interventions for people with psychotic disorders and substance use disorders.

Another important thing we learned was that these folks needed meaningful goals in their lives. The idea that they would just say no to alcohol and drugs and take their medications like they were prescribed was too superficial and didn't work. What mattered to them was safe housing, a job, and that they had some friends who didn't use drugs—what we'd now call social determinants that can have a greater impact on outcomes than any specific treatment.

What we learned flew in the face of everything I'd learned in my training about addiction. What I'd been taught was wrong. People didn't need to be sober for three, six, or twelve months before they

my story

got a job. People who actively used were often successful at work, and *that* became the motivation to decrease the substance use.

As for what works? Interventions must be modified to recognize that the person has a co-occurring disorder(s)—from family, work, choice of and approaches to medications, counseling, and housing options. At every step, you need to take both disorders into account.

The second thing is that people with co-occurring disorders recover over time, and our data shows the process continued for the whole sixteen years. What the people we studied want is what everyone wants. People recover over time and in idiosyncratic patterns. Some will work on their relationships with their family first. For others it's getting a job, and for someone else it's cutting down the heroin. It differs by the person and their disorders, drugs, skills, strengths, and aspirations. They want what everyone wants. They want to control their problems and care for themselves. They want to have a safe place to live, a job, and friends who help them and don't give them drugs. They want to have a good quality of life and some hope.

my story

OVERVIEW

Worldwide, the prevalence of schizophrenia and other psychotic disorders (e.g., schizoaffective disorder, schizophreniform disorder, etc.) is roughly 1 percent. This does not include people who experience psychotic symptoms in response to substance-induced or medically induced conditions, such as hallucinations associated with alcohol and benzodiazepine withdrawals or intoxication with PCP, hallucinogens, and many other substances.

Lifetime rates of coexisting substance use disorders in people with schizophrenia range from 47 to 70 percent, not including tobacco. Substance use in this population is associated with increased rates of hospitalization, violence, incarceration, homelessness, HIV and hepatitis infections, and poor treatment adherence. Common substances used by people with schizophrenia are nicotine and alcohol, followed by cannabis and cocaine. Tobacco use is especially prevalent, with rates ranging between 70 to nearly 90 percent. Heavy smoking (i.e., more than forty cigarettes/day) is also high. In recent years, the high potency, low cost, and easy availability of opioids have made these substances of increased concern for people with psychotic disorders, especially for nonhabitual users, where one or two bags of fentanyl can prove fatal.

Even though people with psychotic disorders run the spectrum in terms of overall functional ability, the schizophrenia spectrum disorders are chief among those considered severe/serious and persistent mental illness, severe/serious and persistent illness, or severe/serious mental illness.

It is in this group that the movement for integrated treatment first took root, based on the realization that traditional substance use programs and mental health programs did not adequately address clinical and psychosocial needs. This push for integrated treatment now includes primary care (i.e., medical) as well, which is accomplished through the creation of behavioral health–enhanced patient-centered medical homes (PCMH) and behavioral health homes (BHH). The intent here is to decrease the lifespan disparity between people with severe mental disorders and the general population, which is a difference of fifteen to twenty-four years. The causes for this abysmal health outcome are multifactorial and include several preventable causes of morbidity and mortality, such as high rates of smoking, obesity, drug and alcohol use, elevated cholesterol and other lipid abnormalities, and sedentary lifestyle. The largest contributor to the mortality gap is coronary artery disease. Given that many medications are associated with weight gain and metabolic syndrome, interest and concern surround the question of how medications may worsen this lifespan disparity.

Integrated psychiatric and substance use treatment for people with schizophrenia and other serious and persistent mental illness is now included as an evidence-based practice in medicine. To enhance adherence, it is recommended that treatment be located within a single facility and team of providers. Core components of integrated treatment for people with schizophrenia spectrum and substance use disorders may include:

- Psychosocial interventions
  - o Motivational enhancement
  - o Harm reduction strategies
  - o Skills training
  - o Dual-focused self-help and other 12-step and non-12-step community-based supports
  - o Peer supports
- Medication
  - o To manage the symptoms of schizophrenia
  - o To manage withdrawal syndromes
  - o To decrease substance use and urges to use
- Case management strategies
  - o Assertive community treatment teams (ACTT)
  - o Targeted case management
  - o Case management through other agencies, which might include in-home nursing services

Treatment for people with schizophrenia spectrum disorders is often located in community mental health centers and not-for-profit clinics. Some of these may be state run, while others will receive a mixture of state and federal funds combined with fee-for-service payment.

In addition to integrated substance use and mental health services, attention to routine medical evaluation and follow-up is crucial to improve overall health outcomes. Newer models of medical integration include behavioral health PCMHs, which can be collocated within a mental health clinic or federally qualified health care center (FQHC).

SPECIAL CONSIDERATIONS

People with schizophrenia spectrum disorders can present with a wide range of functional abilities, as well as challenges. This continuum includes people with rich work, home, and social connections, and others who may live in the margins of society, where pressing concerns involve poverty, homelessness, exposure to violence, substance use, and involvement with the legal system.

Cognitive Challenges

At present, there are no specific markers for schizophrenia, and it is likely that what is currently included in the spectrum represents multiple conditions, and there is substantial overlap with other diagnoses. These are neuropsychiatric disorders with related cognitive and functional impairments that can range from subtle to severe.

Problem areas can include difficulty with focus, attention, the ability to switch between tasks, as well as with processing multistep undertakings, negotiating social situations, and dealing with complex systems (e.g., housing, health care, disability, legal, etc.).

For clinicians unfamiliar with people with cognitive impairments and the negative symptoms of schizophrenia, it is easy to label client behavior as nonadherent or willful when they habitually miss appointments or don't follow through with things they said they'd do. Strategies to address cognitive deficits and the negative symptoms of schizophrenia may include:

- Neuropsychological testing to identify and clarify strengths and deficits and assist in developing effective interventions
- Use of occupational therapy assessment and treatment to clarify areas to develop along with strategies to make that happen. This can cover a broad range of skills, from helping identify a person's areas of interest to increased competence in the kitchen
- Use of case management/care management services, such as targeted case management and ACTT services, especially for people with frequent hospitalization who struggle to maintain their basic needs in the community
- Use of peer mentors and mutual self-help groups
- Family psychoeducation and enhancement of the person's natural supports, including use of the faith communities and wellness programs
- Identification of skills the person needs, such as how to practice drug refusal, maintain a safe and clean home, manage finances, and so forth
- Skills training that works with identified cognitive processing issues, such as breaking down tasks into their component parts and practicing until the skill is learned
- Careful attention to the selection of medications to enhance functioning and minimize side effects that could negatively impact memory, focus, level of alertness, and other cognitive processes

Social Issues

People with schizophrenia spectrum disorders experience high rates of social problems. These range from family disintegration and limited, or absent, social supports to homelessness, poverty, and legal problems. In addition, because of cognitive deficits that may be associated with the individual's disorder, negotiating complex systems, such as obtaining and maintaining disability, low-income housing, and adequate food, may prove impossible for some to manage and maintain without assistance.

Engagement with Treatment

For people with co-occurring substance use and schizophrenia, treatment engagement is often a process. This can be complicated by the person's inability to acknowledge that they have a mental illness (i.e., anosognosia). Anosognosia is often cited as the reason why a person discontinues their medication. "I'm not sick. I don't need this. Why would I take it?" One strategy to address anosognosia is to identify what it is the person wants versus what it is you as a clinician think they need. If they are homeless and they want help with that (but not with their drinking or drug use or with the voices they hear), then assistance with housing is the best way to start. Through the use of motivational and harm reduction strategies, this "meet the person where they're at" approach provides the possibility of helping the person move forward in other areas of recovery. It may be that they will never take the medication for schizophrenia, but if those pills help them focus at work, they'll give them a try.

DIAGNOSTIC ISSUES

As with other co-occurring substance use and mental disorders, teasing apart the history is essential to clarify diagnoses. The clinician wants to know which came first: the use of alcohol and/or drugs, or the development of psychotic symptoms. In theory, one would think this is straightforward. In practice, it is often unclear, even after a thorough assessment. Schizophrenia, which has its typical onset in the late teens and early twenties, can have a significant prodromal phase, free from any evidence of psychosis. One study used childhood home movies and asked viewers to identify which child would go on to develop schizophrenia. Based on withdrawn and odd behaviors, the viewers were able to accurately do this, well above what could be expected from chance alone.

It can be difficult to identify the underlying cause of psychotic symptoms, as they can be attributed to a psychotic disorder, such as schizophrenia; the effects of drugs, alcohol, and various medical conditions; or a combination of factors. The importance of clarifying what may be substance or medically related is both a challenge and important. When people with psychotic disorders are in crisis, they can have serious medical conditions, such as dangerously low blood sugar or alcohol withdrawal, which are overlooked or attributed to their mental disorder. Historical, clinical, and physical findings can help clarify the diagnoses:

- Did the psychotic symptoms (e.g., voices, visions, disorganization) precede the substance use problem?
- At what age did the person first experience psychotic symptoms?
- Does the person have psychotic symptoms when they don't use substances?
- Are the psychotic symptoms typical for a schizophrenia spectrum disorder?
  - Auditory hallucinations are the most frequent hallucinatory experience in schizophrenia.
  - Visual and tactile hallucinations, while they can occur in schizophrenia, are more suggestive of a substance-induced psychosis, withdrawal state, or other medically induced delirium. This would be especially true with a person who normally hears voices but has now started to see things.

- Substance-induced psychotic symptoms more frequently include positive symptoms of schizophrenia, such as hallucinations, delusions, and disorganized speech and behavior. Negative symptoms (e.g., low motivation, diminished speech, lack of interest, blunted emotional range) are less typical.

- Are the timing and onset of psychotic symptoms directly related to the ingestion of or withdrawal from drugs or alcohol?

- Does the person have an underlying medical condition that could cause the psychotic symptoms?

- Are the symptoms compatible with syndromes related to medications the person takes, such as a lithium toxicity delirium or anticholinergic delirium, as can be seen from overtaking many psychiatric medications or can even occur with prescribed dosages?

- Screening tests:

  - Urine toxicology can detect substances that may account or contribute to the psychotic symptoms

  - Liver function tests may indicate the presence of chronic alcohol use or the presence of infectious disease related to intravenous drug use, such as hepatitis C

  - Elevated ammonia levels seen in heavy drinkers can account for confusion and delirious states

- Do physical findings or complaints indicate an altered physiological (i.e., medical or drug-induced) state?

  - Dilated or pinpoint pupils

  - Nystagmus (i.e., visible rhythmic movements of the eyes), which is often seen in certain intoxication states, such as with PCP and ketamine. This can also be associated with serotonin syndrome

  - Flushed or bone-dry skin

  - Elevations in blood pressure and pulse

  - Elevated temperature

  - Hyperexcitable reflexes

  - Muscle rigidity

  - Pain

  - Abdominal distension

  - Complaints of constipation

  - Inability to urinate

  - Catatonia

- Do the patient, family, or other reporters provide information that the symptoms are typical for the person's psychiatric disorder, or do they indicate that something different is going on?

• Has the person used substances that can cause psychotic symptoms? This is a growing and rapidly changing list that will include many substances that may not show up on standard toxicology screens, such as synthetic cannabis (K-2, Spice) and various amphetamine-type stimulants, such as bath salts, which are sold under a broad variety of names. This also includes the misuse of prescription medications, as well as many over-the-counter sleep and cold medications.

Drugs That Can Cause Psychotic Symptoms

Drug	Comments
Alcohol	Psychosis possible when intoxicated, as well as common in severe withdrawal states (e.g., hallucinosis and delirium tremens). Rarely associated with persistent psychosis, as seen in some instances of alcoholic dementia (e.g., Korsakoff's dementia)
Barbiturates	Psychosis possible when intoxicated and in withdrawal states
Benzodiazepines	Psychosis possible when intoxicated and in withdrawal states
Cannabis and synthetic cannabis (K-2, Spice)	Psychosis possible when intoxicated, including rare cases of persistent psychosis. Synthetic cannabis is associated with more extreme psychosis. Also, cannabis is frequently treated or "dipped" in substances such as formaldehyde, which can cause a prolonged delirium (up to six months)
Hallucinogens (LSD, psilocybin/magic mushrooms, peyote)	Hallucinations and delusions when intoxicated. Rare cases of persistent psychosis that can last for weeks to months
Inhalants (nitrous oxide, toluene, other solvents)	All associated with psychotic symptoms when intoxicated. Solvents implicated in persistent psychotic states
MDMA (Ecstasy)	Psychosis common when intoxicated
NMDA antagonists (PCP, ketamine)	Psychosis during intoxication that may persist for weeks or even months in the case of PCP (which is often combined with cannabis)
Opioids (heroin, methadone, oxycodone, fentanyl)	Hallucinations when intoxicated. Rare cases of persistent psychosis with smoked heroin. Rare cases of withdrawal-related psychosis, which can be protracted (weeks to months)
Steroids	Psychosis possible, along with typical behavioral and mood changes (e.g., "roid rage")
Stimulants (cocaine, ADHD medication, bath salts, methamphetamine)	Psychosis possible when intoxicated (e.g., all forms of hallucinations and delusions, including extreme paranoia and grandiosity). Psychosis can persist for weeks after the last use
Over-the-counter cold medications (dextromethorphan)	Many over-the-counter medications, when taken in higher than recommended doses, can cause hallucinations, disorientation, and dissociative symptoms

Medical Conditions That Can Cause Psychotic Symptoms

Medical Condition	Comments
Infectious diseases	HIV/AIDs, bacterial or viral meningitis, high-fever states, Lyme disease, syphilis, urinary tract infections
Neoplasms (tumors/cancers)	Certain hormone-secreting tumors, certain lung cancers
Electrolyte abnormalities	Many disturbances in electrolyte balance can manifest as confusion or delirium, such as dangerously low sodium
Metabolic and nutritional abnormalities	B12 deficiency, hypoglycemia (low blood sugar), hyperglycemia (elevated blood sugar), hypoxia (inadequate oxygen in the blood), hypercarbia (increased CO_2 levels)
Medication toxicities	An extensive number of medications can cause toxic and delirious states, both alone and in combination with other medications, illicit drugs, and alcohol. This includes lithium, anticholinergic medications, sedative hypnotics, opioids, anticonvulsants, anti-Parkinson's medications, antivirals, antiarrhythmics, steroids, antidepressants, and many others
Endocrine abnormalities (hormonal)	Hyper- or hypothyroidism, hyperadrenalism
Dementia (neurocognitive disorders)	All neurocognitive disorders, such as Alzheimer's disease, can be associated with delusions and hallucinations. In some, such as Lewy body disease, this is common
Autoimmune disorders	Lupus, multiple sclerosis
Renal disorders (kidney)	Uremia (elevations in waste products in the blood due to renal failure), urinary tract infections
Hepatic disease (liver)	Hepatic encephalopathy, elevated ammonia levels due to liver disease
Gastrointestinal	Bowel obstruction due to severe constipation
Neurologic conditions	Stroke, seizures (postictal confusion and delirium), multiple sclerosis, head trauma

There is also a growing body of evidence that, in some cases, substance use may hasten or even bring on the development of schizophrenia and related syndromes. Cannabis has been implicated in susceptible individuals who carry a gene variant that codes for a protein involved in the synthesis of dopamine (cyclic O-methyl transferase/COMT). One study that followed 45,000 Swedish army conscripts for fifteen years showed that those who smoked cannabis on a regular basis were six times more likely to have a follow-up diagnosis of schizophrenia. Similar results have been found in other studies.

THE DSM-5 AND SCHIZOPHRENIA SPECTRUM DISORDERS

In the current DSM-5 diagnostic system, psychotic disorders are characterized by abnormalities in the following areas:

- **Delusions:** These are fixed false beliefs that can take many forms:
  - Paranoid (persecutory) delusions: The belief that known, or unknown, persons or entities wish to cause the client harm
  - Grandiose delusions: The belief that a person has special powers or abilities that they do not possess. This can include the belief that they are a famous person, God, or the devil or that they have supernatural powers and/or abilities
  - Erotomanic delusions: The belief that another person—often a famous person—is in love with them. In some instances, the person may have met the object of their delusion, but often they have not
  - Thought insertion and thought broadcasting: The belief that they can read another person's mind or vice versa
  - Thoughts of reference: The belief that there are special messages just for them coming through the television, the newspaper, or another medium
- **Hallucinations:** In schizophrenia spectrum disorders, hallucinations are most frequently auditory (hearing voices), but can also be visual and less frequently tactile (touch) or olfactory (smell).
- **Disorganized thought:** This abnormality will be evidenced in the person's speech patterns and may include:
  - Tangential thoughts and looseness of associations: There is a connection between thoughts, but the overall train rambles and does not come to conclusive points. It's difficult for a listener to follow what the person says.
  - Word salad: This is where there is a disconnection from one utterance to the next. Speech may appear jumbled and nonsensical.
  - Unusual patterns of enunciation, rhyming, echolalia (the repeating of words), or echopraxia (the repeating, or parroting, of another person's behaviors).
- **Disorganized behavior:** These can run the range from idiosyncratic and odd mannerisms to catatonia.
- **Negative symptoms:** Observers note diminished emotional range and response, often referred to as a flat or blunted affect. Negative symptoms can include signs of depression, such as apathy, amotivation, ambivalence, loss of interest, and an inability to experience pleasure. A person with negative symptoms may have no interest in doing anything more than staying at home and watching TV while chain-smoking cigarettes for hours or even days on end.

In the DSM-5, the psychotic disorders include delusional disorder, brief psychotic disorder (symptoms last from one day to one month), schizophreniform disorders (symptoms last from one month to six months), schizophrenia (symptoms have been present for more than six months), and schizoaffective disorder (there is both evidence of a psychotic disorder and a mood disorder, where for at least a two-week period there have been psychotic symptoms without a mood episode). There are also designations for psychotic disorders that can be due to medical conditions and substance/medication-induced psychotic disorders.

Schizophrenia Spectrum Disorders

Disorder	Criterion A*	Time Frame	Other Key Features
Delusional Disorder	Delusions only	At least one month	Never meets criteria for schizophrenia and is typically able to function. Not due to another medical, substance, or mental disorder
Brief Psychotic Disorder	Presence of one or more: delusions, hallucinations, disorganized speech	One day to one month	Not due to another medical, substance, or mental disorder
Schizophreniform Disorder	Presence of two or more, one of which must be: delusions, hallucinations, disorganized speech	One month to six months	Not due to another medical, substance, or mental disorder
Schizophrenia	Presence of one or more: delusions, hallucinations, disorganized speech	At least six months	Not due to another medical, substance, or mental disorder
Schizoaffective Disorder	Presence of two or more, one of which must be: delusions, hallucinations, disorganized speech	Not specified	⊠ Major mood episode (depressive or manic) is concurrent with criterion A symptoms of schizophrenia. ⊠ Delusions or hallucinations without a mood episode must be present for at least two weeks at some point in the illness. ⊠ Not due to another medical, substance, or mental disorder

*Criterion A: Delusions, hallucinations, disorganized speech, disorganized behavior, negative symptoms

ASSESSMENT AND SCREENING TOOLS

Clinician-Rated Dimensions of Psychosis Severity

This eight-item, Likert-type (0 = not present, 4 = present and severe) assessment tool covers the five core symptoms of schizophrenia. Three additional items assess for the presence and severity of cognitive impairment, depression, and mania. It is available through the American Psychiatric Association (www.psychiatry.org/practice/dsm/dsm5/online-assessment-measures#Disorder) and can be used freely by researchers and clinicians as a recommended assessment tool in the DSM-5.

The Positive and Negative Syndrome Scale

A thirty-item clinician-administered instrument, the Positive and Negative Syndrome Scale (PANSS) measures the positive and negative symptoms of schizophrenia. It is widely used in studies evaluating the efficacy of medication and nonmedication therapies for people with psychotic disorders. It takes forty-five to fifty minutes to complete.

The Brief Psychiatric Rating Scale

Developed in the early 1960s, the Brief Psychiatric Rating Scale (BPRS) is a widely used clinician-administered screen for psychiatric disorders, including the presence of psychotic symptoms. The BPRS is based on the clinician's interview and interactions with a client. Most versions contain twenty-four items, which are rated on a scale of 0 (not present) to 7 (extremely severe). It can be given over the course of treatment and used to mark clinical progress. It takes approximately twenty to thirty minutes to complete.

TREATMENT CONSIDERATIONS

Psychotherapies

Assertive Community Treatment Teams. ACTT is an evidenced-based, in-the-community treatment approach to working with people with severe mental illness. It can be especially effective for people who have difficulty engaging in treatment and who have had multiple hospitalizations. It involves the use of a multidisciplinary team that provides integrated treatment and support to clients. ACT teams meet frequently to review cases and share responsibility among team members. Caseloads are kept low (10:1 ratio for case managers) on account of the intensity of services. The majority (ideally 80 percent or more) of services are delivered in the community versus an office or clinic. ACTT provides 24/7 availability. Positive outcomes from ACTT include decreased rates of hospitalization and improved psychosocial outcomes.

Integrated Dual Diagnosis Treatment. Although this book focuses on integrated treatment across all diagnoses, the concept of integrated treatment first took root in working with people with severe and persistent mental illness. Integrated dual diagnosis treatment (IDDT), as studied in this population, is considered an evidence-based approach to help people who have severe mental illness and substance use problems. IDDT is typically provided through agencies and mental health clinics that employ multidisciplinary treatment approaches, often through the use of ACT teams. Key components to the IDDT model include:

- Stage-specific treatment
  - Engagement: This involves the establishment of a relationship with the client. With people with schizophrenia spectrum disorders, this may include various forms of community outreach and literally "meeting the person where they are at."
  - Establishment of treatment goals with the client
  - Interventions that are specific to the person and where they are in their recovery
  - Attention to the person's immediate, intermediate, and longer-range goals
- Attention to basic needs, such as housing and finances
- Motivational interviewing
  - Attention to the person's level of motivation to change high-risk behaviors, including substance use
  - Typically done in one-to-one sessions of varying lengths. Various studies have found three one-hour sessions associated with positive outcomes.
  - Emphasis on empowerment and responsibility
  - Evaluation of the risks and benefits of continued drug and alcohol use (i.e., weighing the pros and cons)
- Cognitive behavior therapy (CBT)
  - CBT strategies assist with recognizing thoughts, emotions, and behaviors associated with craving and relapse.
  - Through cognitive restructuring, CBT can help people identify healthier ways to manage their mental illness, real-life stressors, and cravings. Cognitive restructuring can be used to challenge beliefs about the positive benefits of drug/alcohol use.
  - CBT can help normalize relapses and get the person back on track: "It's not the end of the world. Today's a new day."
  - CBT can be used to model and practice skills through techniques such as role-playing, which can be especially helpful in developing drug refusal skills.
  - CBT can be used to improve overall problem-solving skills.
- Principles of harm reduction and "meeting the person where they are at"
  - Empowering the person in recovery

o Supporting all positive change

- Assertive community outreach, including homeless outreach teams, the use of peer engagement specialists, and other case management approaches
- Comprehensive and multidimensional services and supports that might include:
  o Psychiatric assessment and ongoing treatment, including medication
  o Housing assistance
  o Vocational training, assistance, and support
  o Peer supports
  o Wellness programs
  o Enhancement of natural social supports (e.g., family, friends, faith community)
  o Utilization of mutual self-help programs (e.g., Hearing Voices Network, 12-step groups, Double Trouble in Recovery)
  o Liaison with other providers
  o Liaison with the criminal justice system
  o Access to specialized programs to address specific needs, goals, and priorities (e.g., DBT, eating disorder treatment, CBT for specific anxiety disorders, etc.).

Behavioral Treatment for Substance Abuse in Serious and Persistent Mental Illness (BTSAS). Developed by Alan Bellack, MD, and colleagues, this small-group approach (four to six members, although with some individual components) consists of manualized treatment that includes several integrated features. BTSAS emphasizes the over-learning of a few important skills, such as drug refusal, and adapts the treatment to the individual's specific needs and cognitive abilities. BTSAS has several core components:

- Individual motivational interviewing, in which a specific drug that needs to be addressed is identified
- Contingency management, which uses the results of urine drug screens to provide monetary rewards
- Collaborative goal setting, in which realistic short-term goals are identified
- A harm reduction approach, which works with people at all stages of their drug use
- Social skills training to teach drug refusal and to enhance sober social supports
- Psychoeducation about drug use, unsafe behaviors, and their consequences. This includes learning about mental disorders and specific issues for people with co-occurring substance use problems.
- Relapse prevention training to help people identify high-risk situations, learn how to avoid them, and learn how to manage urges and lapses.

BTSAS is a structured treatment where clients learn the format, which includes a urinalysis, review of goals and goals setting, a review of the prior session, and presentation of new material, which typically includes didactics, discussion, and role-playing around important skills to be learned.

Case Management. Although case management is included as part of the ACTT model and many others, when it is included as an add-on to other treatments, it has been shown to be effective in improving overall care integration and adherence to treatment. People with schizophrenia often have severe problems with motivation, as well as other specific cognitive deficits, that can lead to frustration and treatment failure, especially when the individual must navigate multiple complex systems, such as mental health and substance use agencies, the legal system, welfare and disability agencies, and basic needs, such as housing and grocery shopping. Through a nonclinical lens, this is like having a personal assistant. Specific roles of the case manager can include:

- Identifying needed/desired services and then helping the client navigate systems to put them in place, such as obtaining a primary care physician or nurse practitioner

- Providing care coordination, from setting up appointments to helping with transportation

- Providing assistance and skills training in budgeting so there is adequate food in the house and so critical services, such as rent and utilities, get paid. For people who receive disability income, this could include designation of a representative payee who ensures that bills related to basic needs (e.g., rent, utilities, groceries) are paid each month.

- Working with the client's goals and aspirations to help them more fully realize their lives in the community. This includes assistance with vocational, educational, spiritual, social, and recreational goals.

Peer and Natural Supports

- **Mutual self-help groups:** These can include AA, NA, SMART Recovery, and many other groups, both in-person and/or online.

- **Double Trouble in Recovery and Dual Diagnosis Anonymous Groups:** These 12-step mutual self-help groups are specifically designed for people with both mental illness and substance use disorders. These targeted groups allow individuals to address both their issues with mental illness and their substance abuse. Hundreds of groups meet nationwide, but the organization currently has no central website. For those interested in starting a group, a low-cost electronic manual is available by Howard Vogel, called *Double Trouble in Recovery: Basic Guide*. To find a group, individuals should contact 2-1-1 or the local mental health authority.

- **Peer support specialists:** Over the past decade, the use of peer specialists, which now go by many names (e.g., recovery support specialists, peer navigators), has grown and are often embedded within ACTT, as well as in other case management and outreach services. Peer specialists are people in recovery from mental illness, and from possibly substance use disorders as well, who help others with similar issues.

Peer support specialists differ from traditional case managers in that their role is directly focused on engagement with a client as one person in recovery with another. It is common for peer support specialists to focus on developing the relationship with the client, such as going to a movie or eating a meal together or doing some other more social and less typically treatment-type activity.

Pharmacology

The few studies that look at specific antipsychotic medication for people who have both schizophrenia and substance use disorders generally show improvement in both the symptoms of schizophrenia and the severity of the substance use disorder. These findings, which include decreased substance use and improved function, support the importance of offering pharmacological treatment even when people use illicit drugs and/or alcohol. That said, important factors need to be considered when medications are prescribed:

- Assess the potential for drug interactions and adverse reactions between any medication and the substance(s) the person uses.
  - Sedating antipsychotics, such as quetiapine (Seroquel), increase the risk of respiratory depression in people who use central nervous system depressants, such as opioids and alcohol.
  - Someone who misuses amphetamines or goes through intermittent alcohol or benzodiazepine withdrawal while taking certain antidepressants or antipsychotics will be at an increased risk for seizures.
  - Cocaine is associated with increased adverse cardiac events, which may worsen with the use of medications associated with cardiac conduction delays, such as the prolongation of the QT interval (a measurement of the heart's electrical conduction), which can lead to dangerous arrhythmias and sudden death with medications like ziprasidone (Geodon), methadone, and hydroxyzine (Vistaril).
  - Cigarette smoking, through its effects on the liver, can decrease the blood levels of certain antipsychotic medications by more than 50 percent.
- Keep medication regimens as safe and streamlined as possible. Less is often more. "Start low and go slow."
- The risk of suicidal behavior increases when someone is intoxicated. For people who struggle with recurrent suicidal thoughts and behaviors, it will be important to limit the amounts and types of medication they have.

- Limit the prescribing of medications that can be misused, such as benzodiazepines, opioid pain medications, and stimulants.

- Consider strategies to increase adherence, such as once-a-day dosing or long-acting injectable medications. When needed, case managers and in-home nursing supports can assist with community-based medication management.

- Assess how medications are stored and kept secure. Does the person need a lockbox? Would daily medication delivery improve the chances that the person's medications would not be misused? This precaution could be achieved through an ACT team or other case management model, through an in-home nursing agency, or with a responsible family member.

- Educate patients on the importance of taking medications to treat their psychotic symptoms even if they have lapsed into substance use.

Antipsychotic Medications. The mainstay pharmacological treatments for schizophrenia are the antipsychotic medications, also termed neuroleptics and major tranquilizers, which are divided into two broad classes: the first-generation (typical) and second-generation (atypical) antipsychotics.

First- and Second-Generation Antipsychotics

First-Generation/Typical Antipsychotics	Available as a Long-Acting Decanoate	Second-Generation/ Atypical Antipsychotics	Available as a Long-Acting Decanoate
Chlorpromazine (Thorazine)	No	Aripiprazole (Abilify)	Yes
Fluphenazine (Prolixin)	Yes	Asenapine (Saphris)	No
Haloperidol (Haldol)	Yes	Cariprazine (Vraylar)	No
Loxapine (Loxitane)	No	Clozapine (Clozaril)	No
Molindone (Moban)	No	Iloperidone (Fanapt)	No
Perphenazine (Trilafon)	No	Lurasidone (Latuda)	No
Thioridazine (Mellaril)	No	Olanzapine (Zyprexa)	Yes
Thioxanthene (Navane)	No	Paliperidone (Invega)	Yes
Trifluoperazine (Stelazine)	No	Quetiapine (Seroquel)	No
		Risperidone (Risperdal)	Yes
		Ziprasidone (Geodon)	No

Both classes of antipsychotic medication carry significant risks for side effects and serious adverse reactions, some that can be fatal. Concerning too is the development of movement abnormalities, obesity, and metabolic syndrome.

All these medications are available in pill or capsule form, and several can be given as a rapid-acting injectable, specifically haloperidol (Haldol) and olanzapine

(Zyprexa). These shots are typically used in situations where rapid tranquilization is required to help someone who is severely agitated.

Long-acting decanoate-injectable medications with dosing schedules that stretch between every two to four weeks to three months (each medication has a specific schedule range) are also available for several medications. Because decanoate medications are dosed infrequently, they have higher rates of medication adherence. They carry all the risks and benefits associated with the shorter-acting versions of the medications and can be associated with local reactions at the injection site (pain, redness, swelling).

Side Effects and Adverse Reactions Common with the First-Generation/Typical Antipsychotics

- **Movement abnormalities and dystonia**

  o **Parkinsonism:** This involves the shortening of a person's gait, "the Thorazine shuffle," accompanied by diminished arm swing, muscle stiffness, and a flattened and often depressed-appearing facial expression. This is not to be confused with Parkinson's Disease, which is a progressive neurodegenerative disease. Parkinsonism is an adverse reaction from the medications and is reversible.

  o **Akathisia:** An uncomfortable feeling of restlessness, it can be severe and may manifest with anxious and fidgety behavior and an inability to stay still. This can include foot and arm tapping and rocking. It can be mistaken for the hyperactivity and inattention seen in ADHD.

  o **Acute dystonic reactions:** These are involuntary contractions or muscle spasms. They appear suddenly after administration of an antipsychotic. They are rarely life-threatening but can be disturbing and even painful. They often require emergency treatment with the use of anticholinergic medications, such as diphenhydramine (Benadryl), benztropine (Cogentin), or trihexyphenidyl (Artane). Benzodiazepines may also be used. Examples of dystonic reactions include:

    Torticollis, an intense contraction of the muscles of the neck, often on one side, that results in an asymmetric posture

    Opisthotonic reaction, in which the muscles of the back become rigid and the body arches back

    Oculogyric crisis, where the eyes roll back and remain fixed

    Laryngeal dystonia, which results in difficulty speaking

    Buccolingual crisis, which affects the muscles of the tongue and mouth. This can manifest as grimacing, involuntary protrusion of the tongue, and/or intense contraction of the muscles of the lower face into a fixed smile

  o **Tardive dyskinesia:** This is a common and potentially irreversible involuntary movement abnormality, mostly associated with the older antipsychotics. Tardive dyskinesia typically affects the muscles around the mouth and tongue and can include lip smacking and the unintended protrusion of the tongue.

Although most frequently limited to the face and tongue, it can affect all muscle groups—including the major muscle groups of the arms, legs, and trunk—and become disfiguring and disabling. There are currently two FDA-approved medications for the treatment of tardive dyskinesia, though results with either are not typically robust.

- **Anticholinergic side effects**
  o Dry mouth
  o Urinary retention
  o Decreased ability to sweat (especially worrisome in warm weather when it puts people at risk for heat exhaustion and stroke)
  o In severe cases, confusion and delirium, which can easily be mistaken as a worsening of an underlying psychotic illness

- **Orthostatic changes** involve drops in blood pressure, at times without an adequate increase in pulse, when a person goes from lying down to seated or seated to standing. It results in light-headedness and in more severe instances, the person could fall or faint.

- **Sedation** can be caused by any of the antipsychotic medications, but it is most significant with chlorpromazine (Thorazine) and thioridazine (Mellaril).

Side Effects and Adverse Reactions Common with the Second-Generation/ Atypical Antipsychotics

- **Metabolic syndrome** is caused by the increased appetite and alterations in insulin and glucose metabolism seen with the atypical antipsychotics. It encompasses serious health conditions characterized by weight gain, increased abdominal girth, and elevations in blood pressure, cholesterol, and triglycerides. These changes predispose the person to obesity, type 2 diabetes, hypercholesterolemia, coronary artery disease, and stroke. Metabolic syndrome represents a major health concern and is one factor in the overall poor mortality statistics for people with schizophrenia spectrum disorders.

  Significant weight gain has been reported with all the atypical antipsychotics with the exception of ziprasidone (Geodon). With some medications, such as clozapine (Clozaril) and olanzapine (Zyprexa), weight gain can be a pound or more per week. Other medications, such as risperidone (Risperdal) and quetiapine (Seroquel), have weight gain more on the order of half a pound per week.

- **Sedation** is especially significant with clozapine (Clozaril) and quetiapine (Seroquel) but can occur with any antipsychotic medication.

- **Blood pressure changes:** Can be profound with clozapine (Clozaril)

- **Tardive dyskinesia:** Although this movement abnormality is less common with the second-generation antipsychotics, it can still occur.

Clozapine: Special Considerations, Monitoring, and Concerns. Clozapine (Clozaril, Fazaclo) was the first of the second-generation antipsychotics. It is considered the "gold standard" because a significant number of patients who have not responded or have had an inadequate improvement with other medications will show clinical improvement that in some cases is dramatic.

Clozapine carries the risk for a potentially life-threatening condition— agranulocytosis—in which the bone marrow stops producing white blood cells that are necessary to protect the body from infection. Because of this risk, clozapine is not used as a first-line treatment for schizophrenia but is reserved for individuals who do not respond to other agents. Rates of agranulocytosis run as high as 1 percent, and individuals on clozapine need to be registered and have regular blood counts (CBC) drawn. Initially, draws are weekly, then biweekly, and after six months, if all the results are normal, monthly. Pharmacies are required to verify the blood work results before filling prescriptions.

In addition to the risk of agranulocytosis, clozapine carries a heavy side effect and adverse reaction burden, which can include:

- Seizures, especially when the dose is greater than 600 mg/day
- Sialorrhea (i.e., extreme salivation and drooling): It's common for people to complain of pillow-drenching drool.
- Weight gain and metabolic syndrome, which can be severe
- Orthostatic blood pressure changes: This is often experienced as light-headedness and can increase the risk for falls and fainting.
- Tachycardia (i.e., rapid heart rate): It is common for people on clozapine to have resting heart rates greater than 100 beats per minute.
- Sedation: Often severe and requires a slow titration (i.e., increase of the medication to therapeutic doses) for the person to be able to tolerate it.

How to Monitor for Tardive Dyskinesia

People on antipsychotics, both first- and second-generation, should be monitored for the development of tardive dyskinesia. The standard of care includes the use of the Abnormal Involuntary Movement Scale (AIMS). An AIMS examination should be completed prior to starting or switching antipsychotics and then every six months thereafter. The AIMS exam takes five to ten minutes to perform and can be completed by the prescriber or, with training and adequate supervision, other providers. The AIMS examination is in the public domain and may be freely copied. Performing an AIMS examination follows these steps:

1. At some point before or after the examination, observe the patient for signs of involuntary movement when they are unaware—in the waiting room, for instance.
2. Ask the client to remove their shoes and socks. (This will allow visualization of movement in the toes.)

3. Have the patient sit in a firm chair without arms.

4. Ask the client if they have anything in their mouth (gum, tobacco). If they do, have them remove it, as the chewing could be mistaken for symptoms of tardive dyskinesia.

5. Ask the client if they wear dentures and/or have problems with their teeth. Loose-fitting dentures can lead to mouth movements that look like tardive dyskinesia.

6. Ask the client if they notice any involuntary movements in their mouth, face, lips, hands, feet, or other parts of their body. Ask them to describe those movements and whether they are distressed and/or impaired by them.

7. Have the client sit in the chair with their hands resting on their legs or knees and their feet shoulder-width apart. Visually scan the client from head to toe for any signs of movement.

8. Ask the client to let their arms and hands hang unsupported by their legs. Observe the body for movement.

9. Ask the client to open their mouth and observe the tongue for movements. Do this twice.

10. Ask the client to stick out their tongue. Observe the tongue for unusual movements, such as thrusting or crossing the midline of the mouth.

11. Ask the client to tap their thumb against each of their fingertips in rapid succession. Have them do this for ten to fifteen seconds with one hand and then with the other. Observe movements throughout the body as they do so. This distraction strategy is called activation and will bring out or worsen movements of tardive dyskinesia.

12. Extend and flex the client's left and right arms. Notice signs of rigidity or cogwheeling (where the arm has a jerky ratchet-like quality as it is moved). This type of cogwheel rigidity can be associated with the adverse reaction of parkinsonism.

13. Ask the client to stand. Observe the body for signs of movement.

14. Ask the client to extend their arms in front of their body with their palms facing down. Observe the entire body for movement.

15. Have the client walk a few paces, turn, and then walk back. Observe for normal arm swing and for gait. In people with parkinsonism, the gait may be shuffling in nature, and they may have a restricted or absent arm swing. This may also activate movement associated with tardive dyskinesia.

THE ABNORMAL INVOLUNTARY MOVEMENT SCALE (AIMS)

Client name: _____   Date: _____

ID number: _____   Examiner: _____

Code: 0 = None   1= Minimal   2 = Mild   3 = Moderate   4 = Severe

Instructions: Complete the examination prior to scoring.

_____

Facial and oral movements:

1. Muscles of facial expression (movements of the forehead, around the eyes, cheeks; include grimacing, smiling, blinking)	0	1	2	3	4
2. Lips and around the mouth (puckering, lip-smacking, pouting)	0	1	2	3	4
3. Jaw (biting, grinding, lateral movements, clenching)	0	1	2	3	4
4. Tongue (rate only increases in movement both in and out of the mouth)	0	1	2	3	4

Extremity movements:

5. Upper: Arms, wrists, hands, and fingers. Include slow and rapid movements, snake-like movements. Do not include tremor.	0	1	2	3	4
6. Lower: Legs, feet, toes, ankles. Lateral movements of the knee, foot-tapping, inward and outward movements of the feet, flexing and contracting of the feet	0	1	2	3	4

Trunk movements:

7. Neck, shoulders, hips, torso (rocking, twisting, squirming, pelvic gyrations)	0	1	2	3	4

Overall severity of movements:

8. Severity of abnormal movements	0	1	2	3	4
9. Incapacitation due to abnormal movements	0	1	2	3	4

Client's awareness of movements:

No awareness = 0; Aware, no distress = 1; Aware, mild distress = 2; Aware, moderate distress = 3; Aware, severe distress = 4

10. Client's awareness of movement	0	1	2	3	4

Dental status

11. Current problems with teeth and/or dentures?	Yes	No
12. Are dentures usually worn?	Yes	No

Comments: _____   Examiner's signature: _____   Date/Time: _____

Scoring the AIM Examination

- The AIMS examination is considered positive if there is a score of 2 on any two movements, or a score of 3 or four 4 any single movement.
- The score is not summed (i.e., a score of 1 on five separate movements does not equal 5).
- Add 1 to a score if the client is aware and/or distressed by the movement.

How to Monitor for Metabolic Syndrome

Because a serious risk of metabolic syndrome is associated with the second-generation antipsychotics, it is crucial that routine monitoring is done prior to starting or changing medication and is then ongoing. There are multiple monitoring guidelines. The following recommendations are from the American Diabetes Association and the American Psychiatric Association:

- Assess for personal and family history of obesity, diabetes, high blood pressure, cardiovascular disease, and lipid abnormalities (obtain at baseline and update annually).
- Measure weight and height.
- Calculate BMI at baseline (i.e., before starting medication), monthly for the first three months and then quarterly. Greater frequency may be required if the BMI increases. Free applications for calculating BMI are available, including this one through the CDC: www.cdc.gov/healthyweight/assessing/bmi/index.html.
- Measure waist circumference at baseline, monthly for the first three months and then quarterly.
- Measure fasting lipids (e.g., cholesterol, triglycerides, HDL, LDL) at baseline, then at three months, and every five years. If there are elevations, the frequency should be adjusted.
- Measure fasting blood glucose at baseline, at three months, and then annually. (There is some disagreement in the literature as to whether or not the glucose needs to be a fasting one.)

In addition to the above, it's common for practitioners to also obtain a Hemoglobin A1C, which is a marker for the development of diabetes.

Strategies to Address Weight Gain and Metabolic Syndrome. For people on medications that carry the risk of weight gain and metabolic syndrome, education and early intervention are crucial.

- Address modifiable cardiovascular risk factors and unhealthy lifestyle habits, such as tobacco use, elevated lipids, lack of adequate exercise, and unhealthy and high-calorie diets.
- Educate regarding adequate sleep and sleep hygiene to decrease the risk of sleep apnea, which often accompanies metabolic syndrome.
- Educate family and involved supports about the risk of metabolic syndrome and efforts that can be made to prevent and reverse it should it occur.
- Maintain active medical follow-up and liaison between the psychiatric prescriber and the primary care practitioner. Should someone develop weight gain, elevations in lipids, hypertension, and so forth, these will need to be followed and addressed medically, which might include the use of medications for elevated lipids (i.e., statins) or for type 2 diabetes.
- Consider the use of antipsychotic agents less associated with metabolic syndrome. This could include the use of first-generation medications or ziprasidone (Geodon).

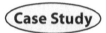

David Gray

David Gray is a twenty-three-year-old, single Caucasian man who is initially evaluated in the emergency room where he has been brought by police on an emergency hold/police request for psychiatric evaluation. He lives with his mother, Lillian Gray, who called 9-1-1 after he threatened to kill himself. She is present for the evaluation and reports that her son has been drinking heavily and using other substances as well. She has several empty packages of a substance that claims to be "plant food." Her son has been purchasing it over the internet.

In the emergency room, David is agitated, red-faced, and aggressive toward staff. He swears, and when the police remove the handcuffs, he lunges for a nurse. A security code is called, and with the assistance of his mother, David agrees to take a shot of haloperidol (Haldol) and lorazepam (Ativan). He calms but appears distracted and admits to hearing the voice of the devil telling him to end his own life. His mood fluctuates rapidly—at times he is sobbing and then laughing and talking rapidly with an odd punctuated cadence where he repeats words. His blood alcohol level is 0.12 (legal limit for driving in his state is 0.08), and his urine toxicology is positive for cannabis. His blood pressure and pulse are elevated and return to normal range with the administration of an additional dose of lorazepam (Ativan).

His mother describes how David has always had emotional problems and how he started to drink, smoke cigarettes, and use cannabis when he was in middle school. "He was always very shy, never made friends, and told me that pot was the only thing that calmed him down." He dropped out of school in the tenth grade. "He just stopped going." He has been hospitalized twice (both times involuntary) with similar presentations and has had two additional emergency room evaluations where he was discharged home with his mother and referred to outpatient treatment. "I tried to get him to keep those appointments, but he won't. He insists there's nothing wrong with him and that all he needs is marijuana." She states he's taken deliberate overdoses in the past, and she's frightened that one day he will take his life.

The family history is significant for a maternal uncle with schizophrenia who committed suicide, and David's father died from cirrhosis after decades of heavy drinking. His mother does not use substances and reports that, other than anxiety over her son, she has no mental health problems.

David's medical history is unremarkable, although he's not been to see a physician, other than in emergency room evaluations, for years. He has no allergies. Blood work obtained in the emergency room is normal except for elevated liver enzymes and an elevated mean corpuscular volume (MCV) on his CBC.

As David's blood alcohol level drops, he continues to display bizarre behavior with pressured speech and rapid shifts in his mood. When asked about suicide, he replies, "I'm a waste of space. What's the point?" He continues to report hearing voices and eventually falls asleep after a dose of tranquilizing medication. He is placed on a CIWA protocol for alcohol withdrawal, and the emergency room psychiatrist makes the determination to hospitalize David on an involuntary basis based on his imminent risk for self-harm and the fact that he is gravely disabled, based on his current level of psychosis, auditory hallucinations telling him to kill himself, agitation, and substance use.

Three days later, David is on an inpatient psychiatric unit. His symptoms of alcohol withdrawal are well-controlled with lorazepam (Ativan) combined with a medication for blood pressure. He has been prescribed risperidone (Risperdal) for his hallucinations and delusional thinking but has refused most doses of this medication. He states, "There's nothing wrong with me. All I need to do is smoke pot. It's the only thing that helps."

He is calmer overall, and no additional emergency doses of injectable tranquilizers have been required. He is able to be interviewed and answers most questions. He states he's been hearing voices since he was fourteen. It is usually the voice of a man he doesn't recognize but thinks is the devil. It often tells him to harm himself or carries on a narrative of derogatory comments about David. "You're worthless, a piece of shit." He states when he's tried to harm himself in the past, it's been at the urging of the voice. He admits to frequent thoughts of self-harm but states he currently has no intention of acting upon them. He denies any thoughts of harming others. He rates his mood as severely depressed (10/10). He rates his level of anxiety as between an 8–10/10. He reports that his goal is to get out of the hospital and go back to smoking "as much pot as I can." He does, however, agree that his drinking has become excessive. "But I didn't need to be in a hospital to stop. I do that all the time on my own."

His mother visits daily. She provides additional information, as well as prior records from his two earlier hospitalizations. She states that her son's mood fluctuates between extreme depression, to where he won't leave his room for weeks and even months at a time, to periods of manic agitation, often accompanied by heavy drug and alcohol use. During those periods, he stops sleeping, becomes loud and hyperverbal, and talks about having special powers. During these episodes, she calls the police because his behavior becomes frightening and at times dangerous, such as getting behind the wheel of a car and driving at high speeds while intoxicated. She believes that even when he is not depressed or manic, he continues to hear voices. He has been arrested on multiple occasions for possession of cannabis and breach of the peace. He's received two DUIs and does not currently have a license. As far as she is aware, he has no history of violence toward anyone but himself, although he has "trashed his room and punched holes in the wall" on multiple occasions. She states that David has never hit her but has threatened to do so multiple times.

Step One: Level of Care Determination and Discussion

The above scenario shows a person with a psychotic disorder who presents to an emergency room with grossly disorganized behavior, hallucinations, delusions, and severe substance use with imminent risk of alcohol withdrawal. He requires inpatient hospitalization both for treatment of withdrawal and to stabilize his symptoms of mania and psychosis.

Beyond the immediate situation, the larger question will be how to engage with him in treatment moving forward. The history of repeated failed referrals to outpatient levels of care will need to be explored and different strategies pursued. His inability to see that anything is wrong (i.e., anosognosia) coupled with his stated goal of continuing to smoke cannabis (i.e., precontemplative stage of change) creates challenges in a common scenario.

For David, it will help to think in terms of staged treatment and short-term, intermediate, and longer-range goals. In cases of imminent safety issues, the short-term goals are focused on crisis stabilization, and inpatient hospitalization is indicated. Once he is out of danger of serious withdrawal and his behavior and thoughts no longer represent an imminent danger to himself or others, he will need to transition to a less restrictive setting.

Currently, in the United States, the average inpatient psychiatric hospitalization is about one week—far too short to do more than stabilize the immediate crisis. The risk here is that without adequate aftercare plans and linkages to treatment, this individual will quickly relapse and require rehospitalization or suffer the consequences of his high-risk behaviors.

Inpatient psychiatric units do aggressive crisis management that starts during the intake. They also focus on aftercare and want their patients to successfully transition to lower levels of care. In this case, treatment could go in a number of directions. David would meet admission criteria for a longer post-acute rehabilitation stay, ideally in a facility that has treatment for people with serious co-occurring disorders. However, with his stated goal of leaving the hospital and his lack of motivation to be abstinent from cannabis, this is unlikely to happen voluntarily. Depending on the state David lives in, his mother, the hospital, or an outside agency might decide to pursue a longer inpatient hospitalization on an involuntary basis. This typically requires going before a probate judge. It might involve a trial on the inpatient unit and additional evaluations by independent psychiatrists. Involuntary commitment processes and procedures vary from state to state.

A less restrictive option that might be acceptable to David would be referral to a state agency or private not-for-profit mental health agency that can provide community-based services, such as an ACT team. Ideally this team would include a peer engagement specialist, case manager/coordinator, substance abuse counselor, psychiatrist or prescribing APRN, and other specialty services, including group and individual therapies for people with co-occurring disorders, housing, and employment services. For this kind of outpatient linkage to succeed, it is best that the initial stages of engagement occur while he is still on the inpatient unit. In an ideal circumstance, this would include completion of the application with in-person meetings with the peer specialist and case manager on the inpatient unit. This would allow David a chance to meet the people he would be working with and hopefully see some benefit to the services offered.

Step Two: Construct the Problem/Need List

Substance Use	Mental Health	Medical
Heavy use of alcohol	Threatened to kill self	No allergies
Use of synthetic cannabis and other substances	Agitated and aggressive	Only medical contact has been through emergency rooms and on psychiatric units
Blood alcohol level of 0.12 several hours after last drink	Labile mood	Blood pressure and pulse elevated
Urine toxicology positive for cannabis	Always "shy" and withdrawn	Elevated liver enzymes and MCV
Cannabis calms him down	Cannabis calms him down	
Began to drink and use cannabis in middle school	Since age fourteen, hears the devil telling him to kill himself	
Father was a heavy drinker who died of cirrhosis	Speaks in an odd cadence	
Two DUIs	Depression rated 10/10	
Multiple arrests	Uncle with schizophrenia committed suicide	
High-risk behaviors when manic and intoxicated	Two prior involuntary hospitalizations	
Wants to keep smoking cannabis daily	Episodes of manic agitation	
	Episodes of sustained depression	
	Hears voices even when not having a mood episode	
	Believes nothing is wrong with him (anosognosia)	
	High-risk behaviors when manic and intoxicated	
	History of overdoses	
	Does not follow up with aftercare plans	

In this case study, both the substance use and mental health problem/need will meet criteria for an inpatient admission. Deciding which diagnosis goes first may have more to do with the type of unit he gets admitted to and how they get reimbursed. For example, a predominantly alcohol detoxification unit would list the substance use issue first, whereas a predominantly psychiatric unit would likely list the mental health problem/need statement first. The few issues in the medical column might call for a separate problem/need statement or be subsumed in the substance use statement.

1. **Active and severe substance use with imminent risk of alcohol withdrawal**, AEB daily drinking, elevated vital signs, daily use of cannabis, and synthetic drugs purchased via the internet; Blood alcohol level of 0.12 several hours after last drink and urine drug screen positive for cannabis; Abnormal labs consistent with heavy drinking

2. **Severe and disabling psychosis and depression with command auditory hallucinations telling him to kill himself**, delusional thinking, disorganized speech, agitation, high-risk behaviors, and severe depression (10/10) and anxiety (8–10/10).

3. **Inadequate medical care**, given that his only contact with medical care has been in acute care settings; Has been on high-risk medications and has multiple high-risk behaviors (e.g., tobacco use, heavy drinking)

Step Three: Establish the Initial Goals/Objectives for Treatment

1. Active and severe substance use with imminent risk of alcohol withdrawal

  a. Short-term goals/objectives:

   i. Client will be treated for signs and symptoms of alcohol withdrawal using the CIWA protocol.

   ii. The patient will be free from all signs of alcohol withdrawal.

  b. Long-term goals:

   i. The patient will be abstinent from alcohol.

   ii. The patient will reduce his cannabis use by 50 percent or more.

2. Severe and disabling psychosis and depression with command auditory hallucinations telling the patient to kill himself

  a. Short-term goals/objectives:

   i. Provide a safe environment.

   ii. Decrease symptoms of manic agitation to where the patient gets at least seven hours of sleep/day and reports a 50 percent or greater reduction in auditory hallucinations.

   iii. The patient will identify at least one positive reason to continue taking medication for his mood and psychotic symptoms.

  b. Long-term goals: The patient will achieve full remission from his symptoms of psychosis and mood swings.

3. Inadequate medical care

  a. Short-term goals/objectives:

   i. Complete a history and physical, including AIMS examination, and obtain routine screening tests, including screens for metabolic syndrome.

   ii. Identify any active medical issues.

  b. Long-term goals: The patient will have a regular outpatient primary care provider and receive regular follow-up for any active problems.

Treatment-and-Recovery Plan

Patient's Name: David Gray	
Date of Birth: 3/3/1997	
Medical Record #: XXX-XX-XXXX	

Level of Care: Adult inpatient detoxification and acute psychiatric unit

ICD-10 Codes	DSM-5 Diagnoses
F10.239	Alcohol withdrawal with alcohol use disorder, severe*
F25.0	Schizoaffective disorder bipolar type
F12.20	Cannabis use disorder, moderate
F17.200	Tobacco use disorder, moderate
Z91.19	Nonadherence to medical treatment

The individual's stated goal(s): "To get out of the hospital and be able to smoke as much pot as I can get my hands on and to not get thrown back in here"

---

1. Problem/Need Statement: Active and severe substance use with imminent risk of alcohol withdrawal

Long-Term Goal: Abstain from alcohol; Decrease cannabis and tobacco consumption and use of other illicit substances by 50 percent or more

Short-Term Goals/Objectives (with target date):

1. Client will be treated for signs and symptoms of alcohol withdrawal using the CIWA protocol. (immediately—8/13/20)
2. The patient will be free from all signs of alcohol withdrawal within five days. (8/17/20)

---

2. Problem/Need Statement: Severe and disabling psychosis and depression with command auditory hallucinations telling the patient to kill himself

Long-Term Goal: The patient will achieve full remission from his symptoms of psychosis and mood swings.

Short-Term Goals/Objectives (with target date):

1. Provide a safe environment. (immediately—8/12/20)
2. Decrease symptoms of manic agitation to where the patient gets at least seven hours of sleep/day and reports a 50 percent or greater reduction in auditory hallucinations. (by third day of admission)
3. The patient will identify at least one positive reason to continue taking medication for his mood and psychotic symptoms. (by day of discharge)

3. Problem/Need Statement: Inadequate medical care
Long-Term Goal: The patient will have a regular outpatient primary care provider and receive regular follow-up for any active problems.
Short-Term Goals/Objectives (with target date):
1. Complete a history and physical, including AIMS examination, and obtain routine screening tests, including screens for metabolic syndrome. (within twenty-four hours of admission)
2. Identify any active medical issues. (within three days of admission)

Interventions					
Treatment Modality	**Specific Type**	**Frequency**	**Duration**	**Problem Number**	**Responsible Person(s)**
Alcohol Detoxification	CIWA protocol	Every shift	Until CIWA score is less than 5, his vital signs have normalized, and Mr. Gray has been tapered off benzodiazepine medication	1	MD/RN staff
Medical	Medication management, including evaluation and management of medical issues	Daily	Daily meeting with prescribing physician	1, 2, 3	MD
Safety Checks	Monitor for self-harm, high-risk behavior, or worsening of withdrawal	Every 15 minutes	To be reassessed daily	1, 2	Nursing and patient-care staff

(Continued)

(Continued)

Individual Therapy	Motivational interviewing	Daily	30–60 minutes	1, 2	Primary clinician

Interventions					
Treatment Modality	**Specific Type**	**Frequency**	**Duration**	**Problem Number**	**Responsible Person(s)**
Group Therapy	Goals setting	Daily	50 minutes	1, 2, 3	Occupational therapist
	Skills group	Daily	50 minutes	1, 2	Activity therapist
	Psycho-education	Daily	50 minutes	1, 2	Nurse practitioner
	Double Trouble in Recovery	Daily	50 minutes	1, 2	Peer specialist
Family	Counseling and liaison	Daily in-person or phone contact with patient's mother	15–30 minutes, longer if needed	1, 2	Social worker, primary nurse
Discharge Planning and Coordination	Referral to local ACT team	As required throughout the admission	As required, with the goal of having at least two meetings between Mr. Gray and a member of the ACT team while he is on the unit	1, 2, 3	Social worker

Identification of strengths: Intelligent and creative, with some willingness to stop drinking

Peer/family/community supports to assist: His mother and the local mental health authority

Barriers to treatment: Risk for relapse after discharge. History of not connecting to outpatient providers

Staff/client-identified education/teaching needs: To help Mr. Gray identify potential advantages to using community supports and to help him understand the connections between his substance use and problems at home and in the community

Assessment of discharge needs/discharge planning: To be free from any signs of alcohol withdrawal and to have no active suicidal urges. To have a clear discharge plan in place with a completed referral to the ACT team

Completion of this treatment-and-recovery plan was a collaborative effort between the client and the following treatment team members:

SIGNATURES		Date/Time:
Client:	I agree with maybe half of what's on here, but I'm signing anyway so I can get out of here, David Gray.	8/12/2020, 2:15 p.m.
Physician:	Mellissa Croft, MD	8/12/2020, 2:20 p.m.
Treatment Plan Completed By:	Jeanette Grace, RN	8/12/2020, 2:22 p.m.
Social Worker:	Tracey Thrall, LCSW	8/12/2020, 3:10 p.m.
Other:	Lillian Gray (David's mother)	8/12/2020, 3:30 p.m.

* In this instance, the code for alcohol withdrawal with alcohol use disorder, severe, <u>without</u> perceptual disturbances has been selected, even though the patient clearly has psychotic symptoms. The rationale is that his psychotic symptoms are likely related to his psychotic disorder and not to an alcohol withdrawal syndrome.

CHAPTER 16

....

Personality Disorders and Co-Occurring Substance Use Disorders

OVERVIEW

Studies place the overall prevalence of personality disorders in the United States at over 9 percent, with the majority of those never seeking or receiving treatment. Rates for Cluster A disorders (paranoid, schizoid, schizotypal) range from 2.1–6.8 percent, Cluster B (borderline, antisocial, narcissistic, histrionic) from 1.5–6.1 percent, and Cluster C (avoidant, dependent, obsessive-compulsive) from 2.6–10.6 percent.

All the personality disorders have high rates of co-occurring substance use disorders and high rates of other mental disorders. Co-occurrence is especially true for people with borderline and antisocial personality disorders, where it is common to have multiple (three or more) comorbid disorders. While fewer in number, people with Cluster B personality disorders are the most likely to seek and receive treatment in any twelve-month period (nearly 50 percent) due to symptoms that can include frequent suicidality, impulsivity, and emotional and behavioral dyscontrol.

THE PERSONALITY DISORDERS

In order to meet DSM-5 criteria for a personality disorder, a person must have a pervasive (stemming back to adolescence or early adulthood) and maladaptive pattern of thinking, feeling, and behaving that involves impaired interpersonal relationships, a distorted view of themselves and the world around them (misperceptions), and for some, problems with impulsivity and emotion regulation. Tremendous overlap can occur between personality disorders, and individuals often have traits of more than one (e.g., someone with borderline personality disorder may have antisocial and narcissistic features).

Cluster A Personality Disorders

- Paranoid Personality Disorder
  - Is suspicious, has trouble trusting, suspects and misperceives the intentions of others, holds grudges, and is quick to anger
- Schizoid Personality Disorder
  - Is emotionally detached, flat, and isolative. Avoids interpersonal relationships. Has minimal interest in sex or other pleasurable pursuits. Is indifferent to praise or criticism
- Schizotypal Personality Disorder
  - Has trouble forming relationships/a lack of close relationships, is characterized by eccentric beliefs and presentation (dress, style of speech), and is prone to distortions. Exhibits ideas of reference (non-delusional), odd thoughts and beliefs, unusual sensory experiences, suspiciousness, anxiety in social settings

Cluster B Personality Disorders

- Antisocial Personality Disorder
  - Exhibits disregard for the rights, safety, property, and feelings of others. Characterized by deceitfulness, impulsivity, and illegal activities. Lacks empathy. Engages in frequent fights/assaults. May be predatory. Can appear charming
- Borderline Personality Disorder
  - Is emotionally vulnerable and impulsive with self-injurious behavior (e.g., cutting, burning). Experiences recurrent suicidality, transient paranoia, and dissociation. Characterized by black-and-white thinking (e.g., people, things, and situations are either all good or all bad). Can experience psychotic symptoms, most typically paranoia, when under stress. Is highly sensitive to rejection from others, both perceived and real. Exhibits high rates of comorbid trauma and PTSD
- Histrionic Personality Disorder
  - Characterized by excessive expressed emotions/dramatic speech and dress. Is provocative and seductive. Requires/seeks to be center of attention. Is dramatic and suggestible

- Narcissistic Personality Disorder
  - o Has a grandiose sense of self. Requires/insists upon admiration. Believes rules do not apply to special people, such as themselves. Fantasizes about power and importance. Lacks empathy. May appear arrogant. Takes advantage of others to achieve own ends

Cluster C Personality Disorders

- Avoidant Personality Disorder
  - o Avoids interpersonal relationships and situations. Feels inadequate, inferior, and judged. Is sensitive to rejection and believes others think negatively of them. Avoids risks
- Dependent Personality Disorder
  - o Needs to be taken care of. Is submissive and clingy. Fears rejection and abandonment. Feels helpless and in constant need of nurturance. Becomes frantic when relationships end
- Obsessive-Compulsive Personality Disorder
  - o Is rigid, orderly, and perfectionistic. Is intolerant of other ways of doing things. Often unable to complete tasks secondary to perfectionism. Characterized by moral inflexibility ("The rules are the rules"). Has trouble discarding even worthless items and is prone to hoarding

Treatment of Co-Occurring Substance Use Disorders and Personality Disorders

Personality disorders encompass a diverse range of presentations. The spectrum of personality disorders runs from people who are socially isolative, emotionally restricted, and globally avoidant to people whose lives are lived in emotional minefields where self-injury and even suicide seem like reasonable options in the face of unbearable suffering.

With borderline personality disorder, evidence-based psychotherapies—DBT in particular—have been well studied with people who have both a personality and substance use disorder. However, once we move away from borderline personality disorder, there are few controlled studies that address specific personality disorders and almost none that examine co-occurring substance use and personality disorders. At the time of this book's publication, there are no FDA-approved medications for any of the personality disorders.

While potentially daunting, this lack of research should not deter the clinician from constructing effective and integrated treatment for individuals with any of the personality disorders. As with all clients, it boils down to the individual and their specific goals and priorities. Things to consider:

- Conduct a thorough assessment.
- Achieve engagement and establish meaningful goals and priorities.

- Based on the assessment, make recommendations for the appropriate level of care.

- Active safety concerns always come first (e.g., suicidality and/or homicidality, serious medical concerns, grave disability, dangerous withdrawal or intoxication states).

- Identify connections between the mental disorder and the substance use. Does someone with avoidant personality disorder turn to alcohol when confronted with a feared situation (i.e., liquid courage)? Does someone with schizotypal disorder use hallucinogens or cannabis to add support for their world view? Does someone with antisocial disorder get into legal difficulties (i.e., commit crimes) when they are under the influence of alcohol or cocaine? Is that something they might want to address?

- Provide psychoeducation by exploring with clients what is known and how improving either the substance use or mental health problem will typically generate positive gain in the other problem.

- Use motivational strategies to help move people in the direction of wanted/desirable change.

- Employ cognitive behavioral techniques to target specific distortions and maladaptive behaviors.

  ○ For someone with avoidant personality disorder, this would include identifying the avoidant behaviors and corresponding thoughts and emotions and then working to consistently and safely expose the individual to those things, people, and situations.

  ○ For someone with paranoid personality disorder, it would involve the identification of misperceptions and the use of objective data to help them challenge their beliefs.

  ○ For someone with obsessive-compulsive personality disorder, it would mean helping them challenge long-held beliefs about behavior and the need to be perfect and have others be perfect, as well as helping them learn that there may indeed be multiple ways to get a job done.

- Treat co-occurring mental disorders.

- Attend to active medical issues.

- Develop and enhance daily wellness routines.

Dialectical Behavior Therapy

DBT, which was developed by Marsha Linehan, PhD, has been shown in numerous controlled studies to be an effective treatment for borderline personality disorder. It decreases suicidal and nonsuicidal self-injurious behavior, decreases rates of hospitalization, and improves quality of life. DBT is also effective in working with a broader range of individuals, including those with co-occurring substance use disorders. It has been studied in people with antisocial personality disorder, including people who are incarcerated, and the results have been positive.

DBT is a manual-based therapy, grounded on the triad of CBT, mindfulness (founded in Zen and other contemplative practices), and dialectics (the recognition that there can be multiple and at times seemingly conflicting truths). The core dialectic in DBT is one of radical acceptance while moving the person to change maladaptive and harmful behaviors and patterns of thought. An example of this core dialectic could include a statement such as "It makes total sense you feel this way, *and* we need to help you find other ways than cutting yourself, or drinking till you pass out, to deal with the phone calls from your mother."

DBT recognizes that people with borderline personality disorder have tremendous difficulty with emotion regulation and can go from feeling okay to suicidal in the flash of a thought. DBT uses CBT and behavioral chain analysis to help the person tease apart what triggers their emotions and problem behaviors. It then identifies skills the person needs to learn and practice that will help them manage painful feelings and that will also help them successfully negotiate real-life situations and relationships. The structure of DBT (as it has been most studied) includes:

1. **Weekly skills-training groups**, which last between one and a half to two hours. These are structured to review material from the prior session, including homework, and then present the new week's material. There are four skills modules: mindfulness, interpersonal effectiveness, emotion regulation, and distress tolerance.

2. **Individual (1:1) DBT therapy**, which is typically weekly. The individual therapy utilizes a diary card, which the patient completes and brings to each session. There is a hierarchy to what will be discussed, based on the presence or absence of suicidal thought or behavior, nonsuicidal self-injury, therapy-interfering behaviors (e.g., missed appointments, excessive demands on the therapist's time, the therapist being unavailable), and quality-of-life-interfering behaviors, such as problematic substance use.

3. **Consultation team:** The DBT clinical team meets weekly to practice the therapy, provide case consultation, and enhance their skills so they can teach the skills more effectively. It is not a business meeting, and in the DBT lingo, it is considered "therapy for the therapist."

4. **Telephone consultation/Coaching call:** The patient has the ability and is encouraged to contact the therapist between sessions when in need of skills coaching. Parameters around acceptable times and reasons to call are established early in the therapy.

5. **Accessory services**, which might include access to a prescribing physician or APRN, case management for some clients, family psychoeducation, mutual self-help groups, and a structure to the treatment environment/facility that supports fidelity to the model. An example of structuring the treatment environment is ensuring that DBT clinicians have their schedules cleared consistently for the nonbillable weekly consultation team.

Pharmacotherapy

As mentioned, there are no FDA-approved medications for personality disorders, so all prescribing for these disorders is "off-label." Medications are often used to target core symptoms and comorbid mental disorders, such as mood instability, irritability, depression, insomnia, anxiety, impulsivity, inattention, and so on. People with co-occurring personality and substance use disorders may well benefit from medication-assisted therapies for tobacco, alcohol, and opioids (Chapters 17–19).

While it is common for individuals with borderline personality disorder to be prescribed multiple psychotropic medications, there is limited evidence to support the efficacy of such strategies to decrease symptoms and improve outcomes. As people with borderline personality disorder often struggle with recurrent suicidality, overdoses are common and often with the prescribed medications. Therefore, any medication strategies need to include their relative safety and attention to quantities prescribed.

Although antidepressants, including SSRIs, are widely prescribed for people with borderline personality disorder, studies have shown disappointing results with their use. There is some concern that these agents might worsen symptoms of irritability and mood instability, especially with people who have co-occurring bipolar spectrum disorders.

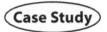

Tracey Race

Tracey Race is a thirty-two-year-old Caucasian woman who is twice divorced and now separated from her third husband. She is a mother of three, who states she is self-referred to get help for her substance use problems and "horrible mood swings" but then adds, "I need to be in treatment or my husband will use my drinking and the pills to take the kids." She currently shares custody of her two daughters with her estranged husband. Her son, born when Tracey was sixteen, was placed in a closed adoption. She works full time from home as an insurance adjuster.

She relates that she had several psychiatric assessments and brief trials of medication and therapy when she was a teenager and in college. "The meds either didn't work, made me gain weight, or made me worse."

Between the ages of eleven and twelve, Tracey was sexually molested by an uncle. The abuse continued for more than a year, although she is unable to remember much about that time. "I don't think I want to remember." When she reported the molestation to her mother, she wasn't believed. However, her uncle was no longer allowed into the home, and this created a rift in her family for which her mother blames Tracey. No charges were ever brought against the uncle. She admits to occasional nightmares related to the abuse but no flashbacks.

She first started to cut herself with a razor or box cutter when she was in junior high. "It wasn't to kill myself, although that's what everyone thinks. It just relieves the stress." She admits to frequent (daily) suicidal thinking, which she says she's experienced since she was thirteen. She has taken several overdoses in the past and describes episodes where she becomes emotionally overwhelmed and will impulsively take "whatever I can get my hands on." She has had two psychiatric hospitalizations, both after overdoses. The first followed the adoption of her son, a decision she still regrets. "My mother made me do it. Said she wouldn't pay for college if I didn't go through with the adoption." The second was when she was a sophomore in college and her boyfriend had broken up with her. Her most recent overdose was three months ago, when her husband served her with divorce papers and revealed that he had been having an affair with a mutual friend. She took a combination of lorazepam (Ativan), OxyContin, and alcohol. She did not seek treatment and slept for two days.

Her first use of alcohol and cannabis was at age thirteen. "My uncle would get me drunk and stoned." She adds, "But I found that the booze and pot helped numb me out and calm the anxiety. It's the same thing with pills (mostly opioids). At least it was in the beginning." She reports binge drinking between half a pint to a pint of hard liquor one to three times per week. She has never been in a detox program and has never had a seizure, although she states her hands sometimes shake in the morning after a binge. At times, she will go months without any alcohol, and her last drink was over a week prior to this evaluation. She smokes cannabis daily and has been taking OxyContin and, recently, heroin/fentanyl (snorted), up to ten bags/day. She has never injected drugs. If she goes more than half a day without opioids, she experiences withdrawal symptoms, which get severe after a day. She has purchased buprenorphine/naloxone (Suboxone) illicitly and hopes to get it prescribed as a result of today's evaluation. She smokes a half-pack of cigarettes daily and has smoked since she was thirteen. She denies habitual use of benzodiazepines or other sedatives.

Her family psychiatric history includes a sister with depression, a brother who is opioid dependent, and her mother, who has been treated for anxiety and depression. Her father is in recovery from an alcohol use disorder.

Her medical history includes asthma, for which she has a rescue inhaler. She has had three live births, one miscarriage, and two abortions. She had a tubal ligation after her last child. She has no allergies. She is not currently on any prescribed medications.

Tracey was born and raised in suburban New York. She is the middle of three children. Her parents divorced when she was nine. She describes her early years as chaotic, with frequent fights between her parents and witnessing her mother get hit by her father when he was drunk. She lived with her mother and had no contact with her father until she went to college.

She did well in school but dropped out as a sophomore in high school when she became pregnant. She subsequently completed high school and attended college, where she achieved a BA in finance and an MBA. She has worked in the insurance industry since graduation and describes her job as stressful but lucrative. She likes working from home but adds that she is socially isolated and can go for weeks on end with direct contact only with her children and her drug dealer. She has no close friends, and her intense mood swings and rage attacks have ended relationships in the past.

She has been married three times. The first when she was twenty. "We fought all the time." She reports the relationship turned physically abusive and ended after eight months. The second marriage was when she was twenty-two and lasted two years. "He was a worse drunk than I was." She remarried when she was twenty-five and has two daughters, Kayla and Erin (ages six and four).

She comes to this evaluation dressed in a business suit and is neatly groomed. She describes her mood as depressed (9 out of 10, with 10 being the worst) and anxious, also a 9 out of 10. While describing intense depression and anxiety, she appears calm and pleasant. She denies experiencing any auditory or visual hallucinations but states she gets paranoid when under stress. She admits to some thoughts of suicide but adds that she has no intention of acting upon them. She also describes frequent urges to cut herself but states that she hasn't done this in several years.

Her vital signs are stable. She is not tremulous and does not appear to be in opioid withdrawal. A dipped urine sample is positive for cannabis and fentanyl. Her breathalyzer is negative.

Step One: Level of Care Determination and Discussion

This case study includes multiple substance use problems, severe mood symptoms, and problem behaviors, including recurrent suicidality and self-injury. It ticks the boxes for borderline personality disorder, but the history of trauma, transient paranoia, depression, and anxiety need further exploration to better assess for the presence or absence of other major diagnoses, such as a major depressive or bipolar spectrum disorder, PTSD, substance-induced mood disorder, and so on. Indeed, if all the symptoms can be related to the recurrent and significant trauma this woman experienced, a PTSD diagnosis could prove a viable option.

In this case, despite active suicidality, the client reports she is unlikely to act on these thoughts and has had them daily for many years. Also, while her use of alcohol is problematic, it has been a week since her last drink, and she has no history or objective findings of withdrawal. Likewise, she is not actively dependent on benzodiazepines. Her stated goal is to get into treatment with the goal of retaining shared custody of her children. She also expresses a desire to be prescribed buprenorphine for opioid replacement therapy, which she views as her most pressing concern. Taking these factors into account, reasonable levels of care would include:

- An IOP that includes opioid replacement therapy along with treatment for her other substance use problems and specialized treatment for her borderline personality disorder and complex trauma. An IOP that offers a dual diagnosis DBT track could be ideal.

- Parallel outpatient treatment, where she receives opioid replacement in an office-based setting, along with treatment and monitoring of her other substance use problems. She would also be admitted to an outpatient DBT program or practice that would include a dual diagnosis focus.

- Integrated outpatient treatment, where she receives opioid replacement therapy and other substance use treatment, along with co-occurring comprehensive DBT and/or trauma-focused therapy in one setting.

Step Two: Construct the Problem/Need List

Substance Use	Mental Health	Medical
Fears she'll lose custody of her children if not in treatment	Molested as a child by an uncle, which when reported, was initially not believed and then not supported	Asthma as a child
Alcohol and cannabis use started at age thirteen	Several psychiatric assessments as a teen and in college	Three live births, one miscarriage, two terminations
Daily use of OxyContin and/or heroin/fentanyl (ten bags)	Multiple unsuccessful medication trials	Tubal ligation
No intravenous drug use	Started cutting herself in junior high, still has urges to cut but has not done so in years	Not tremulous
Experiences opioid withdrawal	Daily thoughts of suicide	Goes into opioid withdrawal within half a day of last use
Binge drinking multiple times per week	Multiple overdoses in the past	
Father with alcohol problem	Two inpatient admissions following overdoses	
No history of withdrawal seizures or delirium	Recent multidrug overdose in which she did not seek help	
Occasional shakiness after heavy drinking	Impulsivity	
Last drink over a week ago	Mood swings and rage attacks	
Has gone for extended periods without alcohol	Chaotic childhood	
Urine positive for opioids and cannabis	Witnessed domestic violence	
Use of benzodiazepines and other sedative hypnotics but not currently	Parents divorced when patient was age nine	
Smokes half a pack of cigarettes/day	Minimal contact with her father	
No history of withdrawal seizures or delirium	Teenage pregnancy, child given up for adoption	
Smokes cannabis daily	Socially isolated	
	No close friends	
	Depressed and anxious	
	Transient stress-related paranoia	

The following three-item list incorporates the majority of Ms. Race's symptoms and helps us focus on what is emergent (frequent and current suicidality and use of fentanyl) and urgent (high-risk drug use), as well as what will be the focus for longer-range treatment (long-standing problems with emotion regulation and mood swings and an extensive trauma history):

1. **Suicidal thoughts and behavior**, AEB daily thoughts of suicide, past history of overdose attempts, and recent overdose in which she did not seek help

2. **Severe and active high-risk substance use problems**, AEB daily opioid use, including fentanyl, binge drinking, and daily cannabis and tobacco use; Experiences opioid withdrawal within half a day of last use

3. **Severe mood swings** with emotional lability, impulsivity, and high levels of depression and anxiety; History of self-injurious—but nonsuicidal—self-harm; Extensive history of trauma

Step Three: Establish the Initial Goals/Objectives for Treatment

1. Suicidal thoughts and behavior, AEB daily thoughts of suicide, past history of overdose attempts, and recent overdose in which she did not seek help

    a. Short-term goals/objectives:

    i. Establish and maintain a safety plan

    ii. Have no active suicidal behavior

    b. Long-term goal: Be free from suicidal thoughts and behaviors

2. Severe and active high-risk substance use problems, AEB daily opioid use, including fentanyl, binge drinking, and daily cannabis and tobacco use; Experiences opioid withdrawal within half a day of last use

    a. Short-term goals/objectives:

    i. Obtain evaluation for and, if appropriate, get started on medication-assisted treatment for opioid dependence

    ii. Eliminate binge-drinking behavior and be in early abstinence for alcohol

    iii. Assess levels of motivation to decrease and/or eliminate cannabis and tobacco use

    b. Long-term goals:

    i. Be abstinent from alcohol

    ii. Be on opioid replacement therapy*

    iii. Be abstinent from tobacco

    iv. Be abstinent from cannabis

    v. Be abstinent from benzodiazepines

3. Severe mood swings, emotional lability, and impulsivity with high levels of depression and anxiety; History of self-injurious—but nonsuicidal—self-harm; Extensive trauma history

    a. Short-term goals/objectives:

        i. Have a 30 percent reduction in depressive and anxious symptoms as measured using a 10-point scale

        ii. Be free from stress-related paranoia and rage attacks

        iii. Practice, and document using her diary card, at least two DBT skills daily

        iv. Complete a more thorough evaluation of trauma and related symptoms

    b. Long-term goals:

        i. Have a stable mood, as measured by self-report

        ii. Experience levels of depression and/or anxiety no greater than a 4 on a 10-point scale

        iii. Be free from thoughts and urges to self-harm

*Due to the high-risk nature of her current opioid use and the risks for both intentional and unintentional overdose, this generates both a short- and long-term goal for Ms. Race to be evaluated and started on medication as soon as possible and to then continue medication.

Treatment-and-Recovery Plan

Patient's Name: Tracey Race
Date of Birth: 12/2/1987
Medical Record #: XXX-XX-XXXX

Level of Care: Outpatient co-occurring DBT with medication management

ICD-10 Codes	DSM-5 Diagnoses
F11.20	Opioid use disorder, moderate
F60.3	Borderline personality disorder
F32.9	Unspecified depressive disorder with anxious distress
F10.20	Alcohol use disorder, moderate
F17.200	Tobacco use disorder, moderate
F12.20	Cannabis use disorder, moderate
Z63.5	Disruption of family by separation or divorce

The individual's stated goal(s): "I want my mood to be stable. I want to be off all street drugs. I want to be a good mother. Eventually, but not yet, I'd like to stop smoking cigarettes."

1. Problem/Need Statement: Suicidal thoughts and behavior, AEB daily thoughts of suicide, history of overdose attempts, and recent multidrug overdose in which she did not seek help

Long-Term Goal: Be free from suicidal thoughts and behaviors

Short-Term Goals/Objectives (target date):
1. Establish and maintain a safety plan (at the time of this evaluation and to be reassessed at each session)
2. Have no active suicidal behavior (current date and ongoing)

2. Problem/Need Statement: Severe and active high-risk substance use problems, AEB daily opioid use, including fentanyl, binge drinking, and daily cannabis and tobacco use; Experiences opioid withdrawal within half a day of last use

Long-Term Goal(s):

1. Be abstinent from alcohol
2. Be on opioid replacement therapy
3. Be abstinent from tobacco
4. Be abstinent from cannabis
5. Be abstinent from benzodiazepines

Short-Term Goals/Objectives (target date):

1. Obtain evaluation for and, if appropriate, get started on medication-assisted treatment for opioid dependence (by the end of today)

2. Eliminate binge-drinking behavior and be in early abstinence for alcohol (today)

3. Assess levels of motivation to decrease and/or eliminate cannabis and tobacco use (two weeks from today)

---

3. Problem/Need Statement: Severe mood swings, emotional lability, and impulsivity with high levels of depression and anxiety; History of self-injurious—but nonsuicidal—harm; Extensive trauma history

Long-Term Goal(s):

1. Have a stable mood, as measured by self-report

2. Experience levels of depression and/or anxiety no greater than a 4 on a 10-point scale

3. Be free from thoughts and urges to self-harm

Short-Term Goals/Objectives (Target date):

1. Have a 30 percent reduction in depressive and anxious symptoms as measured using a 10-point scale (one month from today)

2. Be free from stress-related paranoia and rage attacks (two months from today)

3. Practice, and document using her diary card, at least two DBT skills daily (one month from today)

4. More thoroughly assess history and symptoms of trauma (one month from today)

Interventions					
Treatment Modality	**Specific Type**	**Frequency**	**Duration**	**Problem Number**	**Responsible Person(s)**
Medical	Complete diagnostic evaluation	Upon admission	2 hours	1, 2, 3	MD, RN, Ms. Race
	Medication management to include opioid replacement therapy	At least monthly	20–30 minutes	1, 2, 3	MD and Ms. Race
Individual Therapy	Dual diagnosis–focused DBT and further assessment of trauma	Weekly	Six months to one year (1-hour sessions)	1, 2, 3	DBT therapist and Ms. Race

(Continued)

(Continued)

Interventions					
Treatment Modality	**Specific Type**	**Frequency**	**Duration**	**Problem Number**	**Responsible Person(s)**
Group Therapy	Dual diagnosis–focused DBT skills training	Weekly	Six months to one year (2-hour sessions)	1, 2, 3	DBT skills trainer and Ms. Race
Lab Work	Routine blood work	Upon admission, and as needed	N/A	1, 2, 3	MD and Ms. Race
	Drug screens	Upon admission, and at least monthly	For the duration of treatment	2	MD and Ms. Race
Mutual Self-Help	Of Ms. Race's choosing	At least 2 meetings/ week	Ongoing	2	Ms. Race

Identification of strengths: Intelligent and articulate. Motivated to work on both her substance use and emotional/behavioral difficulties. Has a strong work ethic and finds her job to be an important source of self-respect, financial support, and stability

Peer/family/community supports to assist: Unable to identify any at this time but is willing to explore mutual self-help groups in the community and/or online

Barriers to treatment: Inability to stop using illicit opioids and alcohol

Staff/client-identified education/teaching needs: To understand the risks/benefits of any recommended medications, including buprenorphine for opioid replacement therapy. To understand the principles and goals of DBT

Assessment of discharge needs/discharge planning: To be reassessed at six months and as needed. When goals achieved, can move toward less intensive level of treatment

Completion of this treatment-and-recovery plan was a collaborative effort between the client and the following treatment team members:

SIGNATURES		Date/Time:
Client:	Tracey Race	8/12/2020, 2:15 p.m.
Physician:	Lenore Picano, MD	8/12/2020, 2:20 p.m.
Primary Therapist:	Mildred Forest, LCSW	8/12/2020, 2:22 p.m.

SUBSTANCE-SPECIFIC
TOPICS and TREATMENTS

CHAPTER 17

....

Alcohol

OVERVIEW

More than half of Americans over the age of twelve drink alcohol, and nearly one quarter report binge drinking. Heavy drinking—at least five episodes of binge drinking in a month—is reported by more than seventeen million Americans (6.5 percent). Current alcohol use among youth ages twelve to seventeen is nearly 13 percent, with 7.2 percent reporting binge drinking and 1.5 percent heavy drinking.

> **What's a binge?** For men it is defined as five or more drinks on the same occasion, and for women it's four or more. (This was lowered from five.) Binge drinking is defined as having at least one binge per month.

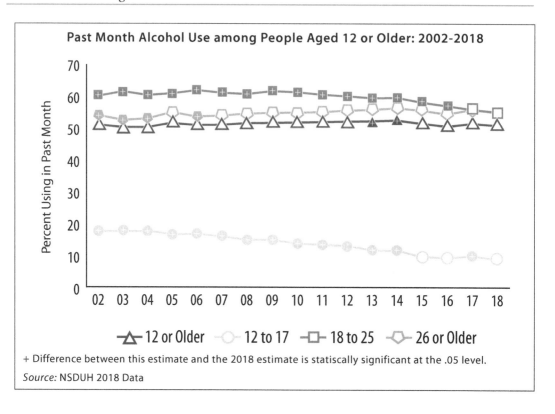

Past Month Alcohol Use among People Aged 12 or Older: 2002–2018

+ Difference between this estimate and the 2018 estimate is statiscally significant at the .05 level.

Source: NSDUH 2018 Data

Alcohol is one of the three leading causes of preventable death in the United States, where eighteen million people meet criteria for alcohol use disorders. Rates of alcohol use disorder are roughly twice as high in men (10–12.4 percent) versus women (4.5–5 percent). The peak ages for developing alcohol use disorders are in the teens through the twenties, but they can occur at any age.

Negative health consequences from alcohol can range from mild to severe, with damage possible to most organ systems and tissues, including the nervous system. Serious health outcomes include alcohol-related dementias (alcohol is a neurotoxin and causes loss of both gray and white matter), liver failure, alcoholic hepatitis, cirrhosis, pancreatitis, ulcers, esophageal varices, and increased rates of stroke and certain cancers. Beyond the impact of alcohol on the body are deaths and injury associated with alcohol-related accidents and the finding that many homicides and suicides are committed while under the influence. According to the National Highway Traffic Safety Administration, there were 10,908 alcohol-related driving fatalities in 2018, which accounted for 29 percent of all vehicular deaths. Finally, while the vast majority of unintentional fatal overdoses in the United States involve opioids, many of those fatalities involve the concomitant use of alcohol or other central nervous system depressants (e.g., benzodiazepines, barbiturates).

Rates of co-occurring alcohol use disorders are high among people with most mental disorders, with worse overall outcomes.

WOMEN AND ALCOHOL

While women have lower rates of alcohol use disorders, there has been a significant upward trend in the past two decades. They achieve higher blood-alcohol levels when consuming the same amount as men, likely due to women weighing less than men on average and having a higher fat-to-water ratio—alcohol is dissolved in water so there is a relatively smaller volume of water in women. They are also more likely to develop serious physical complications from alcohol use, including increased rates of breast cancer. On average, women experience severe negative health outcomes of heavy alcohol use ten years sooner than men (telescoping effect).

The children of women who drink when pregnant have an increased risk for learning and behavioral problems, as well as fetal alcohol problems. Among pregnant women ages fifteen to forty-four, about 10 percent report some alcohol use in the past month, and about 3 percent report binge drinking. These numbers are lower than for nonpregnant women in the same age range.

ASSESSMENT AND DIAGNOSTIC ISSUES

People with mood and anxiety problems are often drawn to alcohol for its short-term emotional benefits. But the longer-term effects of heavy use can lead to a broad range of problems. This becomes part of the co-occurring challenge, as it's often unclear what role the substance use—in this case alcohol—plays in the overall clinical presentation. Alcohol-induced mood and anxiety problems are often impossible to differentiate from nonalcohol variants, especially at intake. A careful history as part of the initial assessment may help clarify which came first: the mental disorder or the substance use problem.

Over time, alcohol problems manifest with a broad range of emotional, behavioral, physical, and cognitive problems. Some of these will resolve over the course of treatment, such as the hallucinosis that can occur with alcohol withdrawal delirium. Others, such as alcohol-related dementia/alcohol neurocognitive disorder (e.g., Korsakoff's syndrome) may be irreversible.

While the assessment of an alcohol use disorder is incorporated into the overall comprehensive assessment (Chapters 2–4), there are some key findings that will help in both assessment and treatment.

Cognitive Examination

People with long-term alcohol use are at increased risk of cognitive impairment due to alcohol's toxic effects on the brain. These deficits range from subtle to severe and may include:

- Problems with short-term memory
- Problems with learning new material
- Confabulation (where the individual makes up a plausible story to cover for what may be lapses in memory)

The cognitive deficits may be subtle or concealed by preserved social function and verbal ease. Also, individuals with alcohol-related neurocognitive disorders may be younger than the average person with a dementia. Therefore, it's important to perform a thorough cognitive evaluation with individuals who have a history of chronic alcohol use. Standardized screens for neurocognitive disorders (dementia)—such as the St. Louis University Mental Status Exam (SLUMS), the Folstein Mini-Mental Status Exam, or the Montreal Cognitive Assessment (MoCA)—would be viable options.

Physical Findings

In addition to the physical symptoms of withdrawal states covered in the following sections, long-term drinkers may display findings on routine or more focused physical examination. These can include:

- An enlarged and/or tender liver
- Tremor
- Psoriasis (dry and flaky patches of skin)
- Broken capillaries on the nose and cheeks (spider veins)
- Red palms
- Jaundice (yellow cast to the skin, often first detected in the whites of the eyes or the underside of the tongue)
- Presence of fluid in the belly (ascites—associated with liver failure and cirrhosis)
- An enlarged spleen
- Clubbed fingers (bulbous enlargement of the ends of the fingers and toes with loss of the normal angle between the nail bed and the surrounding flesh)

Lab Results

- Liver function/enzyme tests (transaminases)
  - Gamma-glutamyl transferase (GGT/GGTP): This is the enzyme that is most closely associated with alcohol use. It remains elevated for three to four weeks after heavy consumption has stopped. With abstinence, it usually returns to normal levels.
  - Elevations in other liver enzymes, including alkaline phosphatase
- Elevated mean corpuscular volume (MCV): This is a measure of the size of the red blood cells and is often elevated in people who have long histories of heavy alcohol consumption.
- Other abnormal labs may include:
  - Increased bilirubin
  - Decreased albumin (a protein associated with liver health and nutritional status)
  - Decreased magnesium

o Decreased potassium

o Increased serum prothrombin time (a measure of the blood's ability to clot)

MODERATE VERSUS HEAVY DRINKING

Based on current dietary guidelines, the amount of alcohol a person can consume and be considered a moderate drinker is:

- Women: on average, no more than one standard drink/day or seven drinks/week
- Men: on average, no more than two standard drinks/day or fourteen drinks/week

Alcohol consumption in excess of these amounts is considered heavy. The current definitions of a standard drink are:

- Five ounces of wine
- Twelve ounces of beer
- One and a half ounces of an eighty-proof liquor, such as vodka, rum, gin, or whiskey

Binge drinking is defined as the rapid consumption of alcohol (i.e., within two hours), in which the blood alcohol level meets or exceeds 0.08 grams/deciliter. For men, this is typically five or more standard drinks, and for women, four or more drinks. Heavy drinking is defined as five or more drinks on five or more days within a thirty-day period.

MILD, MODERATE, AND SEVERE ALCOHOL USE DISORDERS

Alcohol use disorders (formerly alcohol abuse and dependence) are defined by the DSM-5 according to the number of criteria a person meets combined with clinical judgment. The current criteria address cravings, continued use despite negative consequences (e.g., health, occupational, legal, and/or social), unsuccessful attempts to cut down, dangerous activity while intoxicated, and signs and symptoms of tolerance and withdrawal. The number of symptoms, combined with the clinical impression, is used to rate the disorder as mild (two to three symptoms), moderate (four to five), or severe (more than six symptoms).

As with other substances, if withdrawal symptoms are present, the disorder is at least moderate. Other modifiers/specifiers are then added, such as "in early remission" (three to twelve months) or "in late remission" (more than twelve months). These same time frames are used for all substance use disorders.

THE ASSESSMENT OF ALCOHOL WITHDRAWAL

Most people who are alcohol dependent can safely withdraw with minimal intervention. For others, alcohol withdrawal can be severe and even fatal. Symptoms may include seizures, cognitive disturbances (hallucinations and confusion), and dangerous elevations in blood pressure and pulse rate. Behaviors associated with withdrawal can include profound agitation and combativeness that can prove to be a challenge in many settings. The most serious and potentially fatal manifestation of alcohol withdrawal is delirium tremens, which may require admission to an intensive-care setting. People at the greatest risk for serious withdrawal syndromes include:

- People with histories of prior complicated withdrawals (e.g., withdrawal seizures, delirium, hallucinations)
- People with comorbid medical conditions, including heart, liver, and lung diseases
- Older individuals, especially those with longer histories of alcohol use
- Poor nutritional status

Alcohol withdrawal delirium/delirium tremens is a hyperadrenergic state characterized by confusion, hallucinations (often visual), elevated temperature, sweating, rapid pulse, and elevated blood pressure. It can progress rapidly and in some heavy drinkers can begin within hours after the last drink. Withdrawal from alcohol can last up to a week and in some cases longer.

Alcohol withdrawal delirium is a medical emergency that requires inpatient medical stabilization, which will likely include the use of intravenous benzodiazepines, careful monitoring of electrolytes, repletion of vitamins (thiamine and folic acid), and stabilization of blood pressure and pulse.

The Clinical Institute Withdrawal Assessment (CIWA)

The Clinical Institute Withdrawal Assessment (CIWA)—also abbreviated as CIWA-Ar for the revised version—is the most widely used tool to assess severity of alcohol withdrawal. A modified version, the CIWA-B, addresses benzodiazepine withdrawal.

The CIWA is completed by a nurse or other trained clinical observer and incorporates blood pressure and pulse with the following ten symptom domains:

1. Sweating
2. Anxiety
3. Tremor
4. Auditory disturbances
5. Visual disturbances
6. Agitation
7. Nausea
8. Tactile disturbances
9. Headache
10. Orientation and clouding of sensorium

The maximum score possible is a 67. Many facilities that perform detoxification will use protocols and/or guidelines that connect the CIWA to the use of medication. The CIWA is not copyrighted and may be used freely. A score of 15 or greater is associated with an increased risk of serious withdrawal. The higher the score, the greater the risk.

In working with individuals who have co-occurring mental disorders and alcohol withdrawal, clinicians may encounter complicating factors when using the CIWA:

- Is the anxiety from withdrawal or an underlying anxiety disorder?
- Are the visual or auditory disturbances withdrawal or core symptoms of a schizophrenia spectrum disorder?
- Is the tremor new or is it a side effect of lithium or an antipsychotic medication?

A good way to tease this apart is to ask:

- Are these symptoms new or old?
- Have they changed or worsened in the setting of not drinking (since your last drink)?

Regardless, because of the potential seriousness of alcohol withdrawal, when in doubt, err on the side of treating what might be symptoms of withdrawal.

Clinical Institute Withdrawal Assessment for Alcohol, Revised (CIWA-Ar)

Patient: _____ Date: _____ Time: _____

Pulse or heart rate taken for one minute: _____ Blood Pressure: ___/___

Nausea and Vomiting—Ask, "Do you feel sick to your stomach? Have you vomited?" Observation: 0 no nausea and vomiting 1 mild nausea and vomiting 2 3 4 intermittent nausea with dry heaves 5 6 7 constant nausea, frequent dry heaves and vomiting	**Tactile Disturbances**—Ask, "Have you any itching, pins and needles sensations, any burning or numbness, or do you feel bugs crawling on or under your skin?" Observation: 0 none 1 very mild itching, pins and needles, burning or numbness 2 mild itching, pins and needles, burning or numbness 3 moderate itching, pins and needles, burning or numbness 4 moderately severe hallucinations 5 severe hallucinations 6 extremely severe hallucinations 7 continuous hallucinations
Tremor—Arms extended and fingers spread apart. Observation: 0 no tremor 1 not visible, but can be felt fingertip to fingertip 2 3 4 moderate, with patient's arms extended 5 6 7 severe, even with arms not extended	**Auditory Disturbances**—Ask, "Are you more aware of sounds around you? Are they harsh? Do they frighten you? Are you hearing anything that is disturbing to you? Are you hearing things you know are not there?" Observation: 0 not present 1 very mild harshness or ability to frighten 2 mild harshness or ability to frighten 3 moderate harshness or ability to frighten 4 moderately severe hallucinations 5 severe hallucinations 6 extremely severe hallucinations 7 continuous hallucinations

Paroxysmal Sweats—Observation:	Visual Disturbances—Ask, "Does the light appear to be too bright? Is its color different? Does it hurt your eyes? Are you seeing anything that is disturbing to you? Are you seeing things you know are not there?" Observation:
0 no sweat visible	0 not present
1 barely perceptible sweating, palms moist	1 very mild sensitivity
2	2 mild sensitivity
3	3 moderate sensitivity
4 beads of sweat obvious on forehead	4 moderately severe hallucinations
5	5 severe hallucinations
6	6 extremely severe hallucinations
7 drenching sweats	7 continuous hallucinations
Anxiety—Ask, "Do you feel nervous?" Observation:	**Headache, Fullness in Head**—Ask, "Does your head feel different? Does it feel like there is a band around your head?" Do not rate for dizziness or light-headedness. Otherwise, rate severity:
0 no anxiety, at ease	0 not present
1 mildly anxious	1 very mild
2	2 mild
3	3 moderate
4 moderately anxious or guarded, so anxiety is inferred	4 moderately severe
5	5 severe
6	6 very severe
7 equivalent to acute panic states as seen in severe delirium or acute schizophrenic reactions	7 extremely severe
Agitation—Observation:	**Orientation and Clouding of Sensorium**—Ask, "What day is this? Where are you? Who am I?"
0 normal activity	0 oriented and can do serial additions
1 somewhat more than normal activity	1 cannot do serial additions or is uncertain about date
2	2 disoriented for date by no more than two calendar days
3	
4 moderately fidgety and restless	3 disoriented for date by more than two calendar days
5	
6	4 disoriented for place and/or person
7 paces back and forth during most of the interview or constantly thrashes about	
	Total CIWA-Ar Score* _____ **Rater's Initials** _____ ***Maximum possible score 67**
This scale is not copyrighted and can be reproduced freely.	**Source:** Sullivan et al. (1989)

THE TREATMENT OF ALCOHOL WITHDRAWAL

Facilities that treat alcohol withdrawal typically follow written protocols or guidelines combined with clinical judgment. Medically supervised detoxification in most instances involves:

- The use of benzodiazepines to prevent seizures and decrease the autonomic excitability and risk for seizures associated with withdrawal. These may be long-acting agents, such as diazepam (Valium) or chlordiazepoxide (Librium), or medications with shorter half-lives, such as oxazepam (Serax) or lorazepam (Ativan). While typically taken by mouth, in more serious withdrawal syndromes, these will be administered intravenously and in doses large enough to control symptoms.

- Repletion of thiamine (Vitamin B1). This needs to be done prior to the administration of any carbohydrates to prevent the development of a serious complication—Wernicke's encephalopathy—which is characterized by visual disturbances, unsteady gait, and confusion/delirium.

- Repletion of folic acid.

- Some protocols may also use other anticonvulsants to help prevent seizures.

- In severe cases, the person may be placed into a medically induced coma.

PHARMACOTHERAPY

There are currently three FDA-approved medications for the treatment of alcohol use disorder: naltrexone, which is available as a daily medication and long-acting injection (Vivitrol); acamprosate (Campral); and the behavioral aversive disulfiram (Antabuse):

- Naltrexone is an opioid blocker that damps down the behavioral reward experienced with alcohol. It has been shown to decrease cravings for alcohol, as well as for the amount consumed. It is generally safe, but individuals on the long-acting injection should consider wearing a medic alert bracelet should they require emergency analgesia. Because they are on an opioid blocker, the amounts of medication used should they need emergent pain relief could place them at risk for respiratory depression.

- Acamprosate (Campral) is generally well tolerated and has been shown to diminish cravings for alcohol, as well as the number of drinks consumed. It is safe and could be considered for people on psychiatric medications. It has few side effects, the most common being upset stomach or a feeling of bloating or gassiness. Adherence may be difficult as it requires three-times-a-day dosing.

- Disulfiram (Antabuse) is a behavioral aversive that works by preventing the breakdown of alcohol in the body through the inhibition of the enzyme acetaldehyde dehydrogenase. The result is the accumulation of acetaldehyde, which is noxious in high concentrations, and the person experiences unpleasant reactions—

nausea, vomiting, flushing, accelerated heart rate, headache, and confusion. The use of disulfiram should be limited to individuals who are motivated for total abstinence. It's best avoided in people with poor impulse control, especially if they have underlying medical problems, as there have been deaths from respiratory and cardiac complications associated with drinking alcohol when on disulfiram.

CHAPTER 18

....

Tobacco

Overview
Treatment of Tobacco Use Disorders
    Psychosocial Treatments
    Pharmacological Treatments

OVERVIEW

Tobacco use is the number one cause of preventable death in the United States (more than 400,000 annually). It is the leading cause of cancer deaths and greatly increases a person's risk for heart attack, stroke, and chronic obstructive pulmonary disease (COPD). On average, people who smoke die ten years younger than the general population.

The good news is that overall rates of smoking in the United States have diminished from more than 40 percent of the adult population in 1965 to about 20 percent. In 2018, there were 47 million past-month smokers, 27.3 million daily smokers, and 10.8 million who smoked a pack or more per day.

But the above numbers do not reflect the rise in e-cigarettes and vaping. Data sources, such as the Youth Risk Behavior Survey, show that while cigarette use is down, vaping now constitutes a significant source of tobacco use, especially among youth. The 2017 survey of those under eighteen showed 13.2 percent had used a vaped product at least once in the past month.

However, according to NSDUH, rates of daily tobacco use are higher among people with any mental illness than the general population (36.1 percent versus 21.4 percent), as is the number of cigarettes smoked in a month (331 versus 310). Men of all ages have higher rates of tobacco use than women, and quit rates among people with mental illness are lower than the general population. The CDC reports worse statistics, finding that people with mental illness are twice as likely to smoke and represent about one third of smokers.

The National Comorbidity Study, which broke down data by specific diagnoses, reported elevated rates of lifetime smoking among all mental illnesses, with the highest rates found in people with bipolar disorder (68.8 percent), substance use disorders (49 percent), schizophrenia (49.4 percent), GAD (46 percent), and PTSD (46.3 percent). Quit rates are low among people with mental illnesses when compared to the general population.

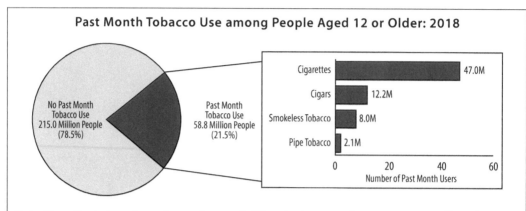

Past Month Tobacco Use among People Aged 12 or Older: 2018

No Past Month Tobacco Use 215.0 Million People (78.5%)

Past Month Tobacco Use 58.8 Million People (21.5%)

Cigarettes 47.0M
Cigars 12.2M
Smokeless Tobacco 8.0M
Pipe Tobacco 2.1M

0   20   40   60
Number of Past Month Users

Note: The estimated numbers of current users of different tobacco products are not mutually exclusive because people could have used more than one type of tobacco product in the past monrh.

Source: NSDUH 2018 Data

Tobacco control programs, which include education, regulation and taxation of tobacco products, efforts to decrease exposure to secondhand smoke, establishment of smoke-free environments, quit lines, and so forth, have shown success in the general population but have had poor outcomes with people who have mental illness. This finding, combined with overwhelming evidence of the negative health outcomes related to tobacco use, underscore the need to address and integrate tobacco reduction into mental health and substance use services.

TREATMENT OF TOBACCO USE DISORDERS

There are effective treatments for tobacco cessation, but they are underutilized in people with mental illness. These include a variety of therapeutic strategies, medications, and decisions made at a governmental or organizational level to increase the likelihood that someone will quit. For smokers with mental illness, certain factors can enhance or diminish the chances of quitting:

- At an organizational level, providers need to make smoking cessation a priority. This will include making sure:
  o Everyone is assessed for tobacco use.
  o Everyone who smokes or uses tobacco is asked about their thoughts/plans for quitting. Motivation and stage of change are assessed upon admission and throughout the course of treatment.
  o Everyone who wishes to quit will be offered treatment to help achieve that goal.
- Cigarette smoking (not the nicotine), through interactions in the liver (i.e., induction of Cytochrome P4501A4), can significantly lower the blood levels of many psychiatric medications, including several antipsychotics. For some, lower

medication levels may be associated with worse psychiatric symptoms, a decrease in medication side effects, or both. This has been identified as one factor that makes smoking cessation more difficult for people on these medications.

- Develop smoke-free environments. This limits the availability of places where people can smoke. Smoke-free zones can include mental health clinics, hospitals, social clubs, and mutual-support settings.

Psychosocial Treatments

There is a wealth of information and support to help people quit smoking, including websites and government-sponsored programs (some of which are funded by tobacco-settlement money):

- Smokefree.gov is a well-organized website that provides education and free resources.
- 1-800-QUIT-NOW is a federal and state initiative that provides free counseling and, in some states, free nicotine patches (and possibly other forms of nicotine replacement, such as gum or lozenges) to help people stop smoking.

Nonpharmacological strategies to help people quit include:

- Education
  - Provide an honest look at smoking's effect on the mind and the body: ten years of lost life; greatly increased risks for heart attack, stroke, and cancer; and increased levels of depression.
  - Educate around potential withdrawal associated with tobacco cessation, including increases in irritability, anxiety, depression, and appetite (which may last a few weeks).
- Motivational enhancement
  - Weigh the pros and cons of smoking: "It calms me down, but I can't stand the way it makes my clothes smell, and my car is like a giant ashtray."
  - Increase the discomfort around smoking.
  - Encourage change talk: "It sounds like you're thinking about quitting. That's awesome. Do you have a quit plan?"
  - Create a quit plan, which includes setting a date and telling friends and family about it.
- Cognitive behavioral approaches, including group, individual, and self-directed strategies
  - Identify triggers for smoking.
  - Introduce a "delay" before lighting up, which involves waiting a certain time period before each cigarette. This delay increases an awareness of the act of smoking and decreases the automatic patterns. "Before you light up, wait

fifteen seconds. You can still have the cigarette, but you have to wait. Then when you're doing that consistently, increase to thirty seconds, then a minute, two minutes, and so forth."

  o Create rules around smoking, such as no smoking in the house and in the car.

  o Create a reward system whereby money saved from not smoking goes to something fun.

  o When the quit plan goes into effect, make certain all tobacco products are out of the house. Avoid situations and people who actively smoke, at least initially.

• Mindfulness training

  o Observe the urge to smoke and let it pass. Or engage in a distracting activity, such as TV, a video game, social media, or something else that will take your mind off lighting up.

  o When you do light up, smoke with complete attention.

Pharmacological Treatments

Several FDA-approved treatments are available to help with smoking cessation. They include various forms of nicotine replacement (patches, gum, lozenges), as well as the medications varenicline (Chantix) and bupropion (Zyban), the latter of which is a low dose of the antidepressant Wellbutrin. The selection of a medication will be influenced by the underlying mental disorder and the potential risks and benefits of the medication.

Tobacco replacement is generally safe, but make certain that the person understands how the medication is to be used and the potential risks should they continue to smoke while on replacement therapy (e.g., palpitations, flushing, nausea). There is also unclear information around e-cigarettes (vaporized nicotine), as it appears these may create nicotine dependence and subsequent smoking, especially for younger people. It is not clear what is contained in the vapor.

The medication varenicline (Chantix), which carries the highest quit rate of the available medications, also has the highest rate of adverse reactions. These can vary from mild to extreme and include intense and unpleasant dreams and increases in suicidal and even homicidal thinking. Its use needs to be carefully weighed, especially in individuals who struggle with emotional instability. One recent study has shown promise with individuals with schizophrenia whose psychiatric symptoms were stable.

Bupropion (Zyban, Wellbutrin) may also be of benefit in smoking cessation. But as with any antidepressant, its potential for manic switching in susceptible individuals needs to be considered.

CHAPTER 19

· ·

Opioids

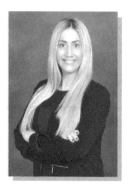

My Story

By Sarah Howroyd, MSW, LCSW

my story

The Golden Child

I grew up in Manchester, Connecticut and am the eldest of three. Both of my parents are educators. I went to Catholic schools and was an A student—a golden child. Things came easy to me as a kid. I didn't have major adverse childhood experiences, though I did have a blood disease. I spent a lot of time in the hospital, and it eventually cost me my spleen, but even there, my mom took a couple years off from work and was with me daily.

Not too much challenged me, even though at seven, I was diagnosed with ADHD. Like a lot of girls with ADHD, I daydreamed. But I hid. The complaint from my teachers was always that I couldn't stop talking, and I'd get an unsatisfactory grade in self-control. Don't bother moving me, teacher. I'll talk to whoever is next to me. I still do. But my parents wouldn't let them put me on stimulants. Those came in college.

In junior high, I began to obsess about my weight. And in seventh or eighth grade, I started with over-the-counter diet pills. In high school, I was involved in community service, worked with the handicapped, and volunteered in the Best Buddy program. I'd party on the weekends, but not excessively. Like most Connecticut teenagers, it was drinking in the woods from red plastic Solo cups. I tried weed, but it made me paranoid. And while I struggled with depression, anxiety, and unrelenting concerns about everything I ate, I continued to excel.

I attended college in Boston and got my bachelor's degree in social work. My junior year I met my fiancé. He was an engineer, and I fell head over heels. We spent our twenties together. And I thought he was the one. We'd get married, have kids. I could see the whole thing and was totally okay with that idea. But my eating disorder had worsened and shifted from bulimia-type symptoms to more severe anorexia with obsessive calorie counting. I had lists of every bite I consumed. Sometimes I'd go an entire day without eating. This was also the era of heroin chic, super model Kate Moss, and the idea that skinnier was better and you couldn't be too thin. The image of beauty for women of my age was an anorexic one.

In November of 2004, my dad was diagnosed with cancer. I got the call and headed to Connecticut with my fiancé. We were in a car accident in Manchester and were brought to the hospital. Our injuries weren't critical enough for an admission, but we were told to follow up with our primary care doctors.

I'm something of a doctor snob—I want one with an ivy league pedigree. And six months before this, I'd gone into the phone book, shopped, and found one with an MIT and Tufts background. She was brilliant. As to my injuries, they weren't severe. I had aches and pains, and my neck and back were sore from whiplash.

As I look back now, there are times in my life when opioids would have been appropriate, like after major surgery. That was not one of them. She started me on an astronomical amount of OxyContin (120 mg/day = 180 morphine equivalents) and put my fiancé on the same amount. There was no informed consent. I asked her if they were habit-forming. She told me they weren't, that only 1 percent got addicted, and that this was the humane, pain-free wave of the future. But it wasn't just OxyContin. Because of my ADHD and problems with anxiety and depression, she also prescribed boatloads of Adderall and Xanax.

And the pills made all my problems disappear. For the first time in my life, all the emotional pain stopped. I didn't obsess over calories or count everything I ate. It was like a hug from Jesus. In my mind, Oxy is the same as heroin. If anything, it was purer than heroin, at least what was available then. The prescriptions continued for two years, and I'd see her every month. She always ran late. I'd wait an hour or more, watch the drug reps come in and out of her office—they even had their own room—see her for five minutes, and get my refills.

In 2006, my fiancé was in a motorcycle accident. As happens with people on opioids, he needed a lot more to handle the pain, and he started to take some of mine. Things spiraled. We began to buy them off the street. And for the first time, our doctor called us in for a pill count. She'd never done it, and I was panic stricken. This was my lifeline. I thought I wasn't going to be able to function. How was I going to be able to do anything? I felt trapped and terrified. In hindsight, she was likely under investigation by the Massachusetts licensing board.

I didn't know at the time that she was on Purdue Pharma's Region Zero List (a list of over 1,800 prescribers suspected by the drug company of over-prescribing OxyContin). I'd learn that years later when I worked with the Connecticut Attorney General in a lawsuit against Purdue.

As to that doctor—whom I liked—she lost her contract with Blue Cross/Blue Shield because of her prescribing and concerns over patients who had overdosed and died. Eventually she surrendered her license and then committed suicide by hanging. In the Massachusetts suit against Purdue, she was personally named.

After the pill count, we were discharged and told by a member of her staff, "I'm sorry we can't see you anymore." We did not see the doctor, and there was no taper.

We had to buy on the street and did it in bulk—one hundred packs of OxyContin 80 mg pills for $3,400. We did this two or three times a week. We went through our savings, retirement accounts, anything of value. It was a dark time. And my family was oblivious. I was still the golden child who got straight A's and lived in Boston with her fiancé.

One night we couldn't get Oxies. I was sick to where it hurt to blink or even breathe. We bought heroin instead. It was a seamless transition. I was so sick that I didn't care. "Just give me it." I sniffed it and soon progressed to needles. It was a move of desperation, and the needles became my preferred method. It was bad, although I did have a healthy fear of overdosing. I kept a diary in my phone and tracked how much I'd taken.

I started to hear about all these kids in Boston who were dying. I knew nothing about addiction at the time. There started to be talk about the combination of opioids and benzos killing people, so I weaned myself off the Xanax. It wasn't horrendous because I was on so many opioids. And my Catholic guilt kicked in. What would my parents think if they knew? My greatest fear was that I'd overdose and die and that it would devastate my family. I think that kept me alive.

But I started to do cocaine. It was never my drug of choice. I'd stay up for three or four days in this induced psychosis. It was during one of these runs that I called my parents and it hit the fan. Their

my story

twenty-seven-year-old golden daughter was crashing. I ended up in the psych ward at Mclean Hospital in Boston, but I was in total denial about my addiction.

When I was discharged, I went out and did the same thing. And three or four months later, I was back in the hospital.

I made the decision to move back to Connecticut. I knew I couldn't stay where I was and get well. My fiancé moved out west. He wanted me to go with him, and I wanted to, but my parents intervened. They knew we were doing drugs together, and the pain and raw fear in their faces held me back. I moved into the home where I grew up and made my first stab at sobriety. I white-knuckled it and did not go on medication-assisted treatment (MAT) then.

Then my dad died, and I found him. I relapsed in the summer of 2012 and went on a run for about six months in Connecticut. It was a very different experience because I didn't have my fiancé to protect me.

I checked myself into a residential program, and it turned out I had endocarditis (an infection on the leaflets of the heart valve). I was admitted into an intensive care unit for a few weeks, where I became septic and almost died. The blood disease I'd had as a child, which cost me my spleen, made the infection much more dangerous.

That's how I got sober. I ended up going into an outpatient program, still without MAT, and for three to five months, I was suicidal. It's not that I wanted to die, I just didn't want to feel that awful. I was depressed from my brain trying to come off opioids. Finally, my mom intervened, and my psychiatrist put me on Suboxone. I also went on Prozac and Wellbutrin, which were very helpful.

I went back to work within a few months of that and threw myself into a 12-step program. I dedicated my life to service. I worked with the Manchester chief of police and started the HOPE initiative that offers treatment versus incarceration to people with drug problems. And today I oversee addiction counseling programs in long-term care facilities. For someone who has felt a lot of stigma over being in recovery, it's nice to have my experience valued. My hope is for anyone else in recovery to have a similar experience of acceptance.

My fiancé did not make it. In 2016, he overdosed and died. I look back now, and I wonder how different our lives would have been. We'd be together with six kids. That's where I go back to now, all the things that can't be undone and the realization that none of this should have happened.

OVERVIEW

America is in its worst, but not first, opioid epidemic. The past thirty years have seen a dramatic rise in the number of Americans with opioid use disorders—now at more than two million people. A recent Youth Risk Behavior Survey of high school students reported that nearly 3 percent of students had tried heroin and/or a fentanyl compound in the past year, and 20 percent had taken prescription drugs, including opioids, without a prescription. And 1 percent of pregnant women admit to the use of illicit opioids.

But it's been the exponential surge in opioid-related overdose deaths, over 400 percent since 1990, that have grabbed headlines and concern. Opioids are implicated in more than 90 percent of unintentional fatal overdoses in the United States. And the number of dead is staggering—over 500,000 in the past decade. Many of these deaths involve polypharmacy, where opioids are combined with other central nervous system depressants, such as alcohol or benzodiazepines (Valium-type drugs). And since 2012, cheap and potent fentanyl compounds, largely produced in China, have added an even greater degree of urgency to the problem.

Reasons for the current epidemic are multiple and include a tremendous rise in prescriptions for narcotic pain medications, the relative low cost and easy access to higher-purity heroin, and now the proliferation of potent and profitable fentanyl. The 2018 NSDUH data showed that over 50 percent of nonmedical painkiller users obtained the opioids for free from friends and relatives, most of whom had prescriptions.

Intravenous use of opioids and other drugs adds another layer of serious and potentially life-threatening health risks, which include infectious diseases such as HIV/AIDs, hepatitis C, cellulitis, bacterial endocarditis (infections on the leaflets of the heart valves), septicemia (blood infections), and limb amputations due to infections and crush injuries.

Once dependent on opioids, people become trapped—they need to obtain an adequate supply to prevent withdrawal (e.g., jonesing, dope sickness). Depending on the availability and their choice of opioid, they may need to dose themselves from once a day (methadone, buprenorphine) to every four to six hours (heroin, fentanyl, oxycodone, hydrocodone, hydromorphone).

People become addicted to opioids in various ways. For some, it starts with prescribed pain medications that they are unable or unwilling to stop. Others enjoy the euphoric effects of opioids, and some with co-occurring mood, anxiety problems, and PTSD find a temporary relief from painful and negative emotions.

Some with chronic pain conditions, who grow tolerant to the effects of opioid medications, may overuse their prescriptions and run out too soon. To prevent a return of symptoms, which have now been complicated by withdrawal syndromes, people are faced with difficult choices, such as buying medication illicitly, finding additional prescribers—so-called doctor shopping—or diverting medications from others who have been given legitimate prescriptions. If they are unable to obtain prescription

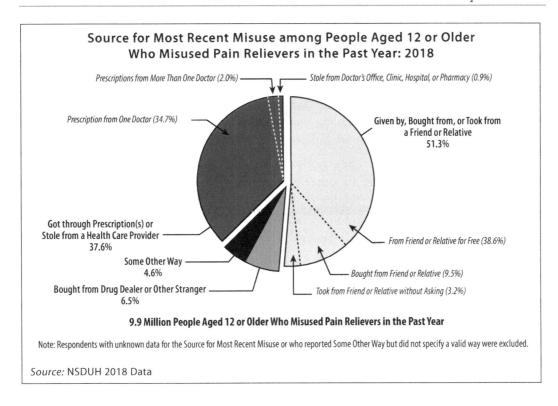

Source for Most Recent Misuse among People Aged 12 or Older Who Misused Pain Relievers in the Past Year: 2018

Prescriptions from More Than One Doctor (2.0%)

Stole from Doctor's Office, Clinic, Hospital, or Pharmacy (0.9%)

Prescription from One Doctor (34.7%)

Given by, Bought from, or Took from a Friend or Relative 51.3%

Got through Prescription(s) or Stole from a Health Care Provider 37.6%

From Friend or Relative for Free (38.6%)

Some Other Way 4.6%

Bought from Friend or Relative (9.5%)

Bought from Drug Dealer or Other Stranger 6.5%

Took from Friend or Relative without Asking (3.2%)

9.9 Million People Aged 12 or Older Who Misused Pain Relievers in the Past Year

Note: Respondents with unknown data for the Source for Most Recent Misuse or who reported Some Other Way but did not specify a valid way were excluded.

Source: NSDUH 2018 Data

medications, they turn to heroin and now fentanyl both to relieve their pain and to prevent withdrawal.

A common pattern of usage starts with pain pills taken orally, then crushed and snorted, and then injected. First experiences with heroin usually involve snorting (insufflation), but in time many people want to experience the more intense high from injecting the drug. Heroin can also be smoked (known as "chasing the dragon").

There is a vast array of available opioids, and people may not understand that the medication they're taking is an opioid and can be habit-forming. This is especially true for some of the newer pain medications, which bind to opioid receptors in the brain, tramadol (Ultram) being one example.

Types of Opioids

Not all opioids are the same. What unifies them is they bind to opioid receptors in the brain and throughout the body. Clinically, it is useful to understand some basic differences between the various agents. These include the relative half-lives of the different compounds (i.e., how long they stay in the body and how frequently people need to be dosed) and their potencies (i.e., milligram for milligram how strong they are when compared to 1 milligram of morphine). The following terms help describe how particular substances work at the opiate receptors in the brain and body:

- **Agonist/pure agonist:** These substances, when taken in higher quantities, have no ceiling effect. With opioids this means that when a pure agonist is taken in a great enough dose, the person will eventually experience respiratory arrest and stop breathing. Examples include heroin, methadone, fentanyl, and morphine.

- **Antagonist (blocker):** These substances bind to the opioid receptor and block it from being available to other substances. They include naltrexone (Revia, Vivitrol) and naloxone (Narcan). These are not opioids, although naloxone is combined with the opioid buprenorphine to make the medications Suboxone and Zubsolv, as well as available generics.

- **Partial agonist:** This substance provides some of the typical opioid effect (e.g., pain relief, prevention of withdrawal symptoms), but when taken in higher doses, it has a ceiling effect and will not lead to respiratory depression unless combined with other central nervous system depressants. They include buprenorphine (Suboxone, Subutex, Zubsolv, Sublocade, Probuphine).

What's the difference between opiates and opioids? Opiates are naturally occurring substances found in the sap of opium poppies (papaver somniferum) and include codeine and morphine. Opioids initially referred to synthetic substances, such as oxycodone, the semisynthetic heroin, fentanyl, hydromorphone, and others. In common usage, however, the term *opioids* includes all substances that act as agonists (i.e., bind to and cause typical effects) on opioid receptors. The diagnoses of opioid use disorders include both naturally derived and synthetic substances.

Opioids

Substance	How Used	Dosing Frequency	Type
Buprenorphine (Subutex, Sublocade)	• Sublingual (under the tongue): Subutex • Injection: Sublocade	Sublingual is once or twice daily, more frequently if used for pain. The injections are monthly.	Partial agonist
Buprenorphine/ naloxone (Suboxone, Zubsolv)	Sublingual	Once or twice daily, more frequently if used for pain	Partial agonist combined with an antagonist
Codeine (Darvon)	Oral	Every 3–6 hours	Pure agonist
Fentanyl (there are now over twenty identified variants of illicit fentanyl)	Transdermal/patch, oral (lozenge), injection	• Oral unclear • Injection every 4 hours • Patch every 72 hours	Pure agonist
Heroin	Snorted, injected, smoked	Every 4–8 hours	Pure agonist
Hydrocodone (Vicodin, Lortab, Lorcet)	Oral	Every 4–6 hours	Pure agonist
Hydromorphone (Dilaudid)	Oral, rectal (suppository), intravenous	Every 3–4 hours	Pure agonist
Methadone (Dolophine, Amidone, Methadose)	Oral	Once a day	Pure agonist
Meperidine (Demerol)	Oral, intravenous	Every 2–3 hours	Pure agonist
Morphine	Oral, intravenous	• Immediate release every 3–4 hours • Slow release every 8–12 hours	Pure agonist
Opium	Smoked	Every 4–6 hours	Pure agonist
Oxycodone (OxyContin, Roxicodone, Percocet, Percodan)	Oral	• Immediate release every 3–4 hours • Sustained release (OxyContin) every 8–12 hours	Pure agonist
Propoxyphene (Darvocet)	Oral	Every 3–4 hours	Pure agonist
Sufentanil	Intravenous	Every 2–4 hours	Pure agonist

OPIOID WITHDRAWAL

Opioid withdrawal states create intense physical and psychological symptoms that perpetuate the compulsive cycle of drug-seeking. For people with long-standing opioid habits, it is no longer about experiencing euphoric highs. Instead, much of their day is focused on doing whatever it takes to prevent withdrawal.

Depending on the substance, withdrawal symptoms can start within a few hours of the last dose. Symptoms can be divided between those that are physically distressing and those that are psychologically distressing. Acute withdrawal symptoms can last from a few days to more than two weeks.

Physical symptoms of opioid withdrawal include:

- Diarrhea
- Cramping (muscles, stomach)
- Achiness (bones, muscles)
- Muscle twitches
- Pupil dilation (mydriasis)
- Yawning
- Runny nose
- Tearing
- Nausea and vomiting
- Hot and cold flashes, sweating
- Gooseflesh (piloerection)

Psychological symptoms of opioid withdrawal include:

- Anxiety
- Intense cravings to use
- Irritability
- Depression
- Restlessness

ASSESSMENT TOOLS

There are several tools used to quantify the severity of withdrawal syndromes. Two that are often used, and at times used together, are the Clinical Opiate Withdrawal Scale (COWS) and Subjective Opiate Withdrawal Scale (SOWS).

Clinical Opiate Withdrawal Scale

The COWS is an eleven-item assessment completed by a clinician. It assesses the severity of changes in pulse rate, sweating, pupil size, restlessness, degree of cramping and achiness, stomach upset/nausea and vomiting, tremors, anxiety and irritability, gooseflesh, and yawning/tearing. It can be performed at intervals to assess improvement, such as what you would want to see upon starting an opioid replacement medication like buprenorphine or methadone. It is reprinted here and is in the public domain.

Clinical Opiate Withdrawal Scale (COWS)

Flow-sheet for measuring symptoms over a period of time during buprenorphine induction.

For each item, write in the number that best describes the patient's signs or symptom. Rate on just the apparent relationship to opiate withdrawal. For example, if heart rate is increased because the patient was jogging just prior to assessment, the increased pulse rate would not add to the score.

Patient's Name: _____ Date: _____				
Buprenorphine induction: Enter scores at time zero, 30 minutes after first dose, 2 hours after first dose, etc.				
Times: _____ _____ _____ _____				
Resting Pulse Rate (*Record beats per minute. Measured after patient is sitting or lying for one minute.*) 0 pulse rate 80 or below 1 pulse rate 81–100 2 pulse rate 101–120 4 pulse rate greater than 120				
Sweating (*Over past ½ hour, not accounted for by room temperature or patient activity*) 0 no report of chills or flushing 1 subjective report of chills or flushing 2 flushed or observable moistness on face 3 beads of sweat on brow or face 4 sweat streaming off face				
Restlessness (*Observation during assessment*) 0 able to sit still 1 reports difficulty sitting still but is able to do so 3 frequent shifting or extraneous movements of legs/arms 5 unable to sit still for more than a few seconds				

Pupil Size 0 pupils pinned or normal size for room light 1 pupils possibly larger than normal for room light 2 pupils moderately dilated 5 pupils so dilated that only the rim of the iris is visible				
Bone or Joint Aches (*If patient was having pain previously, only the additional component attributed to opiates withdrawal is scored.*) 0 not present 1 mild diffuse discomfort 2 patient reports severe diffuse aching of joints/muscles 4 patient is rubbing joints or muscles and is unable to sit still because of discomfort				
Runny Nose or Tearing (*Not accounted for by cold symptoms or allergies*) 0 not present 1 nasal stuffiness or unusually moist eyes 2 nose is running or tearing 4 nose constantly runs or tears streaming down cheeks				
Gastrointestinal (GI) Upset (*Over last ½ hour*) 0 no GI symptoms 1 stomach cramps 2 nausea or loose stool 3 vomiting or diarrhea 5 multiple episodes of diarrhea or vomiting				

Tremor (*Observation of outstretched hands*) 0 no tremor 1 tremor can be felt, but not observed 2 slight tremor is observable 4 gross tremor or muscle twitching				
Yawning (*Observation during assessment*) 0 no yawning 1 yawning once or twice during assessment 2 yawning three or more times during assessment 4 yawning several times/minute				
Anxiety or Irritability 0 none 1 patient reports increasing irritability or anxiousness 2 patient is obviously irritable or anxious 4 patient is so irritable or anxious that participation in the assessment is difficult				
Gooseflesh Skin 0 skin is smooth 3 piloerections of skin can be felt or hairs standing up on arms 5 prominent piloerections				
Total scores with observer's initials				

Scoring key:
5–12 = mild
13–24 = moderate
25–36 = moderately severe
More than 36 = severe withdrawal

The Subjective Opiate Withdrawal Scale

Similar to the COWS, the SOWS is a sixteen-item Likert-based tool completed by the client. It can be useful to complete both instruments and then compare the results. Do they show a similar severity of withdrawal, or is one significantly higher than the other? A downloadable version of the SOWS is available at www.ncbi.nlm.nih.gov/books/NBK143183/bin/annex10-fm2.pdf.

TREATMENT OF OPIOID USE DISORDERS AND MEDICATION-ASSISTED TREATMENT

In our current opioid epidemic, we face rapidly evolving scenarios, such as the introduction of fentanyl into the illicit drug markets and the growing recognition that abstinence-only models are dangerous for people who have opioid use disorders. The reasons for that last statement are as follows. Substance use disorders, regardless of the drug, have high relapse rates on the order of 80 percent over the course of a year. Studies that have looked at detoxification and relapse with opioids show that 50 percent, or more, will misuse within one week of discharge.

Nationwide, we see spikes in fatal overdoses among people who have been opioid free and then use, such as those who have been incarcerated or in abstinence-based residential treatment. The person who has been opioid free has lost some or all of their previous tolerance to opioids, and combined with the potent, available, and inexpensive drugs, both prescription and illicit, what might have been a safe dose when they were a daily user is now lethal. To put that into context, the Drug Enforcement Agency (DEA) reports that approximately 2 mg of fentanyl is what is found in a typical fatal overdose. The average cost of that deadly dose is less than ten dollars.

Which brings us to the current standard of care for opioid use disorders: medication for opioid use disorders, also known as medication-assisted treatment or MAT. At present, this involves the use of longer-acting opioids as replacement therapy—methadone or buprenorphine (Suboxone, Subutex, Zubsolv, Sublocade, and others)—or the opioid blocker naltrexone (Revia, Vivitrol). Studies with the two replacement therapies show strong results with treatment retention and negative drug screens in the 70 to 80 percent range, while there are less robust outcomes with naltrexone.

Information on medications for opioid use disorders needs to be presented to clients in a clear manner. What are the options, and what are the pros and cons of each agent? Next, factor the availability of the various treatment options, their cost, and so forth. Then combine the above with frank discussion about the client's short- and long-term goals. What do they want?

For most individuals who have used opioids for extended periods, abstinence may not be realistic or realistic *right now*. It is important to acknowledge the person's long-term goal of being free of opioids but to also set a more immediate goal of getting them off street drugs or illicitly obtained prescriptions and pursuing an immediate course of opioid replacement therapy.

For people who have achieved abstinence from opioids, relapse rates remain high, especially during that first year. Therapeutic, peer-based, supportive, and possibly pharmacological strategies along with wellness routines can be used to help with relapse prevention.

Opioid Replacement Therapy

In the United States, there are currently two standard forms of opioid replacement therapy: methadone and buprenorphine.

Methadone. Synthesized in 1939 by German scientists, methadone was brought to the United States in 1947 for the treatment of narcotic dependency. It is a DEA Schedule II controlled substance and is a pure opioid agonist with a half-life of 24–36 hours. On account of the long and variable half-life, withdrawal from methadone can be protracted and last from several days to several weeks.

As replacement treatment for opioid use disorders, methadone can only be prescribed through opioid treatment programs (OTP) that are state licensed and approved by SAMHSA. There are approximately 2,000 of these licensed centers nationwide.

The side effects of methadone are similar to other opioids: sedation, nodding, constipation, dry mouth, and urinary retention. Methadone comes with a black box warning for QT prolongation that is dose dependent, and a pretreatment ECG is recommended. Because of this, it's best to avoid other medications that cause cardiac conduction delays, as this adverse reaction can be additive and lead to a dangerous arrhythmia, heart failure, and sudden death.

Recent studies using doses of 120–150 mg per day showed reduced use of illicit opioids and were found to be safe. The current consensus is that 60–100 mg per day is safe and effective. Less than 60 mg per day is associated with increased relapse rates.

Methadone can be dangerous and potentially lethal in overdose or when combined with other sedatives, such as benzodiazepines, other opioids, certain sleeping medications, or alcohol.

Most clinics require daily attendance and include some form(s) of therapy and psychiatric consultation. A list of local opioid treatment programs maintained by SAMHSA can be accessed at https://dpt2.samhsa.gov/treatment/directory.aspx.

Buprenorphine. Buprenorphine is a partial opioid agonist/antagonist that is used alone (Subutex, Sublocade) or in combination with the opioid blocker naloxone (Narcan) under the trade names Suboxone, Zubsolv, and others. By occupying the opioid receptor site, buprenorphine blocks the effects of other opioids, so if a person were to use heroin or most narcotic pain medication while taking buprenorphine, that person would not get the euphoric effect, or the full effect, of the other drug. Buprenorphine is less sedating and does not have the "high" of other opioids, although some people do report a general feeling of well-being, especially when they first start using the medication.

Buprenorphine is taken under the tongue (sublingually) as either a strip or a dissolving tablet. There is also a form that is dissolved in the cheek (Bunavail). Taken in this manner, the naloxone (Narcan) component is inactive. However, should the medication be misused and snorted or injected, the naloxone (Narcan) would precipitate symptoms of withdrawal. Even so, some people have reported snorting the pill form of this medication and have experienced a euphoric high.

Prior to starting buprenorphine, patients should be in active opioid withdrawal in order to prevent the medication from precipitating a withdrawal when it displaces from the receptors the other opioid the patient has been using.

Unlike methadone, buprenorphine does not have to be prescribed through a SAMHSA-designated opioid treatment program. Physicians (MDs and DOs), nurse practitioners, and physician assistants who wish to prescribe buprenorphine for the treatment of opioid use disorders must receive additional education and obtain a special DEA waiver: "the X."

Credentialed professionals can prescribe buprenorphine as opioid replacement therapy through a typical office practice or through a clinic or other program. Initially, patients receive a small prescription for the medication, but when stable, they may receive monthly prescriptions. Typical doses for opioid replacement therapy are 8–24 mg per day of the buprenorphine component. Higher doses can be associated with a greater risk of medication diversion.

Other Medication-Assisted Treatment for Opioid Use Disorders

Another FDA-approved for the treatment of opioid use disorders is the opioid antagonist, naltrexone. As opposed to methadone and buprenorphine (opioid replacement therapies), naltrexone is for individuals who are completely opioid free (at least seven to ten days, possibly longer for longer-acting opioids, such as methadone or buprenorphine). Naltrexone will precipitate withdrawal symptoms if the person is still on opioids.

Naltrexone is available as both a long-acting injection (once a month) or as a daily oral medication. Unlike buprenorphine and methadone, it does not carry a risk of dependence or diversion. No special training is required for a licensed practitioner to prescribe naltrexone.

People who want to be on this medication need to be informed that they will not get the euphoric feeling or pain relief associated with opioids if they use opioids while on naltrexone. And it is possible to fatally overdose with opioids while on naltrexone. This occurs most commonly when someone misses doses of oral naltrexone, are at the end of the injection period for the long-acting formulation, or attempt to override the effects of naltrexone with large doses of opioids. A missed dose of the injection represents a clinical emergency, as the person is now at high risk for relapse, has lost some or all tolerance to opioids, and is not protected by the blocker.

Adverse reactions reported with naltrexone include liver toxicity, fatigue, loss of appetite, injection-site reactions with the long-acting formulation, and an allergic pneumonia, which has also been reported with the injectable.

It is recommended that patients on the long-acting injection wear a medical bracelet to alert emergency personnel in the event they are unconscious. If opioids are required for acute pain management, such as might be needed after an accident, this might require a supervised medical setting.

OVERDOSE RESCUE KITS

Most states have passed legislation to allow easier access to the overdose-reversal medication, naloxone (Narcan). Distribution of naloxone to people with opioid use disorders should be considered a standard of care. Most states also allow family members and others to obtain naloxone both with and without a prescription. It's best to check your state's department of public health or similar agency to understand the rules that apply.

Naloxone (Narcan) is a potent opioid antagonist that, when injected into a muscle (intramuscular injection) or blood vessel (intravenous injection) or inhaled, reverses an opioid overdose. Naloxone (Narcan) is short acting and, depending on what someone took and how much, a second dose or even more may be required.

Brief trainings on the use of naloxone should be provided along with the medication. At a minimum, you'd like people to know:

- What naloxone (Narcan) is and how it works
- How to recognize an overdose
- How to administer the drug, which will vary based on the form (inhaled—mist or spray—versus various injections)
- How to activate the emergency medical response (Give the first dose and then call 9-1-1. Stay on the phone until instructed to hang up.)
- What to do after administering the drug (Stay with the person, when they start to wake, roll them onto their side in the "rescue position" to decrease the risk of aspiration if they should vomit.)
- Legal issues, such as good Samaritan legislation in your state (This is important information for those who use drugs with friends in that event that someone overdoses, a common scenario. People run away due to fear of negative legal consequences. Many states have protections that will prevent arrest if a person reverses an overdose and calls 9-1-1. There is state-to-state variability, so it's important to pass on accurate information to your clients.)

PREGNANCY, BREASTFEEDING, AND OPIOID USE DISORDERS

Opioid use disorders occur most frequently in adolescents and young adults. As a result, it is important to understand some basics on how to help a woman who is opioid dependent manage a pregnancy and the postpartum period.

Although it is understandable for a pregnant woman to want to be off all drugs and medication throughout her pregnancy and while breastfeeding, it is not always realistic. The standard of care for an opioid-dependent pregnant woman is to be on replacement therapy.

Abrupt discontinuation of opioids should be avoided, as this is associated with miscarriage, preterm labor, and fetal distress. More ominous are high rates of relapse, overdose, and death. Research shows that pregnancy outcomes (miscarriages, premature delivery, lower birth weights) are worse for women who go on and off opioids through the course of their pregnancy. This makes sense because the unborn child is going in and out of withdrawal along with the mother.

In instances where a woman wishes to be opioid free throughout her pregnancy, the following strategies may help to diminish risks of relapse and harm to her and her unborn child:

- More frequent clinical contact and check-ins
- Informed consent about the relative risks and benefits of replacement therapy versus risks of relapse to her and her unborn child
- Slow taper off current opioid medication
- Open door "Plan B" should she wish to go on replacement therapy

Opioid Replacement Therapy During Pregnancy

For women with moderate or severe opioid use disorders, the standard of care is to remain on or get on some form of opioid replacement therapy. While neither methadone nor buprenorphine have an FDA indication for the treatment of opioid use disorders in pregnancy, there is an abundant literature to support their use through the course of pregnancy and ongoing. Opioid replacement during pregnancy includes the following benefits:

- Decreased relapse rates
- Decreased overdose rates and related morbidity and mortality
- Lower HIV and hepatitis infections to the mother and transmission to the newborn
- Better obstetrical care
- Reduced fetal mortality
- Increased fetal growth
- Increased likelihood that the infant will go home with the mother

A large study that compared outcomes with methadone and buprenorphine, the Maternal Opioid Treatment: Human Experimental Research (MOTHER), showed slightly higher treatment retention for women on methadone and decreased preterm labor and less severe neonatal abstinence syndrome (a withdrawal syndrome) with buprenorphine.

General guidelines for pregnant women on opioid replacement therapy include the following:

- If a woman is on opioid replacement therapy, she should stay on that agent (either methadone or buprenorphine). Typically if a woman is on combined buprenorphine/naloxone, she will be switched to a buprenorphine-only medication.

- Frequent and regular clinical contacts are important between the pregnant woman and the clinical program through which she receives the opioid replacement therapy.

- Ongoing liaison should occur between the prescriber of the opioid replacement therapy and the obstetrical provider(s).

- The woman's partner should be included in the treatment process and receive education about the risks and benefits of opioid replacement therapy. If the partner is actively using illicit substances and/or alcohol, this needs to be addressed, as it may well trigger the pregnant woman to relapse.

- The woman should understand all the risks related to being on opioid replacement therapy throughout pregnancy, as well as the risks of tapering off, including a greatly increased risk for relapse with illicit narcotics.

  o The woman should understand that her baby will be at risk for a neonatal abstinence syndrome (a withdrawal syndrome that may require medical management following delivery).

  o The woman should be aware that children born to mothers who are opioid dependent are at an increased risk for sudden infant death syndrome and that close pediatric supervision is recommended.

- Federal legislation under the Child Abuse Prevention and Treatment Act (CAPTA) mandates that newborns who display signs of substance-related syndromes, such as neonatal abstinence, be reported to a state's child protective services. Therefore, it's crucial to communicate what this means in your state and what measures can be done to lessen any negative consequences. This will involve creation of a safe plan of care, which is most frequently a written document that outlines what treatment a woman is in, who her providers are, and such.

Opioid Replacement Therapy During Breastfeeding (Lactation)

Both methadone and buprenorphine are detected in breast milk, although in low concentrations. The recommendation is that if a woman wishes to breastfeed, the benefits of doing so outweigh the risks.

CHAPTER 20

Selected Topics for Other Substances

OVERVIEW

SAMHSA's 2018 NSDUH data found that nearly one in five Americans had used an illicit substance in the past year (19.4 percent). This represents an increase from the 2015 and 2016 numbers and was mostly driven by cannabis use. Second were prescription pain relievers, with 3.6 percent reporting nonprescribed use. A few notable trends in the use of illicit substances include:

- The introduction of fentanyl and fentanyl analogs into the illicit drug market: Evidence for this is seen in the numbers of samples adulterated with fentanyl confiscated by law enforcement and the growing acknowledgment that most of what is currently sold as heroin is either adulterated with fentanyl or is fentanyl with no heroin.

    o Fentanyl adulteration in pills sold illicitly: Counterfeit medications that appear to be benzodiazepines or prescription pain medications, such as

OxyContin and others, have been widely reported and documented in law enforcement confiscations.

o Fentanyl adulteration of cocaine, including crack cocaine: Much of the increase in stimulant-related deaths (threefold over the past few years) is related to co-administration of fentanyl, whether intended or not.

o Growing concerns about the potential for fentanyl adulteration of cannabis

- A resurgence in cocaine use with a reported 1.9 million past-month users in 2018.

Past-Year Use of Illicit or Misuse of Prescription Drugs Among People Twelve or Older

Substance	Numbers	Percent
All illicit drugs	53.2 million	19.4
Marijuana (including hashish)	43.5 million	15.9
Inhalants	2 million	0.7
Psychotherapeutics*	16.9 million	6.2
Hallucinogens**	5.6 million	2
Cocaine	5.5 million	2
Methamphetamine	1.9 million	0.7
Heroin	808,000	0.3
Stimulants other than methamphetamine, such as amphetamines and methylphenidate (Ritalin)	5.1 million	1.9
Tranquilizers or sedatives (including benzodiazepines and prescription sleeping medications)	6.4 million	2.4
Benzodiazepines	5.4 million	2
Pain Relievers (oxycodone, hydrocodone, tramadol, prescription fentanyl, and others)	9.9 million	3.6

Source: NSDUH 2018 Data

*Psychotherapeutics include prescription painkillers, tranquilizers, sedatives, and stimulants (including methamphetamine).

** Hallucinogens in this survey include LSD, PCP, Ecstasy (MDMA/Molly) and related compounds, peyote, mescaline, ketamine, *salvia divinorum,* and psilocybin mushrooms.

COCAINE

Cocaine, derived from the leaves of the coca plant, can be taken orally, snorted, smoked (crack, freebase), and injected. It is highly habit-forming due to its strong effects on the brain's dopamine reward system. Studies on primates and other mammals have dramatically demonstrated this. When given the choice between food and cocaine, test animals consistently push the bar for cocaine and ignore food.

Cocaine is a central nervous system stimulant that increases heart rate, suppresses appetite, and provides the user with feelings of increased energy, euphoria, and confidence. The effects of cocaine are short acting, from fifteen minutes to an hour.

Negative health outcomes from cocaine include damage to the heart (myocardial ischemia) from vasospasm combined with increased heart rate and elevated blood pressure (cardiac workload). These effects are especially notable when alcohol is combined with cocaine, where it forms cocaethylene, which is associated with increased cardiac toxicity. With heavy use, cocaine is associated with sudden cardiac death and stroke.

The method of cocaine use also carries specific risks, from bloody noses and destruction of nasal cartilage from inhalation, to abscesses, increased rates of HIV/ AIDs and hepatitis B and C with intravenous use; to burns, shortness of breath, chest pain, and lung spasm with smoked (crack, freebase) cocaine.

While the opioid overdose statistics have grabbed headlines, it's important to note that every year over 10,000 Americans die from cocaine-related overdoses. While these numbers had declined, there has been an alarming increase since 2012.

Cocaine Withdrawal/Crash

After a binge, users of cocaine often experience a "crash" or comedown. This crash is characterized by:

- Tiredness that can be extreme, as people may have gone a day or more with little or no sleep
- Vivid dreams
- Sleep disturbance (too much or too little)
- Increased appetite
- Depressed and/or anxious mood (can be severe)
- Suicidality

Pharmacological Treatments

At present, there are no FDA-approved treatments for cocaine use disorders. However, studies conducted with people who have both cocaine use disorders and a co-occurring mental disorder show that, when the mental disorder is well controlled, the severity and frequency of cocaine use diminishes. Numerous medications are being and have been assessed off-label for potential benefits in diminishing cravings and relapses. Among those are:

- Topiramate (Topamax)
- Gabapentin (Neurontin)
- Diclofenac (Baclofen)
- Amantadine (Symmetrel)

STIMULANTS, INCLUDING BATH SALTS

Stimulants (psychostimulants) other than cocaine and caffeine include prescription medications for ADHD—methylphenidate (Ritalin, Concerta), amphetamines, and mixed amphetamine salts (Adderall, Vyvanse)—and a large number of synthetic compounds that go by a variety of names, including "bath salts" and "plant food." Typical effects of stimulants may include:

- Increased energy
- Diminished appetite
- Decreased sleep
- Increased alertness
- Increased concentration
- Increased heart rate and blood pressure
- Increased anxiety
- Increased irritability

With heavy use or in high dosages, additional symptoms of paranoia and psychosis have been reported, often with extreme disturbances in behavior and confusion (toxic delirium).

Issues Specific to Bath Salts and Related Compounds

Many stimulants contain the compound 3,4-methylmethcathinone/MDPV (mephedrone). Despite legislative attempts to ban these substances, they continue to be sold and used. Emergent situations related to their use can present with symptoms of agitation, confusion, psychosis (at times persistent), elevations in blood pressure and pulse, dilated pupils (mydriasis), tremors, seizures, and organ failure (liver and kidney). Deaths due to MDPV toxicity have been reported.

Treatment for MDPV toxicity is supportive and includes the use of sedatives, including intravenous administration of drugs like diazepam (Valium) to help manage the confusion and agitation delirium. If psychotic features (hallucinations and/or delusions) are prominent, rapid-acting tranquilizers have been used.

Withdrawal syndromes from stimulants are similar to those with cocaine. They can include dysphoria, tiredness, excessive sleepiness, vivid dreams, and cravings to use.

CANNABIS

Second to alcohol, cannabis is the most used mind-altering drug in the United States, both in the general population and with people who have co-occurring mental disorders. It is associated with increased psychotic symptoms in people with schizophrenia and an increased frequency of mania, psychosis, suicide attempts, and overall illness severity in people who have bipolar disorder. Significant evidence now indicates that marijuana use may precipitate psychosis in susceptible individuals. In multiple large studies, the use of cannabis has been associated with much greater (six- to sevenfold) rates of psychotic disorders, as well as earlier onset of psychotic disorders. It appears that for some susceptible individuals, this relationship between cannabis and schizophrenia may have a genetic underpinning related to a gene that codes for an enzyme involved in dopamine synthesis. Conceptually, it's as if marijuana switches on the illness (an epigenetic phenomenon). What is not known is whether cessation of cannabis in these same people might eventually lead to symptom resolution.

Attitudes and policies toward cannabis, which contains over one hundred active compounds, are undergoing significant change because many states have legalized medical marijuana, a few have legalized recreational use for people over the age of twenty-one, and many more are considering it. In contrast, the federal government and the DEA continue to consider cannabis an illegal Schedule I controlled substance.

Due to its Schedule I status, which the federal government defines as having no acceptable medical use and high potential for abuse, there have been few well-controlled studies of cannabis. In states where it is legal, indications for medical marijuana are not based on rigorous double-blind studies at this time. The most prescribed indication is for chronic pain. Here there can be some clear advantages in terms of risk versus benefit, certainly over the opioids and possibly over nonsteroidal medications, such as ibuprofen and naproxen, that can have significant GI and renal adverse effects.

With the shift in attitudes and development of study protocols for various conditions, including PTSD, we should see the emergence of new information and hopefully clearer directives around the therapeutic risks and benefits of cannabinoids.

Pharmacological Treatments

To date, there are no FDA-approved medications for the treatment of cannabis use disorders.

Synthetic Cannabis (Incense, Spice, K-2)

Sold under different names, and typically marked "not for human consumption," there has been a tremendous growth in the use of synthetic intoxicating drugs. While many of these have been banned and designated illegal, they continue to be popular, especially among teens and young adults. In addition to the relative availability of these substances—they can be purchased over the internet, at gas stations, and at head shops—many are drawn to them because they pass undetected on standard drug screens. Special tests are available, and one study that looked at urine samples from juvenile probation departments showed positive rates of synthetic cannabis of more than 30 percent.

Synthetic cannabis is a mixture of plant material with laboratory-produced chemicals. It acts on the cannabinoid receptors in the brain. However, unlike natural cannabis, which contains tetrahydrocannabinol (THC), the synthetic compounds are more potent (100–800 times) and are full agonists that can create a much more dramatic drug effect. Effects can include:

- Euphoria, relaxation
- Agitation
- Confusion and changes in perception, altered sense of time, delirium
- Anxiety
- Depression
- Nausea and vomiting
- Increased pulse and blood pressure
- Hallucinations, including command auditory hallucinations, as well as visual and tactile hallucinations
- Paranoia
- Red eyes
- Seizures (rarely reported)

Treatment of Synthetic Cannabis Toxicity

Emergency rooms have seen a marked rise in people admitted in psychotic and agitated states having used synthetic cannabis, often combined with alcohol and other substances. The diagnostic picture is often complicated because synthetic cannabis does not show up on most routine drug screens. Treatment is supportive and may involve the use of sedatives and possibly tranquilizers (neuroleptics/antipsychotics) to help manage symptoms of agitation and psychosis.

HALLUCINOGENS

Hallucinogens are compounds that cause changes in perception to where the user experiences phenomena beyond the range of what is considered normal consciousness. The effects of hallucinogens vary, with some more associated with psychedelic experiences (tripping) and others leading to out-of-body/dissociative or confused/delirious states. Some substances, such as the "club drug" MDMA (3,4-methylenedioxy-*N*-methylamphetamine)—also known as Ecstasy or XTC—have both stimulant and hallucinogenic properties and also provide users with a sense of increased connectivity to others (i.e., they are empathogenic). Negative consequences from hallucinogens are often related to the intoxication stage, when judgment may be impaired. Persistent psychotic states can also be associated with hallucinogens, some of which last on the order of weeks, months, or even longer, especially with PCP. Hallucinogens include:

- Lysergic acid (LSD)
- Psilocybin mushrooms (magic mushrooms)
- Peyote

- Mescaline
- Ayahuasca (a combination of plants used in some South American religious and shamanistic traditions, including the Church of Santo Daime)
- MDMA (3,4-methylenedioxy-*N*-methylamphetamine), also known as Ecstasy, XTC, Molly, or Mandy
- Phencyclidine (PCP)
- *Datura stramonium* (jimsonweed/the devil's cucumber)
- Ketamine
- *Salvia divinorum*

OVER-THE-COUNTER MEDICATIONS

Clinicians need to be aware that some substances found in over-the-counter cold/ flu and sleeping medications, as well as nutritional supplements, can be misused as intoxicants. Among these are dextromethorphan, diphenhydramine, ephedrine, and pseudoephedrine.

Dextromethorphan

Found in many cold and cough preparations, dextromethorphan is typically combined with acetaminophen (Tylenol). At normal doses, this compound has minimal psychoactive properties. However, in higher doses, it creates a dissociated hallucinogenic effect, sometimes referred to as "robo-tripping" because of its association with the over-the-counter medication Robitussin*.

Because dextromethorphan is typically combined with other ingredients, such as acetaminophen (Tylenol), it carries significant risk for liver and kidney toxicity when taken in the high doses required to induce hallucinosis. Habitual users report withdrawal symptoms that can include lethargy, fatigue, nightmares, insomnia, and depression. Some states have restricted the sale of dextromethorphan-containing compounds, but it is not currently a controlled substance.

Diphenhydramine

Diphenhydramine, found in some cold preparations and over-the-counter sleep aids, has been used recreationally for its sedating and, in much higher than recommended doses, hallucinatory properties. Because of its strong anticholinergic properties, typical side effects include:

- Dry mouth
- Blurry vision
- Constipation
- Urinary retention
- Drowsiness

Symptoms of diphenhydramine toxicity can include:

- Hallucinations
- Agitation
- Palpitations
- Bowel obstruction
- Seizure
- Coma
- Death

Ephedrine and Pseudoephedrine

Ephedrine and pseudoephedrine, which are found in the traditional Chinese medicine herb Ma huang (*Ephedra sinica*), are included in many cold, asthma, and flu medications. Because ephedrine can be used in the manufacture of methamphetamine, legislation has limited the use of ephedrine and requires the recording of information identifying all individuals who purchase compounds containing ephedrine. Once sold over the counter, compounds with ephedrine must now be specifically requested from the pharmacist.

INTERNET ISSUES

Clinicians need to be aware that many clients research and obtain mind-altering substances through the internet. Numerous websites and blogs are devoted to specific drugs and to the cultures of "tripping" and to being a "hallucinaut." The internet is also a rich source of material on ways to fool/pass a drug test. Finally, millions of Americans purchase their prescription medications from other countries where they are substantially less expensive.

Clinically, this plays out different ways, and clinicians should encourage a discussion with their clients about any and all substances they have used, are using, and are thinking about trying. Here are a few things to consider:

- Substances that are controlled in this country but are sold over the counter in other countries, such as Canada, Mexico, Japan, India, and Russia: The range here is tremendous and includes benzodiazepines, opioids, sedative hypnotics, and stimulants.
- Substances that are not on the market in this country: There are many medications used throughout the world that are not approved or for sale in this country. These include tranquilizers, sedatives, and painkillers, many of which have tremendous potential for misuse, abuse, and physiologic dependence and associated withdrawal symptoms and syndromes.

- Substances that are incorrectly labeled: Here it is the ultimate case of "buyer beware." The internet purchaser must rely on the seller's honesty regarding the substance they have purchased.

- Substances of uncertain strength and purity: Especially worrisome with the current rates of fentanyl adulteration.

- Substances that have been specifically banned in this country, such as flunitrazepam (Rohypnol or "roofies"), an ultra-fast-acting benzodiazepine and amnestic agent that has been associated with date rape.

- Component ingredients for substances, such as plants used in the production of the hallucinogen Ayahuasca.

- Faking drug tests: The internet has a seemingly limitless array of products, blogs, and websites devoted to passing drug tests. These sites often include the sale of compounds and devices used to confound tests, as well as techniques to slip warm, drug-free urine into the cup when providing a sample.

When faced with the dizzying number of substances available through the internet and varying points of view being expressed, it is important to be open and willing to learn about whatever over-the-counter, nutritional, and/or internet-purchased substances someone has obtained. This starts in the assessment and continues over the course of treatment. One approach, when faced with an unknown substance, is to start with an internet search. Here it is helpful to obtain multiple resources, which include:

- Consumer-driven sites
  - Ask your clients which sites they use.
  - See which sites have the most hits for the topic you have searched.
  - See what has been written about the substance on Wikipedia.org and erowid. org. These sources often include a treasure trove of links to related articles, websites, and blogs.
- Professional websites
  - WebMD (webmd.com)
  - PubMed (pubmed.ncbi.nlm.nih.gov)
- Governmental websites
  - Substance Abuse and Mental Health Services Administration (SAMHSA.gov)
  - Drug Enforcement Agency (DEA.gov)
  - Centers for Disease Control and Prevention (CDC.gov)

Resources and References

For your convenience, the resources in this book are available for download at www.pesi.com/atkins

Chapter 1: Co-Occurring Basics: Overview, Terms, Key Concepts, and a Bit of History

RESOURCES

The American Psychiatric Association and *The Diagnostic and Statistical Manual of Mental Disorders, Fifth Edition* (DSM-5): The DSM-5 is the current psychiatric diagnostic manual in the United States. Updates and corrections, as well as downloadable assessment measures and articles related to the DSM-5, are available on their website

(www.DSM5.org).

The American Society of Addiction Medicine (ASAM): This professional organization comprises physicians and other addiction specialists. They support research and education around substance use disorders, treatment, and prevention

(www.asam.org).

The Food and Drug Administration (FDA): This organization approves and oversees pharmaceutical medications in the United States. Copies of all package inserts, warnings, prescribing updates, and so on are available through their website

(www.fda.gov).

The National Alliance on Mental Illness (NAMI): The largest advocacy organization for families of people with mental illness offers up-to-date information, peer and family support, and clear and concise articles on a broad range of topics, mostly related to mental health and psychiatric disorders but some pertaining to co-occurring and substance use disorders as well

(www.nami.org).

The National Committee for Quality Assurance (NCQA): This private nonprofit organization is focused on improving the quality of health care. They accredit health plans and other organizations and promote continuous quality improvement practices

(www.ncqa.org).

The Substance Abuse and Mental Health Services Administration (SAMHSA): SAMHSA is the governmental agency tasked with overseeing the public health efforts to address mental health and substance abuse in the United States. They are part of the Department of Health and Human Services. Their vision statement is recovery-based and focuses on prevention, treatment, and overall well-being.

The SAMHSA website is easy to search and contains a wealth of information, including treatment guidelines, DVDs, and materials for people in recovery, as well as for family members. Most of SAMHSA's publications can be downloaded or ordered for free. They also maintain a mailing list where all new publications are announced and offered to the public

(www.samhsa.gov).

a. The National Registry of Evidence-Based Programs and Practices (NREPP): This is SAMHSA's easily searchable database with hundreds of evidence-based interventions (www.nrepp.samhsa.gov/Index.aspx).

b. The National Survey on Drug Use and Health (NSDUH): This survey provides national and state data on tobacco, alcohol, and drug use (https://nsduhweb.rti.org).

U.S. Department of Health and Human Services: Agency for Healthcare Research and Quality (AHRQ)

a. National Guideline Clearinghouse (NGC): The NGC is a public resource for evidence-based practice guidelines. It is easily searchable and includes guidelines for medical, mental, and substance use disorders (www.guideline.gov).

b. Patient-Centered Medical Home Resource Center: This site provides information regarding primary care practices that have transformed the organization and delivery of primary care (www.pcmh.ahrq.gov).

The World Health Organization (WHO): The mission of this organization is to allow people across the globe to obtain the highest possible level of health

(www.who.org).

REFERENCES

American Psychiatric Association. (2000). *Diagnostic and statistical manual of mental disorders* (4th ed.). https://dsm.psychiatryonline.org/doi/book/10.1176/appi.books.9780890420249.dsm-iv-tr

American Psychiatric Association. (2013). *Diagnostic and statistical manual of mental disorders* (5th ed.). https://dsm.psychiatryonline.org/doi/book/10.1176/appi.books.9780890425596

Atkins, C. (2014). *Co-Occurring Disorders; Integrated Assessment, Treatment of Substance Use and Mental Disorders.* PESI Publishing and Media.

Center for Substance Abuse Treatment. (2015). *Substance abuse treatment for persons with co-occurring disorders.* Treatment Improvement Protocol (TIP) Series 42. DHHS Publication No. (SMA) 05-3992. Substance Abuse and Mental Health Services Administration. https://www.ncbi.nlm.nih.gov/books/NBK64197/

Croghan, T. W., & Brown, J. D. (2010). *Integrating mental health treatment into the patient-centered medical home.* (Prepared by Mathematica Policy Research under Contract No. HHSA290200900019I TO2.) AHRQ Publication No. 10-0084-EF. Agency for Healthcare Research and Quality. https://pcmh.ahrq.

gov/sites/default/files/attachments/Integrating%20Mental%20Health%20 and%20Substance%20Use%20Treatment%20in%20the%20PCMH.pdf

Drake, R. E., Essock, S. M., Shaner, A., Carey, K. B., Minkoff, K., Kola, L., Lynde, D., Osher, F. C., Clark, R. E., & Rickards, L. (2001). Implementing dual diagnosis services for clients with severe mental illness. *Psychiatric Services, 52*(4), 469–476. https://doi.org/10.1176/appi.ps.52.4.469

Drake, R. E., & Wallach, M. A. (2000). Dual diagnosis: 15 years of progress. *Psychiatric Services, 51*(9), 1126–1129. https://doi.org/10.1176/appi. ps.51.9.1126

Brunton, L., Chabner, B., & Knollman, B. (Eds.). (2011). *Goodman & Gilman's: The pharmacological basis of therapeutics* (12th ed.). McGraw-Hill.

Minkoff, K. (2001). Best practices: Developing standards of care for individuals with co-occurring psychiatric and substance use disorders. *Psychiatric Services, 52*(5), 597–599. https://doi.org/10.1176/appi.ps.52.5.597

The National Council for Community Behavioral Healthcare. (April 2009). *Behavioral health/primary care integration and the person-centered healthcare home.* https://www.thenationalcouncil.org/wp-content/uploads/2018/10/ BehavioralHealthandPrimaryCareIntegrationandthePCMH-2009. pdf?daf=375ateTbd56

O'Brien, C. P., Charney, D. S., Lewis, L., Cornish, J. W., Post, R. M., Woody, G. E., Zubieta, J.-K., Anthony, J. C., Blaine, J. D., Bowden, C. L., Calabrese, J. R., Carroll, K., Kosten, T., Rounsaville, B., Childress, A. R., Oslin, D. W., Pettinati, H. M., Davis, M. A., DeMartino, R., … Weisner, C. (2004). Priority actions to improve the care of persons with co-occurring substance abuse and other mental disorders: A call to action. *Biological Psychiatry, 56*(10), 703–713. https://doi.org/10.1016/j.biopsych.2004.10.002

Substance Abuse and Mental Health Services Administration. (2019). *Key substance use and mental health indicators in the United States: Results from the 2018 National Survey on Drug Use and Health* (HHS Publication No. PEP19-5068, NSDUH Series H-54). Center for Behavioral Health Statistics and Quality, Substance Abuse and Mental Health Services Administration. https://www.samhsa.gov/ data/sites/default/files/cbhsq-reports/NSDUHNationalFindingsReport2018/ NSDUHNationalFindingsReport2018.pdf

Substance Abuse and Mental Health Services Administration. (2013). SAMHSA's working definition of recovery: 10 guiding principles of recovery. https://store. samhsa.gov/sites/default/files/d7/priv/pep12-recdef.pdf

Substance Abuse and Mental Health Services Administration, Health Resources and Services Administration. (May 2012). *Behavioral health homes for people with mental health and substance use conditions.* https://www.samhsa.gov/find-help/treatment

Chapters 2 through 6: The Comprehensive Assessment through Treatment-and-Recovery Plans

Resources

The MacArthur Violence Risk Assessment Study: This study was conducted by the MacArthur Research Network on Mental Health and the Law to ascertain the risk of violence for individuals discharged from psychiatric hospitals (https://macarthur.virginia.edu/risk.html).

References

American Psychiatric Association. (2013). *Diagnostic and statistical manual of mental disorders* (5th ed.). https://dsm.psychiatryonline.org/doi/book/10.1176/appi.books.9780890425596

American Psychiatric Association. (2000). *Diagnostic and statistical manual of mental disorders* (4th ed.). https://dsm.psychiatryonline.org/doi/book/10.1176/appi.books.9780890420249.dsm-iv-tr

Babor, T. F., Higgins-Biddle, J. C., Saunders, J. B., & Monteiro, M. G. (2001). *AUDIT: The Alcohol Use Disorders Identification Test.* (2nd ed.). World Health Organization, Department of Mental Health and Substance Dependence. https://whqlibdoc.who.int/hq/2001/WHO_MSD_MSB_01.6a.pdf?ua=1

Bachmann, S. (2018). Epidemiology of suicide and the psychiatric perspective. *International Journal of Environmental Research and Public Health, 15*(7), 1425. https://doi.org/10.3390/ijerph15071425

Ewing, J. A. (1984). Detecting alcoholism: The CAGE Questionnaire. *JAMA, 252*(14), 1905–1907. https://doi.org/10.1001/jama.1984.03350140051025

Hedegaard, H., Curtin, S. C., & Warner, M. (2018). *Suicide mortality in the United States, 1999–2017.* NCHS Data Brief, No. 330. National Center for Health Statistics. https://www.cdc.gov/nchs/data/databriefs/db330-h.pdf

Joint Commission. (2013). *A practical guide to documentation in behavioral health care* (4th ed.). Joint Commission Resources.

Joint Commission. *2012 behavioral health care requirements.* (Only available through the Joint Commission)

Kitchens, J. M. (1994). Does this patient have an alcohol problem? *JAMA, 272*(22), 1782–1787. https://doi.org/10.1001/jama.1994.03520220076034

Scott, C. L., & Resnick, P. J. (2013). Evaluating psychotic patients' risk of violence: A practical guide. *Current Psychiatry, 12*(5), 29–32.

Chapter 7: Levels of Care

RESOURCES

The American Society of Addiction Medicine (ASAM): This medical society is dedicated to increasing access to and improving the quality of addiction treatment (www.asam.org).

Alcoholics Anonymous (AA): This international mutual-aid program is intended to help people achieve sobriety using a 12-step approach (https://aa.org).

Narcotics Anonymous (NA): Based on the principles of AA, this organization is intended to help individuals with drug problems achieve abstinence (https://na.org).

REFERENCES

Bond, G. R., Drake, R. E., & Becker, D. R. (2008). An update on randomized controlled trials of evidence-based supported employment. *Psychiatric Rehabilitation Journal, 31*(4), 280–290. https://doi.org/10.2975/31.4.2008.280.290

Bond, G. R., Drake, R. E., Mueser, K. T., & Latimer, E. (2001). Assertive community treatment for people with severe mental illness: Critical ingredients and impact on patients. *Disability Management, Health Outcomes, 9*(3), 141–159. https://doi.org/10.2165/00115677-200109030-00003

Center for Substance Abuse Treatment. (2006). *Definitions and terms relating to co-occurring disorders*. COCE Overview Paper 1. DHHS Publication No. (SMA) 06-4163. Substance Abuse and Mental Health Services Administration; Center for Mental Health Services. https://centerforchildwelfare.org/kb/mentalhealth/COD_Definitions.pdf

Copeland, M. E. (1997). *Wellness recovery action plan*. Peach Press.

Davidson, L., Tondora, J., O'Connell, M. J., Kirk Jr, T., Rockholz, P., & Evans, A. C. (2007). Creating a recovery-oriented system of behavioral healthcare: Moving from concept to reality. *Psychiatric Rehabilitation Journal, 31*(1), 23–31. https://doi.org/10.2975/31.1.2007.23.31

Kidd, S. A., George, L., O'Connell, M., Sylvestre, J., Kirkpatrick, H., Browne, G., & Thabane, L. (2010). Fidelity and recovery-orientation in assertive community treatment. *Community Mental Health, 46*(4), 342–350. https://doi.org/10.1007/s10597-009-9275-7

Kolsky, G. D. (2006, November 1). *Current state AOD agency practices regarding the use of patient placement criteria (PPC)—an update*. www.asam.org/docs/publications/survey_of_state_use_of_ppc_nasadad-2006.pdf?Status=Master&sfvrsn=2

Mee-Lee, D. (Ed.). (2013). *The ASAM criteria: Treatment criteria for addictive, substance-related, and co-occurring conditions* (3rd ed.). The Change Companies.

Mueser, K. T., Corrigan, P. W., Hilton, D. W., Tanzman, B., Schaub, A., Gingerich, S., Essock, S. M., Tarrier, N., Morey, B., Vogel-Scibilia, S., & Herz, M. I. (2002). Illness management and recovery: A review of the research. *Psychiatric Services, 53*(10), 1272–1284. https://doi.org/10.1176/appi.ps.53.10.1272

Randall, G. E., Wakefield, P. A., & Richards, D. A. (2012). Fidelity to assertive community treatment program standards: A regional survey of adherence to standards. *Community Mental Health, 48*(2), 138–149. https://doi.org/10.1007/s10597-010-9353-x

Teague, G. B., Bond, G. R., & Drake, R. E. (1998). Program fidelity in assertive community treatment: Development and use of a measure. *American Journal of Orthopsychiatry, 68*(2), 216–232. https://doi.org/10.1037/h0080331

Watts, J., & Priebe, S. (2003). A phenomenological account of users' experiences of assertive community treatment. *Bioethics, 16*(5), 339–454. https://doi.org/10.1111/1467-8519.00301

Wholey, D. R., Zhu, X., Knoke, D., Shah, P., Zellmer-Bruhn, M., & Witheridge, T. F. (2012). The teamwork in assertive community treatment (TACT) scale: Development and validation. *Psychiatric Services, 63*(11), 1108–117. https://doi.org/10.1176/appi.ps.201100338

Chapter 8: Key Psychotherapies, Mutual Self-Help, and Natural and Peer Supports

REFERENCES

Beck, J. (2011). *Cognitive behavioral therapy: Basics and beyond* (2nd ed.). The Guilford Press.

Davis, M., Eshelman, E. R., & McKay, M. (2008). *The relaxation and stress reduction workbook*. New Harbinger Publications.

Kabat-Zinn, J. (1990). *Full catastrophe living: Using the wisdom of your body and mind to face stress, pain, and illness*. Delta.

Kabat-Zinn, J. (2005). *Wherever you go, there you are*. Hyperion.

Marlatt, A. (1998). *Harm reduction: Pragmatic strategies for managing high-risk behaviors*. The Guilford Press.

McKay, M., Davis, M., & Fanning, P. (1997). *Thoughts and feelings: Taking control of your mood and your life: A workbook of cognitive behavioral techniques*. New Harbinger Publications.

Miller, W. R., & Rollnick, S. (2002). *Motivational interviewing: Preparing people for change* (2nd ed.). The Guilford Press.

Nhat Hanh, T. (1999). *The miracle of mindfulness: An introduction to the practice of meditation*. Beacon Press.

Chapter 9: Wellness and Resilience

REFERENCES

Atkins, C. (2019). The Science of Sleep. *PARADE.*

Bhui, K., Dinos, S., Galant-Miecznikowska, M., de Jongh, B., & Stansfeld, S. (2016). Perceptions of work stress causes and effective interventions in employees working in public, private, and non-governmental organisations: A qualitative study. *BJPsych Bulletin, 40*(6), 318–325. https://doi.org/10.1192/pb.bp.115.050823

Centers for Disease Control and Prevention. (2018). *Physical activity guidelines for Americans* (2nd ed.). https://health.gov/paguidelines/second-edition/pdf/Physical_Activity_Guidelines_2nd_edition.pdf

Centers for Disease Control and Prevention. (2019, September 12). *New CDC obesity prevalence maps: Nine states report obesity rates at or above 35 percent.* https://www.cdc.gov/media/releases/2019/s0912-obesity-prevalence-maps.html

Donnelly, J. E., Blair, S. N., Jakicic, J. M., Manore, M. M., Rankin, J. W., & Smith, B. K. (2009). Appropriate physical activity intervention strategies for weight loss and prevention of weight regain for adults. *Medicine & Science in Sports & Exercise, 41*(2), 459–471. https://doi.org/10.1249/MSS.0b013e3181949333

Holt-Lunstad, J., Smith, T. B., & Layton, J. B. (2010). Social relationships and mortality risk: A meta-analytic review. *PLoS Medicine, 7*(7), Article e1000316. https://doi.org/10.1371/journal.pmed.1000316

Hooker, S. A., Masters, K. S., & Park, C. L. (2018). A meaningful life is a healthy life: A conceptual model linking meaning and meaning salience to health. *Review of General Psychology, 21*(1), 11–24. https://doi.org/10.1037/gpr0000115

Huang, P. L. (2009). A comprehensive definition for metabolic syndrome. *Disease Models & Mechanisms, 2*(5–6), 231–237. https://doi.org/10.1242/dmm.001180

Laville, M., Segrestin, B., Alligier, M., Ruano-Rodríguez, C., Serra-Majem, L., Hiesmayr, M., Schols, A., La Vecchia, C., Boirie, Y., Rath, A., Neugebauer, E. A. M., Garattini, S., Bertele, V., Kubiak, C., Demotes-Mainard, J., Jakobsen, J. C., Djurisic, S., & Gluud, C. (2017). Evidence-based practice within nutrition: What are the barriers for improving the evidence and how can they be dealt with? *Trials, 18*, Article 425. https://doi.org/10.1186/s13063-017-2160-8

Martin, C. K., Church, T. S., Thompson, A. M., Earnest, C. P., & Blair, S. N. (2009). Exercise dose and quality of life: A randomized controlled trial. *Archives of Internal Medicine, 169*(3), 269–278. https://doi.org/10.1001/archinternmed.2008.545

Neale, E. P., & Tapsell, L. C. (2019). Perspective: The evidence-based framework in nutrition and dietetics: Implementation, challenges, and future directions. *Advances in Nutrition, 10*(1), 1–8. https://doi.org/10.1093/advances/nmy113

Pelchat, M. L. (2009). Food addiction in humans. *The Journal of Nutrition, 139*(3), 620–622. https://doi.org/10.3945/jn.108.097816

Persson, P. B., & Bondke Persson, A. (2017). Hunger, craving and appetite. *Acta Physiologica, 221*(1), 3–5. https://doi.org/10.1111/apha.12917

Southwick, S., & Charney, D. (2012). *Resilience: The science of mastering life's greatest challenges.* Cambridge University Press.

Swift, D. L., Lavie, C. J., Johannsen, N. M., Arena, R., Earnest, C. P., O'Keefe, J. H., Milani, R. V., Blair, S. N., & Church, T. S. (2013). Physical activity, cardiorespiratory fitness, and exercise training in primary and secondary coronary prevention. *Circulation Journal, 77*(2), 281–292. https://doi.org/10.1253/circj.CJ-13-0007

Umberson, D., & Montez, J. K. (2015). Social relationships and health: A flashpoint for health policy. *Journal of Health and Social Behavior, 51*(Suppl. 1), S54–S66. https://doi.org/10.1177/0022146510383501

Wing, R. R., Lang, W., Wadden, T. A., Safford, M., Knowler, W. C., Bertoni, A. G., Hill, J. O., Brancati, F. L., Peters, A., Wagenknecht, L., & the Look AHEAD Research Group. (2011). Benefits of modest weight loss in improving cardiovascular risk factors in overweight and obese individuals with type 2 diabetes. *Diabetes Care, 34*(7), 1481–1486. https://doi.org/10.2337/dc10-2415

Yang, Y. C., Boen, C., Gerken, K., Li, T., Schorpp, K., & Harris, K. M. (2016). Social relationships and physiological determinants of longevity across the human life span. *Proceedings of the National Academy of Sciences, 113*(3), 578–583. https://doi.org/10.1073/pnas.1511085112

Chapter 10: Co-Occurring Attention-Deficit/Hyperactivity Disorder and Related Disorders

RESOURCES

Attention Deficit Disorder Association: This nonprofit organization maintains an excellent website geared toward parents, people with ADHD, and clinicians. It includes information and links to downloadable screening tools, including the SNAP-IV (https://add.org/resources/).

Adult ADHD Self-Report Scale-V1.1 (ASRS-V1.1): Downloadable files for both the six-item screening tool and full eighteen-question symptom checklist are available through Harvard's webpage for the National Comorbidity Survey (www.hcp.med.harvard.edu/ncs/asrs.php).

REFERENCES

Blix, O., Dalteg, A., & Nilsson, P. (2009). Treatment of opioid dependence and ADHD/ADD with opioid maintenance and central stimulants. *Heroin Addiction and Related Clinical Problems, 11*, 5–14.

Carpentier, P. J., van Gogh, M. T., Knapen, L. J. M., Buitelaar, J. K., & De Jong, C. A. J. (2011). Influence of attention deficit hyperactivity disorder and conduct disorder on opioid dependence severity and psychiatric comorbidity in chronic methadone-maintained patients. *European Addiction Research, 17*(1), 10–20. https://doi.org/10.1159/000321259

Charach, A., Yeung, E., Climans, T., & Lillie, E. (2011). Childhood attention-deficit/hyperactivity disorder and future substance use disorders: Comparative meta-analyses. *Journal of the American Academy of Child & Adolescent Psychiatry, 50*(1), 9–21. https://doi.org/10.1016/j.jaac.2010.09.019

Daigre, C., Ramos-Quiroga, J. A., Valero, S., Bosch, R., Roncero, C., Gonzalvo, B., Nogueira, M., & Casas, M. (2009). Adult ADHD Self-Report Scale (ASRS-v1.1) symptom checklist in patients with substance use disorders. *Actas Españolas Psiquiatria, 37*(6), 299–305.

Dakwar, E., Mahony, M. A., Pavlicova, M., Glass, M. A., Brooks, M. D., Mariani, J. J., Grabowski, J., & Levin, F. R. (2012). The utility of attention-deficit/hyperactivity disorder screening instruments in individuals seeking treatment for substance use disorders. *Journal of Clinical Psychiatry, 73*(11), 1372–1378. https://doi.org/10.4088/JCP.12m07895.

Faraone, S. V., Wilens, T. E., Petty, C., Antshel, K., Spencer, T., & Biederman, J. (2007). Substance use among ADHD adults: Implications of late onset and subthreshold diagnoses. *The American Journal on Addictions, 16*(S1), 24–34. https://doi.org/10.1080/10550490601082767

Kessler, R. C., Adler, L., Barkley, R., Biederman, J., Conners, C. K., Demler, O., Faraone, S. V., Greenhill, L. L., Howes, M. J., Secnik, K., Spencer, T., Ustun, B., Walters, E. E., & Zaslavsky, A. M. (2006). The prevalence and correlates of adult ADHD in the United States: Results from the National Comorbidity Survey Replication. *American Journal of Psychiatry, 163*(4), 716–723. https://doi.org/10.1176/ajp.2006.163.4.716

Knop, J., Penick, E. C., Nickel, E. J., Mortensen, E. L., Sullivan, M. A., Murtaza, S., Jensen, P., Manzardo, A. M., & Gabrielli, W. F. (2009). Childhood ADHD and conduct disorder as independent predictors of male alcohol dependence at age 40. *Journal of Studies on Alcohol and Drugs, 70*(2), 169–177. https://doi.org/10.15288/jsad.2009.70.169

Levin, F. R., Evans, S. M., Brooks, D. J., Kalbag, A. S., Garawi, F., & Nunes, E. V. (2006). Treatment of methadone-maintained patients with adult ADHD: Double-blind comparison of methylphenidate, bupropion, and placebo. *Drug Alcohol Dependence, 81*(2), 137–148. https://doi.org/10.1016/j.drugalcdep.2005.06.012

McAweeney, M., Rogers, N. L., Huddleston, C., Moore, D., & Gentile, J. P. (2010). Symptom prevalence of ADHD in a community residential substance abuse treatment program. *Journal of Attention Disorders, 13*(6), 601–608. https://doi.org/10.1177/1087054708329973

The MTA Cooperative Group. (1999). A 14-month randomized clinical trial of treatment strategies for attention-deficit/hyperactivity disorder. *Archives of General Psychiatry, 56*(12), 1073–1086. https://doi.org/10.1001/archpsyc.56.12.1073

Murphy, P., & Schachar, R. (2000). Use of self-ratings in the assessment of symptoms of attention deficit hyperactivity disorder in adults. *American Journal of Psychiatry, 157*(7), 1156–1159. https://doi.org/10.1176/appi.ajp.157.7.1156

Roy, A. (2008). The relationships between attention-deficit/hyperactive disorder (ADHD), conduct disorder (CD) and problematic drug use (PDU). *Drugs: Education, Prevention and Policy, 15*(1), 55–75. https://doi.org/10.1080/09687630701489481

Safren, S. A., Otto, M. W., Sprich, S., Winett, C. L., Wilens, T. E., & Biederman, J. (2005). Cognitive-behavioral therapy for ADHD in medication-treated adults with continued symptoms. *Behaviour Research and Therapy, 43*(7), 831–842. https://doi.org/10.1016/j.brat.2004.07.001

Sandra Kooij, J. J., Marije Boonstra, A., Swinkels, S. H. N., Bekker, E. M., De Noord, I., & Buitelaar, J. K. (2008). Reliability, validity, and utility of instruments for self-report and informant report concerning symptoms of ADHD in adult patients. *Journal of Attention Disorders, 11*, 445–458. https://doi.org/10.1177/1087054707299367

Schubiner, H., Tzelepis, A., Milberger, S., Lockhart, N., Kruger, M., Kelley, B. J., & Schoener, E. P. (2000). Prevalence of attention-deficit/hyperactivity disorder and conduct disorder among substance abusers. *Journal of Clinical Psychiatry, 61*(4), 244–251. https://doi.org/10.4088/JCP.v61n0402

Sepúlveda, D. R., Thomas, L. M., McCabe, S. E., Cranford, J. A., Boyd, C. J., & Teter, C. J. (2011). Misuse of prescribed stimulant medication for ADHD and associated patterns of substance use: Preliminary analysis among college students. *Journal of Pharmacy Practice, 24*(6), 551–560. https://doi.org/10.1177/0897190011426558

Solanto, M. V., Marks, D. J., Wasserstein, J., Mitchell, K., Abikoff, H., Alvir, J. M. J., & Kofman, M. D. (2010). Efficacy of meta-cognitive therapy for adult ADHD. *American Journal of Psychiatry, 167*(8), 958–968. https://doi.org/10.1176/appi.ajp.2009.09081123

Warden, D., Riggs, P. D., Min, S. J., Mikulich-Gilbertson, S. K., Tamm, L., Trello-Rishel, K., & Winhusen, T. (2012). Major depression and treatment response in adolescents with ADHD and substance use disorder. *Drug and Alcohol Dependence, 120*(1–3), 214–219. https://doi.org/10.1016/j.drugalcdep.2011.08.001

Wilens, T. E., Martelon, M., Joshi, G., Bateman, C., Fried, R., Petty, C., & Biederman, J. (2011). Does ADHD predict substance-use disorders? A 10-year follow-up study of young adults with ADHD. *Journal of the American Academy of Child & Adolescent Psychiatry, 50*(6), 543–553. https://doi.org/10.1016/j.jaac.2011.01.021

Wilens, T. E., & Morrison, N. R. (2011). The intersection of attention-deficit/hyperactivity disorder and substance abuse. *Current Opinions in Psychiatry, 24*(4), 280–285. https://doi.org/10.1097/YCO.0b013e328345c956

Winhusen, T. M., Lewis, D. F., Riggs, P. D., Davies, R. D., Adler, I. A., Sonne, S., & Somoza, E. C. (2011). Subjective effects, misuse, and adverse effects of osmotic-release methylpenidate treatment in adolescent substance abusers with attention-deficit/hyperactivity disorder. *Journal of Child and Adolescent Psychopharmacology, 21*(5), 455–463. https://doi.org/10.1089/cap.2011.0014

Chapter 11: Depressive Disorders and Co-Occurring Substance Use Disorders

REFERENCES

Blanco, C., Alegría, A. A., Liu, S. M., Secades-Villa, R., Sugaya, L., Davies, C., & Nunes, E. V. (2012). Differences among major depressive disorder with and without co-occurring substance use disorders and substance-induced depressive disorder: Results from the National Epidemiologic Survey on Alcohol and Related conditions. *Journal of Clinical Psychiatry, 73*(6), 865–873. https://doi.org/10.4088/JCP.10m06673

Brewer, J. A., Bowen, S., Smith, J. T., Marlatt, G. A., & Potenza, M. N. (2010). Mindfulness-based treatment for co-occurring depression and substance use disorders: What can we learn from the brain? *Addiction, 105*(10), 1698–1706. https://doi.org/10.1111/j.1360-0443.2009.02890.x

Busto, U. E., Sykora, K., & Sellers, E. M. (1989). A clinical scale to assess benzodiazepine withdrawal. *Journal of Clinical Psychopharmacology, 9*(6), 412–416. https://doi.org/10.1097/00004714-198912000-00005

Delgadilo, J., Godfrey, C., Gilbody, S., & Payne, S. (2013). Depression, anxiety and comorbid substance use: Association patterns in outpatient addictions treatment. *Mental Health and Substance Use, 6*(1), 59–75. https://doi.org/10.1080/17523281.2012.660981

Hides, L., Carroll, S., Catania, L., Cotton, S. M., Baker, A., Scaffidi, A., & Lubman, D. I. (2009). Outcomes of an integrated cognitive behavior therapy (CBT) treatment program for co-occurring depression and substance misuse in young people. *Journal of Affective Disorders, 121*(1–2), 169–174. https://doi.org/10.1016/j.jad.2009.06.002

Hides, L., Samet, S., & Lubman, D. I. (2010). Cognitive behaviour therapy (CBT) for the treatment of co-occurring depression and substance use: Current evidence and directions for future research. *Drug and Alcohol Review, 29*(5), 508–517. https://doi.org/10.1111/j.1465-3362.2010.00207.x

Hunter, S. B., Watkins, K. E., Hepner, K. A., Paddock, S. M., Ewing, B. A., Osilla, K. C., & Perry, S. (2012). Treating depression and substance use: A randomized controlled trial. *Journal of Substance Abuse Treatment, 43*(2), 137–151. https://doi.org/10.1016/j.jsat.2011.12.004

Iovieno, N., Tedeschini, E., Bentley, K. H., Evins, A. E., & Papakostas, G. I. (2011). Antidepressants for major depressive disorder and dysthymic disorder in patients with comorbid alcohol use disorders: A meta-analysis of placebo-controlled randomized trials. *Journal of Clinical Psychiatry, 72*(8), 1144–1151. https://doi.org/10.4088/JCP.10m06217

Langås, A. M., Malt, U. F., & Opjordsmoen, S. (2013). Independent versus substance-induced major depressive disorders in first-admission patients with substance use disorders: An exploratory study. *Journal of Affective Disorders, 144*(3), 279–283. https://doi.org/10.1016/j.jad.2012.10.008

Lydecker, K. P., Tate, S. R., Cummins, K. M., McQuaid, J., Granholm, E., & Brown, S. A. (2010). Clinical outcomes of an integrated treatment for depression and substance use disorders. *Psychology of Addictive Behaviors, 24*(3), 453–465. https://doi.org/10.1037/a0019943

Lyness, J. M. (2011). Clinical manifestations and diagnosis of depression. *UpToDate.* Retrieved September 3, 2020, from https://somepomed.org/articulos/contents/mobipreview.htm?33/15/34032

Marmorstein, N. R. (2011). Associations between subtypes of major depressive episodes and substance use disorders. *Psychiatry Research, 186*(2–3), 248–253. https://doi.org/10.1016/j.psychres.2010.10.003

Osilla, K. C., Hepner, K. A., Muñoz, R. F., Woo, S., & Watkins, K. (2009). Developing an integrated treatment for substance use and depression using cognitive-behavioral therapy. *Journal of Substance Abuse Treatment, 27*(4), 412–420. https://doi.org/10.1016/j.jsat.2009.04.006

Pettinati, H. M., O'Brien, C. P., & Dundon, W. D. (2013). Current status of co-occurring mood and substance use disorders: A new therapeutic target. *American Journal of Psychiatry, 170*(1), 23–30. https://doi.org/10.1176/appi.ajp.2012.12010112

Schukit, M. A., Smith, T. L., & Kalmijn, J. (2013). Relationships among independent major depressions, alcohol use, and other substance use and related problems over 30 years in 397 families. *Journal of Studies on Alcohol and Drugs, 74*(2), 271–279. https://doi.org/10.15288/jsad.2013.74.271

The Workgroup on Major Depressive Disorder. (2013). *Practice guideline for the treatment of patients with major depressive disorder* (3rd ed.). https://psychiatryonline.org/pb/assets/raw/sitewide/practice_guidelines/guidelines/mdd.pdf

Chapter 12: Bipolar Disorder and Co-Occurring Substance Use Disorders

RESOURCES

The Depression and Bipolar Support Alliance: This is a peer-directed, not-for-profit organization for people with mood disorders (www.dbsalliance.org).

REFERENCES

Atkins, C. (2007). *The bipolar disorder answer book: Answers to more than 275 of your most pressing questions.* Sourcebooks.

Brown, E. S., Carmody, T. J., Schmitz, J. M., Caetano, R., Adinoff, B., Swann, A. C., & Rush, A. J. (2009). A randomized, double-blind, placebo-controlled pilot study of naltrexone in outpatients with bipolar disorder and alcohol dependence. *Alcoholism: Clinical and Experimental Research, 33*(11), 1863–1869. https://doi.org/10.1111/j.1530-0277.2009.01024.x

Duffy, A., Horrocks, J., Milin, R., Doucette, S., Persson, G., & Grof, P. (2012). Adolescent substance use disorder during the early stages of bipolar disorder: A prospective high-risk study. *Journal of Affective Disorders, 142*(1–3), 57–64. https://doi.org/10.1016/j.jad.2012.04.010

Farren, C. K., Hill, K. P., & Weiss, R. D. (2012). Bipolar disorder and alcohol use disorder: A review. *Current Psychiatry Reports, 14*(6), 659–666. https://doi.org/10.1007/s11920-012-0320-9

Farren, C. K., & McElroy, S. (2010). Predictive factors for relapse after an integrated inpatient treatment program for unipolar depressed and bipolar alcoholics. *Alcohol and Alcoholism, 45*(6), 527–533. https://doi.org/10.1093/alcalc/agq060

Frank, E., Kupfer, D. J., Thase, M. E., Mallinger, A. G., Swartz, H. A., Fagiolini, A. M., Grochocinski, V., Houck, P., Scott, J., Thompson, W., & Monk, T. (2005). Two-year outcomes for interpersonal and social rhythm therapy in individuals with bipolar I disorder. *Archives of General Psychiatry, 62*(9), 996–1004. https://doi.org/10.1001/archpsyc.62.9.996

Lam, D. H., Watkins, E. R., Hayward, P., Bright, J., Wright, K., Kerr, N., Parr-Davis, G., & Sham, P. (2003). A randomized controlled study of cognitive therapy for relapse prevention for bipolar affective disorder: Outcome of the first year. *Archives of General Psychiatry, 60*(2), 145–152. https://doi.org/10.1001/archpsyc.60.2.145

Large, M., Sharma, S., Compton, M. T., Slade, T., & Nielssen, O. (2011). Cannabis use and earlier onset of psychosis: A systematic meta-analysis. *Archives of General Psychiatry, 68*(6), 555–561. https://doi.org/10.1001/archgenpsychiatry.2011.5

McGorry, P. (2011). Transition to adulthood: The critical period for pre-emptive disease-modifying care for schizophrenia and related disorders. *Schizophrenia Bulletin, 37*(3), 524–530. https://doi.org/10.1093/schbul/sbr027

Merikangas, K. R., Akiskal, H. S., Angst, J., Greenberg, P. E., Hirschfeld, R. M., Petukhova, M., & Kessler, R. C. (2007). Lifetime and 12-month prevalence of bipolar spectrum disorder in the National Comorbidity Survey replication. *Archives of General Psychiatry, 64*(5), 543–552. https://doi.org/10.1001/archpsyc.64.5.543

Miklowitz, D. J., George, E. L., Richards, J. A., Simoneau, T. L., & Suddath, R. L. (2003). A randomized study of family-focused psychoeducation and pharmacotherapy in the outpatient management of bipolar disorder. *Archives of General Psychiatry, 60*(9), 904–912. https://doi.org/10.1001/archpsyc.60.9.904

Salloum, I. M., Cornelius, J. R., Daley, D. C., Kirisci, L., Himmelhoch, J. M., & Thase, M. E. (2005). Efficacy of valproate maintenance in patients with bipolar disorder and alcoholism: A double-blind placebo-controlled study. *Archives of General Psychiatry, 62*(1), 37–45. https://doi.org/10.1001/archpsyc.62.1.37

Salloum, I. M., & Thase, M. E. (2000). Impact of substance abuse on the course and treatment of bipolar disorder. *Bipolar Disorders, 2*(3), 269–280. https://doi.org/10.1034/j.1399-5618.2000.20308.x

Schimmelmann, B. G., Conus, P., Cotton, S., Kupferschmid, S., McGorry, P. D., & Lambert, M. (2012). Prevalence and impact of cannabis use disorders in adolescents with early onset first episode psychosis. *European Psychiatry, 27*(6), 463–469. https://doi.org/10.1016/j.eurpsy.2011.03.001

Swann, A. C. (2010). The strong relationship between bipolar and substance-use disorder. *Annals of the New York Academy of Science, 1187*(1), 276–293. https://doi.org/10.1111/j.1749-6632.2009.05146.x

Tolliver, B. K., DeSantis, S. M., Brown, D. G., Prisciandaro, J. J., & Brady, K. T. (2012). A randomized, double-blind, placebo-controlled trial of acamprosate in alcohol-dependent individuals with bipolar disorder: A preliminary report. *Bipolar Disorders, 14*(1), 54–63. https://doi.org/10.1111/j.1399-5618.2011.00973.x

Tolliver, B. K., & Hartwell, K. J. (2012). Implications and strategies for clinical management of co-occurring substance use in bipolar disorder. *Psychiatric Annals, 42*(5), 190–197. https://doi.org/10.3928/00485713-20120507-07

Weiss, R. D., Griffin, M. L., Jaffee, W. B., Bender, R. E., Graff, F. S., Gallop, R. J., & Fitzmaurice, G. M. (2009). A "community friendly" version of integrated group therapy for patients with bipolar disorder and substance dependence: A randomized controlled trial. *Drug and Alcohol Dependence, 104*(3), 212–219. https://doi.org/10.1016/j.drugalcdep.2009.04.018

Weiss, R. D., Griffin, M. L., Kolodziej, M. E., Greenfield, S. F., Najavits, L. M., Daley, D. C., Doreau, H. R., & Hennen, J. A. (2007). A randomized trial of integrated group therapy versus group drug counseling for patients with bipolar disorder and substance dependence. *American Journal of Psychiatry, 164*(1), 100–107. https://doi.org/10.1176/ajp.2007.164.1.100

Chapter 13: Anxiety Disorders and Co-Occurring Substance Use Disorders

REFERENCES

Baker, A. L., Thornton, L. K., Hiles, S., Hides, L., & Lubman, D. I. (2012). Psychological interventions for alcohol misuse among people with co-occurring depression or anxiety disorders: A systematic review. *Journal of Affective Disorders, 139*(3), 217–229. https://doi.org/10.1016/j.jad.2011.08.004

Fatséas, M., Denis, C., Lavie, E., & Auriacombe, M. (2010). Relationship between anxiety disorders and opiate dependence—a systematic review of the literature: Implications for diagnosis and treatment. *Journal of Substance Abuse Treatment, 38*(3), 220–230. https://doi.org/10.1016/j.jsat.2009.12.003

Magidson, J. F., Liu, S. M., Lejuez, C. W., & Blanco, C. (2012). Comparison of the course of substance use disorders among individuals with and without generalized anxiety disorder in a nationally representative sample. *Journal of Psychiatric Research, 46*(5), 659–666. https://doi.org/10.1016/j.jpsychires.2012.02.011

Marmorstein, N. R. (2012). Anxiety disorders and substance use disorders: Different associations by anxiety disorder. *Journal of Anxiety Disorders, 26*(1), 88–94. https://doi.org/10.1016/j.janxdis.2011.09.005

Merikangas, K. R., & Swanson, S. A. (2009). *Comorbidity in anxiety disorders.* In M. B. Stein & T. Steckler (Eds.), *Behavioral neurobiology of anxiety and its treatment* (pp. 37–59). Springer.

Reedy, A. R., & Hall, J. A. (2008). Treatment issues with substance use disorder clients who have mood or anxiety disorders. *Mental Health and Substance Use: Dual Diagnosis, 1*(1), 44–53. https://doi.org/10.1080/17523280701741738

Smith, J. P., & Book, S. W. (2010). Comorbidity of generalized anxiety disorder and alcohol use disorders among individuals seeking outpatient substance abuse treatment. *Addictive Behaviors, 35*(1), 42–45. https://doi.org/10.1016/j.addbeh.2009.07.002

Watkins, K. E., Hunter, S. B., Burnam, M. A., Pincus, H. A., & Nicholson, G. (2005). Review of treatment recommendations for persons with a co-occurring affective or anxiety and substance use disorder. *Psychiatric Services, 56*(8), 913–926. https://doi.org/10.1176/appi.ps.56.8.913

Watkins, K. E., Hunter, S. B., Wenzel, S. L., Tu, W., Paddock, S. M., Griffin, A., & Ebener, P. (2004). Prevalence and characteristics of clients with co-occurring disorders in outpatient substance abuse treatment. *The American Journal of Drug and Alcohol Abuse, 30*(4), 749–764. https://doi.org/10.1081/ADA-200037538

Wolitzky-Taylor, K., Bobova, L., Zinbarg, R. E., Mineka, S., & Craske, M. G. (2012). Longitudinal investigation of the impact of anxiety and mood disorders in adolescence on subsequent substance use disorder onset and vice versa. *Addictive Behaviors, 37*(8), 982–985. https://doi.org/10.1016/j.addbeh.2012.03.026

Chapter 14: Posttraumatic Stress Disorder and Co-Occurring Substance Use Disorders

RESOURCES

International Society for Traumatic Stress Studies (ISTSS): This organization shares information about the effects of trauma and also discusses initiatives to reduce the impact of traumatic stressors and their immediate and long-term consequences (www.istss.org).

The National Center for PTSD (U.S. Department of Veterans Affairs): This rich resource provides access to free online trainings, many of which offer continuing education (CE) and continuing medical education (CME) credits (www.ptsd.va.gov/index.asp).

REFERENCES

Benish, S., Imel, Z. E., & Wampold, B. E. (2008). The relative efficacy of bona fide psychotherapies for treating post-traumatic stress disorder: A meta-analysis of direct comparisons. *Clinical Psychology Review, 28*(5), 746–758. https://doi.org/10.1016/j.cpr.2007.10.005

Berenz, E. C., & Coffey, S. F. (2012). Treatment of co-occurring posttraumatic stress disorder and substance use disorders. *Current Psychiatry Reports, 14*(5), 469–477. https://doi.org/10.1007/s11920-012-0300-0

Bisson, J., & Andrew, M. (2007). Psychological treatment of post-traumatic stress disorder (PTSD). *Cochrane Database of Systematic Reviews.* https://doi.org/10.1002/14651858.CD003388.pub3

Bliese, P. D., Wright, K. M., Adler, A. B., Cabrera, O., Castro, C. A., & Hoge, C. W. (2008). Validating the Primary Care Posttraumatic Stress Disorder Screen and the Posttraumatic Stress Disorder Checklist with soldiers returning from combat. *Journal of Consulting and Clinical Psychology, 76*(2), 272–281. https://doi.org/10.1037/0022-006X.76.2.272

Brady, K. T., Back, S. E., & Coffey, S. F. (2004). Substance abuse and posttraumatic stress disorder. *Current Directions in Psychological Science, 13*(5), 206–209. https://doi.org/10.1111/j.0963-7214.2004.00309.x

Bradley, R., Greene, J., Russ, E., Dutra, L., & Westen, D. (2005). A multidimensional meta-analysis of psychotherapy for PTSD. *American Journal of Psychiatry, 162*(2), 214–227. https://doi.org/10.1176/appi.ajp.162.2.214

Breslau, N., Peterson, E. L., Kessler, R. C., & Schultz, L. R. (1999). Short screening scale for DSM-IV post-traumatic stress disorder. *American Journal of Psychiatry, 156*(6), 908–911. https://doi.org/10.1176/ajp.156.6.908

Brewin, C. R. (2005). Systematic review of screening instruments for adults at risk of PTSD. *Journal of Traumatic Stress, 18*(1), 53–62. https://doi.org/10.1002/jts.20007

Coffey, S. F., Schumacher, J. A., Brady, K. T., & Cotton, B. D. (2007). Changes in PTSD symptomatology during acute and protracted alcohol and cocaine abstinence. *Drug and Alcohol Dependence, 87*(2–3), 241–248. https://doi.org/10.1016/j.drugalcdep.2006.08.025

Department of Veterans Affairs and Department of Defense. (2017). VA/DOD clinical practice guideline for the management of posttraumatic stress disorder. https://www.healthquality.va.gov/guidelines/MH/ptsd/VADoDPTSDCPGFinal.pdf

Donovan, B., Padin-Rivera, E., & Kowaliw, S. (2001). "Transcend" initial outcomes from a posttraumatic stress disorder/substance abuse treatment program. *Journal of Traumatic Stress, 14*(4), 757–772. https://doi.org/10.1023/A:1013094206154

Eftekhari, A., Ruzek, J. I., Crowley, J. J., Rosen, C. S., Greenbaum, M. A., & Karlin, B. E. (2013). Effectiveness of national implementation of prolonged exposure therapy in Veterans Affairs care. *JAMA Psychiatry, 70*(9), 949–955. https://doi.org/10.1001/jamapsychiatry.2013.36

Ferri, M., Amato, L., & Davoli, M. (2006). Alcoholics Anonymous and other 12-step programmes for alcohol dependence. *Cochrane Database of Systematic Reviews.* https://doi.org/10.1002/14651858.CD005032.pub2

Foa, E. B., Keane, T. M., Friedman, M. J., & Cohen, J. A. (Eds.). (2009). *Effective treatments for PTSD: Practice guidelines from the International Society for Traumatic Stress Studies* (2nd ed.). The Guilford Press.

Greyber, L., Dulmus, C. N., & Cristalli, M. E. (2012). Eye movement desensitization reprocessing, posttraumatic stress disorder, and trauma: A review of randomized controlled trials with children and adolescents. *Child Adolescent Social Work Journal, 29*(5), 409–425. https://doi.org/10.1007/s10560-012-0266-0

Harrington, T., & Newman, E. (2007). The psychometric utility of two self-report measures of PTSD among women substance users. *Addictive Behaviors, 32*(12), 2788–2798. https://doi.org/10.1016/j.addbeh.2007.04.016

Johnson, B. A., Rosenthal, N., Capece, J. A., Wiegand, F., Mao, L., Beyers, K., McKay, A., Ait-Daoud, N., Anton, R. F., Ciraulo, D. A., Kranzler, H. R., Mann, K., O'Malley, S., & Swift, R. M. (2007). Topiramate for treating alcohol dependence—a randomized controlled trial. *JAMA, 298*(14), 1641–1651. https://doi.org/10.1001/jama.298.14.1641

Johnson, B. A. (2008). Update on neuropharmacological treatments for alcoholism: Scientific basis and clinical findings. *Biochemical Pharmacology, 75*(1), 34–35. https://doi.org/10.1016/j.bcp.2007.08.005

Kessler, R. C., Chiu, W. T., Demler, O., & Walters, E. E. (2005). Prevalence, severity, and comorbidity of 12-month DSM-IV disorder in the National Comorbidity Survey Replication. *Archives of General Psychiatry, 62*(6), 617–627. https://doi.org/10.1001/archpsyc.62.6.617

Killeen, T., Hien, D., Campbell, A., Brown, C., Hansen, C., Jiang, H., Kristman-Valente, A., Neuenfeldt, C., Rocz-de la Luz, N., Sampson, R., Suarez-Morales, L., Wells, E., Brigham, G., & Nunes, E. (2008). Adverse events in an integrated trauma-focused intervention for women in community substance abuse treatment. *Journal of Substance Abuse Treatment, 35*(3), 304–311. https://doi.org/10.1016/j.jsat.2007.12.001

Killeen, T., Back, S. E., & Brady, K. T. (2011). The use of exposure-based treatment among individuals with PTSD and co-occurring substance use disorders: Clinical considerations. *Journal of Dual Diagnosis, 7*(4), 194–206. https://doi.org/10.1080/15504263.2011.620421

Krystal, J. H., & Neumeister, A. (2009). Noradrenergic and serotonergic mechanisms in the neurobiology of posttraumatic stress disorder and resilience. *Brain Research, 1293*, 13–23. https://doi.org/10.1016/j.brainres.2009.03.044

Monson, C. M., Schnurr, P. P., Resick, P. A., Friedman, M. J., Young-Xu, Y., & Stevens, S. P. (2006). Cognitive processing therapy for veterans with military-related posttraumatic stress disorder. *Journal of Consulting and Clinical Psychology, 74*, 898–907. https://doi.org/10.1037/0022-006X.74.5.898

Najavits, L. M. (2002). *Seeking safety: A treatment manual for PTSD and substance abuse.* The Guilford Press.

Najavits, L. M., Weiss, R. D., Shaw, S. R., & Muenz, L. R. (1998). "Seeking safety": Outcome of a new cognitive-behavioral psychotherapy for women with posttraumatic stress disorder and substance dependence. *Journal of Traumatic Stress, 11*(3), 437–456. https://doi.org/10.1023/A:1024496427434

Norman, S. B., Myers, U. S., Wilkins, K. C., Goldsmith, A. A., Hristova, V., Huang, Z., McCullough, K. C., & Robinson, S. K. (2012). Review of biological mechanisms and pharmacological treatments of comorbid PTSD and substance use disorder. *Neuropharmacology, 62*(2), 542–551. https://doi.org/10.1016/j.neuropharm.2011.04.032

Pae, C. U., Lim, H. K., Peindl, K., Ajwani, N., Serretti, A., Patkar, A. A., & Lee, C. (2008). The atypical antipsychotics olanzapine and risperidone in the treatment of posttraumatic stress disorder: A meta-analysis of randomized, double-blind, placebo-controlled clinical trials. *International Clinical Psychopharmacology, 23*(1), 1–8. https://doi.org/10.1097/YIC.0b013e32825ea324

Powers, M. B., Halpern, J. M., Ferenschak, M. P., Gillihan, S. J., & Foa, E. B. (2010). A meta-analytic review of prolonged exposure for posttraumatic stress disorder. *Clinical Psychology Review, 30*(6), 635–641. https://doi.org/10.1016/j.cpr.2010.04.007

Ravindran, L. N., & Stein, M. B. (2009). Pharmacotherapy of PTSD: Premises, principles, and priorities. *Brain Research, 1293*, 24–39. https://doi.org/10.1016/j.brainres.2009.03.037

Resick, P. A., & Schnicke, M. (1996). *Cognitive processing therapy for rape victims: A treatment manual.* Sage Publications.

Simpson, T. L., Stappenbeck, C. A., Varra, A. A., Moore, S. A., & Kaysen, D. (2012). Symptoms of posttraumatic stress predict craving among alcohol treatment seekers: Results of a daily monitoring study. *Psychology of Addictive Behaviors, 26*(4), 724–733. https://doi.org/10.1037/a0027169

Southwick, S., & Charney, D. (2012). *Resilience: The science of mastering life's greatest challenges.* Cambridge University Press.

Torchalla, I., Nosen, L., Rostam, H., & Allen, P. (2012). Integrated treatment programs for individuals with concurrent substance use disorders and trauma experiences: A systematic review and meta-analysis. *Journal of Substance Abuse Treatment, 42*(1), 65–77. https://doi.org/10.1016/j.jsat.2011.09.001

van Dam, D., Vedel, E., Ehring, T., & Emmelkamp, P. M. (2012). Psychological treatments for concurrent posttraumatic stress disorder and substance use disorder: A systematic review. *Clinical Psychology Review, 32*(3), 202–214. https://doi.org/10.1016/j.cpr.2012.01.004

Chapter 15: Schizophrenia, Other Psychotic Disorders, and Co-Occurring Substance Use Disorders

REFERENCES

Andréasson, S., Engström, A., Allebeck, P., & Rydberg, U. (1987). Cannabis and schizophrenia a longitudinal study of Swedish conscripts. *The Lancet, 330*(8574), 1483–1486. https://doi.org/10.1016/S0140-6736(87)92620-1

Batkin, S. I., Meszaros, Z. S., Strutynski, K., Dimmock, J. A., Leontieva, L., Ploutz-Snyder, R., Canfield, K., & Drayer, R. A. (2009). Medical comorbidity in patients with schizophrenia and alcohol dependence. *Schizophrenia Research, 107*(2–3), 139–146. https://doi.org/10.1016/j.schres.2008.10.016

Beebe, L. H., Smith, K., Burk, R., McIntyre, K., Dessieux, O., Tavakoli, A., & Velligan, D. (2012). Motivational intervention increases exercise in schizophrenia and co-occurring substance use disorders. *Schizophrenia Research, 135*(1–3), 204–205. https://doi.org/10.1016/j.schres.2011.12.008

Bellack, A. S., Bennett, M. E., & Gearon, J. S. (2007). *Behavioral treatment for substance abuse in people with serious and persistent mental illness: A handbook for mental health professionals.* Routledge.

Bellack, A. S., Bennett, M. E., Gearon, J. S., Brown, C. H., & Yang, Y. (2006). A randomized clinical trial of a new behavioral treatment for drug abuse in people with severe and persistent mental illness. *Archives of General Psychiatry, 63*(4), 426–432. https://doi.org/10.1001/archpsyc.63.4.426

Brunette, M. F., Asher, D., Whitley, R., Lutz, W. J., Wieder, B. L., Jones, A. M., & McHugo, G. J. (2008). Implementation of integrated dual disorders treatment: A qualitative analysis of facilitators and barriers. *Psychiatric Services, 59*(9), 989–995. https://doi.org/10.1176/ps.2008.59.9.989

Drake, R. E., Essock, S. M., Shaner, A., Carey, K. B., Minkoff, K., Kola, L., Lynde, D., Osher, F. C., Clark, R. E., & Rickards, L. (2001). Implementing dual diagnosis services for clients with severe mental illness. *Psychiatric Services, 52*(4), 469–476. https://doi.org/10.1176/appi.ps.52.4.469

Drake, R. E., McHugo, G. J., Clark, R. E., Teague, G. B., Xie, H., Miles, K., & Ackerson, T. H. (1998). Assertive community treatment for patients with co-occurring severe mental illness and substance use disorder: A clinical trial. *American Journal of Orthopsychiatry, 68*(2), 201–215. https://doi.org/10.1037/h0080330

Drake, R. E., Mueser, K. T., Brunette, M. F., & McHugo, G. J. (2004). A review of treatments for people with severe mental illnesses and co-occurring substance use disorders. *Psychiatric Rehabilitation Journal, 27*(4), 360–374. https://doi.org/10.2975/27.2004.360.374

Drake, R. E., O'Neal, E. L., & Wallach, M. A. (2008). A systematic review of treatments of psychosocial research on psychosocial interventions for people with co-occurring substance use disorders: A review of specific interventions. *Journal of Substance Abuse Treatment, 34*(1), 123–138. https://doi.org/10.1016/j.jsat.2007.01.011

Drake, R. E., & Wallach, M. A. (2000). Dual diagnosis: 15 years of progress. *Psychiatric Services, 51*(9), 1126–1129. https://doi.org/10.1176/appi.ps.51.9.1126

Fergusson, D. M., Horwood, L. J., & Ridder, E. M. (2005). Tests of causal linkages between cannabis use and psychotic symptoms. *Addiction, 100*(3), 354–366. https://doi.org/10.1111/j.1360-0443.2005.01001.x

Hasnain, M., Vieweg, W. V. R., Fredrickson, S. K., Beatty-Brooks, M., Fernandez, A., & Pandurangi, A. K. (2008). Clinical monitoring and management of the metabolic syndrome in patients receiving atypical antipsychotic medications. *Primary Care Diabetes, 3*(1), 5–15. https://doi.org/10.1016/j.pcd.2008.10.005

Hawthorne, W. B., Folsom, D. P., Sommerfeld, D. H., Lanouette, N. M., Lewis, M., Aarons, G. A., Conklin, R. M., Solorzano, E., Lindamer, L. A., & Jeste, D. V. (2012). Incarceration among adults who are in the public mental health system: Rates, risk factors, and short-term outcomes. *Psychiatric Services, 63*(1), 26–32. https://doi.org/10.1176/appi.ps.201000505

Himelhoch, S., McCarthy, J. F., Ganoczy, D., Medoff, D., Kilbourne, A., Goldberg, R., Dixon, L., & Blow, F. C. (2009). Understanding associations between serious mental illness and hepatitis C virus among veterans: A national multivariate analysis. *Psychosomatics, 50*(1), 30–37. https://doi.org/10.1176/appi.psy.50.1.30

Horsfall, J., Cleary, M., Hunt, G. E., & Walter, G. (2009). Psychosocial treatments for people with co-occurring severe mental illnesses and substance use disorders (dual diagnosis): A review of the empirical evidence. *Harvard Review of Psychiatry, 17*(1), 24–34. https://doi.org/10.1080/10673220902724599

Kay, S. R., Fiszbein, A., & Opler, L. A. (1987). The positive and negative syndrome scale (PANSS) for schizophrenia. *Schizophrenia Bulletin, 13*(2), 261–276. https://doi.org/10.1093/schbul/13.2.261

Koola, M. M., McMahon, R. P., Wehring, H. J., Liu, F., Mackowick, K. M., Warren, K. R., Feldman, S., Shim, J.-C. & Kelly, D. L. (2012). Alcohol and cannabis use and mortality in people with schizophrenia and related psychotic disorders. *Journal of Psychiatric Research, 46*(8), 987–993. https://doi.org/10.1016/j.jpsychires.2012.04.019

Lybrand, J., & Caroff, S. (2009). Management of schizophrenia with substance use disorders. *Psychiatric Clinics of North America, 32*(4), 821–833. https://doi.org/10.1016/j.psc.2009.09.002

Magura, S. (2008). Effectiveness of dual focus mutual aid for co-occurring substance use and mental health disorders: A review and synthesis of the "double trouble" in recovery evaluation. *Substance Use & Misuse, 43*(12–13), 1904–1926. https://doi.org/10.1080/10826080802297005

Matusow, H., Guarino, H., Rosenblum, A., Vogel, H., Uttaro, T., Khabir, S., Rini, M., Moore, T., & Magura, S. (2013). Consumers' experiences in dual focus mutual aid for co-occurring substance use and mental health disorders. *Substance Abuse Research and Treatment, 7*, 39–47. https://doi.org/10.4137/SART.S11006

McHugo, G. J., Drake, R. E., Xie, H., & Bond, G. R. (2012). A 10-year study of steady employment and non-vocational outcomes among people with serious mental illness and co-occurring substance use disorders. *Schizophrenia Research, 138*(2–3), 233–239. https://doi.org/10.1016/j.schres.2012.04.007

Mueser, K. T., Drake, R. E., Sigmon, S. C., & Brunette, M. F. (2005). Psychosocial interventions for adults with severe mental illnesses and co-occurring substance use disorders: A review of specific interventions. *Journal of Dual Diagnosis, 1*(2), 57–82. https://doi.org/10.1300/J374v01n02_05

Mueser, K. T., Glynn, S. M., Cather, C., Zarate, R., Fox, L., Feldman, J., Wolfe, R., & Clark, R. E. (2009). Family intervention for co-occurring substance use and severe psychiatric disorders: Participant characteristics and correlates of initial engagement and more extended exposure in a randomized controlled trial. *Addictive Behaviors, 34*(10), 867–877. https://doi.org/10.1016/j.addbeh.2009.03.025

Overall, J. E., & Gorham, D. R. (1962). The Brief Psychiatric Rating Scale (BPRS). *Psychological Reports, 10*(3), 799–812. https://doi.org/10.2466/pr0.1962.10.3.799

Ross, S., & Peselow, E. (2012). Co-occurring psychotic and addictive disorders: Neurobiology and diagnosis. *Clinical Neuropharmacology, 35*(5), 235–243. https://doi.org/10.1097/WNF.0b013e318261e193

Schmidt, L. M., Hesse, M., & Lykke, J. (2011). The impact of substance use disorders on the course of schizophrenia—a 15-year follow-up study: Dual diagnosis over 15 years. *Schizophrenia Research, 130*(1–3), 228–233. https://doi.org/10.1016/j.schres.2011.04.011

Smelson, D. A., Dixon, L., Craig, T., Remolina, S., Batki, S. L., Niv, N., & Owen, R. (2008). Pharmacological treatment of schizophrenia and co-occurring substance use disorders. *CNS Drugs, 22*(11), 903–916. https://doi.org/10.2165/00023210-200822110-00002

Tenhula, W. N., Bennett, M. E., & Strong Kinnaman, J. E. (2009). Behavioral treatment of substance abuse in schizophrenia. *Journal of Clinical Psychology, 65*(8), 831–841. https://doi.org/10.1002/jclp.20613

Tiet, Q. Q., & Mausbach, B. (2007). Treatments for patients with dual diagnosis: A review. *Alcoholism Clinical and Experimental Research, 31*(4), 513–536. https://doi.org/10.1111/j.1530-0277.2007.00336.x

Tsai, J., Bond, G. R., Salyers, M. P., Godfrey, J. L., & Davis, K. E. (2010). Housing preferences and choices among adults with mental illness and substance use disorders: A qualitative study. *Community Mental Health, 46*(4), 381–388. https://doi.org/10.1007/s10597-009-9268-6

Vincent, P. C., Bradizza, C. M., Carey, K. B., Maisto, S. A., Stasiewicz, P. R., Connors, G. J., & Mercer, N. D. (2011). Validation of the revised Problems Assessment for Substance Using Psychiatric Patients. *Addictive Behaviors, 36*(5), 494–501. https://doi.org/10.1016/j.addbeh.2011.01.024

Vogel, H. S., Knight, E., Laudet, A. B., & Magura, S. (1998). Double trouble in recovery: Self-help for people with dual diagnoses. *Psychiatric Rehabilitation Journal, 21*(4), 356–364. https://doi.org/10.1037/h0095288

Ziedonis, D. M., Smelson, D., Rosenthal, R. N., Batki, S. L., Green, A. I., Henry, R. J., Montoya, I., Parks, J., & Weiss, R. D. (2005). Improving the care of individuals with schizophrenia and substance use disorders: Consensus recommendations. *Journal of Psychiatric Practice, 11*(5), 315–339. https://doi.org/10.1097/00131746-200509000-00005

Chapter 16: Personality Disorders and Co-Occurring Substance Use Disorders

RESOURCES

Behavioral Tech: This organization trains mental health care providers and treatment teams in the use of compassionate and scientifically valid treatments for individuals with complex and severe mental disorders (www.behavioraltech.org).

DBT Self-Help: This consumer-owned-and-operated site provides information on DBT skills for current participants and graduates of DBT (www.dbtselfhelp.com).

National Education Alliance for Borderline Personality Disorder (NEABPD): This organization aims to provide education, increase public awareness, decrease stigma, and increase quality of life of those affected by borderline personality disorder (www.borderlinepersonalitydisorder.com).

Treatment and Research Advancements for Borderline Personality Disorder (TARA4BPD): This not-for-profit agency provides advocacy and support for families and people with borderline personality disorder (www.tara4bpd.org).

REFERENCES

American Psychiatric Association. (2001). *Practice guideline for the treatment of patients with borderline personality disorder.* American Psychiatric Association Publishing.

Dimeff, L., & Koerner, K. E. (2007). *Dialectical behavior therapy in clinical practice: Applications across disorders and settings.* The Guilford Press.

Gunderson, J. (2011). Borderline personality disorder. *New England Journal of Medicine, 364*(21), 2037–2042. https://doi.org/10.1056/NEJMcp1007358

Ingenhoven, T., Lafay, P., Rinne, T., Passchier, J., & Duivenvoorden, H. (2010). Effectiveness of pharmacotherapy for severe personality disorders: Meta-analyses of randomized controlled trials. *Journal of Clinical Psychiatry, 71*(1), 14–25. https://doi.org/10.4088/jcp.08r04526gre

Koerner, K. (2011). *Doing dialectical behavior therapy: A practical guide.* The Guilford Press.

Lenzenweger, M. F., Lane, M. C., Loranger, A. W., & Kessler, R. C. (2007). DSM-IV personality disorders in the National Comorbidity Survey Replication. *Biological Psychiatry, 62*(6), 553–564. https://doi.org/10.1016/j.biopsych.2006.09.019

Lieb, K., Völlm, B., Rücker, G., Timmer, A., & Stoffers, J. M. (2010). Pharmacotherapy for borderline personality disorder: Cochrane systematic review of randomised trials. *British Journal of Psychiatry, 196*(1), 4–12. https://doi.org/10.1192/bjp.bp.108.062984

Linehan, M. (1993). *Cognitive-behavioral treatment of borderline personality disorder.* The Guilford Press.

Linehan, M. (1993). *Skills training manual for treating borderline personality disorder.* The Guilford Press.

Linehan, M., Dimeff, L. A., Reynolds, S. K., Comtois, K. A., Welch, S. S., Heagerty, P., & Kivlahan, D. R. (2002). Dialectical behavior therapy versus comprehensive validation therapy plus 12-step for the treatment of opioid dependent women meeting criteria for borderline personality disorder. *Drug and Alcohol Dependence, 67*(1), 13–26. https://doi.org/10.1016/S0376-8716(02)00011-X

Linehan, M., Schmidt, H., Dimeff, L. A., Craft, J. C., Kanter, J., & Comtois, K. A. (1999). Dialectical behavior therapy for patients with borderline personality disorder and drug-dependence. *American Journal on Addictions, 8*(4), 279–292. https://doi.org/10.1080/105504999305686.

McKay, M., Wood, J. C., & Brantley, J. (2007). *Dialectical behavior therapy skills workbook: Practical DBT exercises for learning mindfulness, interpersonal effectiveness, emotion regulation, and distress tolerance.* New Harbinger Publications.

Oldham, J. M. (2005). Guideline watch: Practice guideline for the treatment of borderline personality disorder. *Focus: The Journal of Lifelong Learning in Psychiatry, 3*(3), 396–400. https://doi.org/10.1176/foc.3.3.396

Trull, T. J., Stepp, S. D., & Durrett, C. A. (2003). Research on borderline personality disorder: An update. *Current Opinion in Psychiatry, 16*(1), 77–82. https://doi.org/10.1097/00001504-200301000-00015

Chapter 17: Alcohol

RESOURCES

Adult Children of Alcoholics: This is a mutual self-help group for people who grew up in alcoholic and otherwise dysfunctional households that utilizes a 12-step approach (www.adultchildren.org).

Al-Anon and Alateen: This is a mutual self-help group for friends and families of problem drinkers that utilizes a 12-step approach (www.al-anon.alateen.org).

Alcoholics Anonymous: This international mutual-aid program is intended to help alcoholics achieve sobriety using a 12-step approach (https://aa.org).

National Institute on Alcohol Abuse and Alcoholism: This governmental agency supports and conducts research on the impact of alcohol use on human health and well-being (www.niaaa.nih.gov).

SMART Recovery: This non-12-step mutual self-help organization emphasizes empowerment as a means of gaining independence from addictive behaviors (www.smartrecovery.org).

U.S. Department of Agriculture and U.S. Department of Health and Human Services *Dietary Guidelines for Americans*: Chapter 3 of this document provides information regarding the recommended use of alcohol, as well as its contraindications (https://health.gov/sites/default/files/2020-01/DietaryGuidelines2010.pdf).

U.S Department of Transportation, National Highway Traffic Safety Administration (NHTSA): This federal agency provides information on alcohol-related driving fatalities (https://www.nhtsa.gov).

REFERENCES

Busto, U. E., Sykora, K., & Sellers, E. M. (1989). A clinical scale to assess benzodiazepine withdrawal. *Journal of Clinical Psychopharmacology, 9*(6), 412–416. https://doi.org/10.1097/00004714-198912000-00005

Foy, A., March, S., & Drinkwater, V. (1988). Use of an objective clinical scale in the assessment and management of alcohol withdrawal in a large general hospital. *Alcoholism: Clinical and Experimental Research, 12*(3), 360–364. https://doi.org/10.1111/j.1530-0277.1988.tb00208.x

Mayo-Smith, M. F., Beecher, L. H., Fischer, T. L., Gorelick, D. A., Guillaume, J. L., Hill, A., Jara, G., Kasser, C., & Melbourne, J. (2004). Management of alcohol withdrawal delirium: An evidence-based practice guideline. *Archives of Internal Medicine, 164*(13), 1405–1412. https://doi.org/10.1001/archinte.164.13.1405

Sachdeva A., Chandra, M., Choudhary, M., Dayal, P., & Anand, K. S. (2016). Alcohol-related dementia and neurocognitive impairment: A review study. *International Journal of High Risk Behaviors and Addiction, 5*(3), Article e27976. https://doi.org/10.5812/ijhrba.27976

Skinner, H. A., & Sheu, W. J. (1982). Reliability of alcohol use indices. The Lifetime Drinking History and the MAST. *Journal of Studies on Alcohol and Drugs, 43*(11), 1157–1170. https://doi.org/10.15288/jsa.1982.43.1157

Sullivan, J. T., Sykora, K., Schneiderman, J., Naranjo, C. A., & Sellers, E. M. (1989). Assessment of alcohol withdrawal: The revised Clinical Institute Withdrawal Assessment for Alcohol Scale (CIWA-Ar). *British Journal of Addiction, 84*(11), 1353–1357. https://doi.org/10.1111/j.1360-0443.1989.tb00737.x

U.S. Department of Transportation, National Highway Traffic Safety Administration. (October 2019). *2018 fatal motor vehicle crashes: Overview*. Report No. DOT HS 812 826. https://crashstats.nhtsa.dot.gov/Api/Public/ViewPublication/812826

Chapter 18: Tobacco

RESOURCES

Centers for Disease Control and Prevention—Vital Signs Telebriefing on Cigarette Smoking among Adults with Mental Illness: This site provides a press briefing transcript on the use of cigarettes among individuals with mental illness (www.cdc.gov/media/releases/2013/t0205_smoking_mentally_ill.html).

Smokefree.gov: This well-organized website provides a wealth of information along with free resources.

1-800-QUIT-NOW: This federal/state initiative provides free counseling and, in some states, free nicotine patches to help people stop smoking.

REFERENCES

Lasser, K., Boyd, J. W., Woolhandler, S., Himmelstein, D. U., McCormick, D., & Bor, D. H. (2000). Smoking and mental illness: A population-based prevalence study. *JAMA, 284*(20), 2606–2610. https://doi.org/10.1001/jama.284.20.2606

Substance Abuse and Mental Health Services Administration. (2013, February 6). *Smoking and mental illness: The NSDUH report.* https://www.samhsa.gov/data/sites/default/files/NSDUH093/NSDUH093/sr093-smoking-mental-illness.htm

Williams, J. M., Willett, J. G., & Miller, G. (2013). Viewpoint: Partnership between tobacco control programs and offices of mental health needed to reduce smoking rates in the United States. *JAMA Psychiatry, 70*(12), 1261–1262. https://doi.org/10.1001/jamapsychiatry.2013.2182

Chapter 19: Opioids

REFERENCES

American College of Obstetricians and Gynecologists (ACOG) Committee on Health Care for Underserved Women. (2012). ACOG Committee Opinion No. 524: Opioid abuse, dependence, and addiction in pregnancy. *Obstetrics and Gynecology, 119*(5), 1070–1076. https://doi.org/10.1097/AOG.0b013e318256496e

Atkins, C. (2018). *Opioid Use Disorders: A Holistic Guide to Assessment, Treatment & Recovery.* PESI Publishing and Media.

Back, S. E., Lawson, K. M., Singleton, L. M., & Brady, K. T. (2011). Characteristics and correlates of men and women with prescription opioid dependence. *Addictive Behaviors, 36*(8), 829–834. https://doi.org/10.1016/j.addbeh.2011.03.013

Back, S. E., Payne, R. L., Simpson, A. N., & Brady, K. T. (2010). Gender and prescription opioids: Findings from the National Survey on Drug Use and Health. *Addictive Behaviors, 35*(11), 1001–1007. https://doi.org/10.1016/j.addbeh.2010.06.018

Brady, K. T., Back, S. E., & Greenfield, S. F. (Eds.). (2009). *Women and addiction: A comprehensive handbook.* The Guilford Press.

Center for Substance Abuse Treatment. (2004). *Clinical guidelines for the use of buprenorphine in the treatment of opioid addiction.* Treatment Improvement Protocol (TIP) Series 40. DHHS Publication No. (SMA) 04-3939. Substance Abuse and Mental Health Services Administration. https://www.ncbi.nlm.nih.gov/books/NBK64245/

De Maeyer, J., Vanderplasschen, W., & Broekaert, E. (2010). Quality of life among opiate-dependent individuals: A review of the literature. *International Journal of Drug Policy, 21*(5), 364–380. https://doi.org/10.1016/j.drugpo.2010.01.010

Fareed, A., Casarella, J., Amar, R., Vayalapalli, S., & Drexler, K. (2010). Methadone maintenance dosing guideline for opioid dependence: A literature review. *Journal of Addictive Diseases, 29*(1), 1–14. https://doi.org/10.1080/10550880903436010

Glover, S., & Girion, L. (2013, August 11). OxyContin maker closely guards its list of suspect doctors. *Los Angeles Times.* https://www.latimes.com/local/la-me-rx-purdue-20130811-story.html

Hall, A. J., Logan, J. E., Toblin, R. L., Kaplan, J. A., Kraner, J. C., Bixler, D., Crosby, A. E., & Paulozzi, L. J. (2008). Patterns of abuse among unintentional pharmaceutical overdose fatalities. *JAMA, 300*(22), 2613–2620. https://doi.org/10.1001/jama.2008.802

Jones, H. E., Kaltenbach, K., Heil, S. H., Stine, S. M., Coyle, M. G., Arria, A. M., O'Grady, K. E., Selby, P., Martin, P. R., & Fischer, G. (2010). Neonatal abstinence syndrome after methadone or buprenorphine exposure. *New England Journal of Medicine, 363*(24), 2320–2331. https://doi.org/10.1056/NEJMoa1005359

Jones, H. E., Tuten, M., & O'Grady, K. E. (2011). Treating the partners of opioid-dependent pregnant patients: Feasibility and efficacy. *American Journal of Drug and Alcohol Abuse, 37*(3), 170–178. https://doi.org/10.3109/00952990.2011.563336

Kakko, J., Heilig, M., & Sarman, I. (2008). Buprenorphine and methadone treatment of opiate dependence during pregnancy: Comparison of fetal growth and neonatal outcomes in two consecutive case series. *Drug and Alcohol Dependence*, 96(1–2), 69–78. https://doi.org/10.1016/j.drugalcdep.2008.01.025

Krupitsky, E., Nunes, E. V., Ling, W., Illeperuma, A., Gastfriend, D. R., & Silverman, B. L. (2011). Injectable extended-release naltrexone for opioid dependence: A double-blind, placebo-controlled, multicentre randomised trial. *The Lancet, 377*(9776), 1506–1513. https://doi.org/10.1016/S0140-6736(11)60358-9

Lacroix, I., Berrebi, A., Garipuy, D., Schmitt, L., Hammou, Y., Chaumerliac, C., Lapeyre-Mestre, M., Montastruc, J.-L., & Damase-Michel, C. (2011). Buprenorphine versus methadone in pregnant opioid-dependent women: A prospective multicenter study. *European Journal of Clinical Pharmacology, 67*(10), 1053–1059. https://doi.org/10.1007/s00228-011-1049-9

McLellan, A. T., & Turner, B. (2008). Prescription opioids, overdose deaths, and physician responsibility. *JAMA, 300*(22), 2672–2673. https://doi.org/10.1001/jama.2008.793

Minozzi, S., Amato, L., Bellisario, C., Ferri, M., & Davoli, M. (2013). Maintenance agonist treatments for opiate-dependent pregnant women. *Cochrane Database of Systematic Reviews.* https://doi.org/10.1002/14651858.CD006318.pub3

Substance Abuse and Mental Health Services Administration. (2012). *An introduction to extended-release injectable naltrexone for the treatment of people with opioid dependence.* DHHS Publication No. (SMA) 12-4682. https://store.samhsa.gov/sites/default/files/d7/priv/sma12-4682.pdf

Trafton, J. A., Humphreys, K., Harris, A. H., & Oliva, E. (2007). Consistent adherence to guidelines to improve opioid dependent patients' first year outcomes. *Journal of Behavioral Health Services and Research, 34*(3), 260–271. https://doi.org/10.1007/s11414-007-9074-2

Unger, A., Jung, E., Winklbaur, B., & Fischer, G. (2010). Gender issues in the pharmacotherapy of opioid-addicted women: Buprenorphine. *Journal of Addictive Diseases, 29*(2), 217–230. https://doi.org/10.1080/10550881003684814

Wesson, D. R., & Ling, W. (2003). The Clinical Opiate Withdrawal Scale (COWS). *Journal of Psychoactive Drugs, 35*(2), 253–259. https://doi.org/10.1080/02791072.2003.10400007

Chapter 20: Selected Topics for Other Substances

REFERENCES

Agrawal, A., Nurnberger Jr, J. I., Lynskey, M. T., & Study, T. B. (2011). Cannabis involvement in individuals with bipolar disorder. *Psychiatry Research, 185*(3), 459–61. https://doi.org/10.1016/j.psychres.2010.07.007

Benotsch, E. G., Koester, S., Martin, A. M., Cejka, A., Luckman, D., & Jeffers, A. J. (2014). Intentional misuse of over-the-counter medications, mental health, and polysubstance use in young adults. *Journal of Community Health, 39*(4), 688–695. https://doi.org/10.1007/s10900-013-9811-9

The Centers for Disease Control and Prevention. (2011, May 18). Emergency department visits after use of a drug sold as "bath salts"—Michigan, November 13, 2010–March 31, 2011. *Morbidity and Mortality Weekly Report, 60*(19), 624–627. https://www.cdc.gov/mmwr/preview/mmwrhtml/mm6019a6.htm

The Centers for Disease Control and Prevention. (2018, August 31). *2018 annual surveillance report of drug-related risks and outcomes—United States.* https://www.cdc.gov/drugoverdose/pdf/pubs/2018-cdc-drug-surveillance-report.pdf

Eden Evins, A., Green, A. I., Kane, J. M., & Murray, R. M. (2012). The effect of marijuana use on the risk for schizophrenia. *Journal of Clinical Psychiatry, 73*(11), 1463–1468. https://doi.org/10.4088/JCP.12012co1c

Fergusson, D. M., Horwood, L. J., & Ridder, E. M. (2005). Tests of causal linkages between cannabis use and psychotic symptoms. *Addiction, 100*(3), 354–366. https://doi.org/10.1111/j.1360-0443.2005.01001.x

Jerry, J., Collins, G., & Streem, D. (2012). Synthetic legal intoxicating drugs: The emerging "incense" and "bath salt" phenomenon. *Cleveland Clinic Journal of Medicine, 79*(4), 258–264. https://doi.org/10.3949/ccjm.79a.11147

Kariisa M., Scholl, L., Wilson, N., Seth, P., & Hoots, B. (2019). Drug overdose deaths involving cocaine and psychostimulants with abuse potential—United States, 2003–2017. *Morbidity and Mortality Weekly Report, 68*(17), 388–395. https://www.cdc.gov/mmwr/volumes/68/wr/mm6817a3.htm

Large, M., Sharma, S., Compton, M. T., Slade, T., & Nielssen, O. (2011). Cannabis use and earlier onset of psychosis. *Archives of General Psychiatry, 68*(6), 555–561. https://doi.org/10.1001/archgenpsychiatry.2011.5

Loeffler, G., Penn, A., & Ledden, B. (2012). "Bath salt"-induced agitated paranoia: A case series. *Journal of Studies on Alcohol and Drugs, 73*(4), 706. https://doi.org/10.15288/jsad.2012.73.706

Murphy, C. M., Dulaney, A. R., Beuhler, M. C., & Kacinko, S. (2013). "Bath salts" and "plant food" products: The experience of one regional U.S. poison center. *Journal of Medical Toxicology, 9*(1), 42–48. https://doi.org/10.1007/s13181-012-0243-1

Pierre, J. M. (2011). Cannabis, synthetic cannabinoids, and psychosis risk: What the evidence says. *Current Psychiatry, 10*(9), 49–58.

Prosser, J. M., & Nelson, L. S. (2012). The toxicology of bath salts: A review of synthetic cathinones. *Journal of Medical Toxicology, 8*(1), 33–42. https://doi.org/10.1007/s13181-011-0193-z

Ross, E. A., Reisfield, G. M., Watson, M. C., Chronister, C. W., & Goldberger, B. A. (2012). Psychoactive "bath salts" intoxication with methylenedioxypyrovalerone. *American Journal of Medicine, 125*(9), 854–858. https://doi.org/10.1016/j.amjmed.2012.02.019

Ross, E. A., Watson, M., & Goldberger, B. (2011). "Bath salts" intoxication. *New England Journal of Medicine, 365*(10), 967–968. https://doi.org/10.1056/NEJMc1107097

Salloum, I. M., Cornelius, J. R., Douaihy, A., Kirisci, L., Daley, D. C., & Kelly, T. M. (2005). Patient characteristics and treatment implications of marijuana abuse among bipolar alcoholics: Results from a double blind, placebo-controlled study. *Addictive Behaviors, 30*(9), 1702–1708. https://doi.org/10.1016/j.addbeh.2005.07.014

van Rossum, I., Boomsma, M., Tenback, D., Reed, C., & van Os, J. (2009). Does cannabis use affect treatment outcome in bipolar disorder? A longitudinal analysis. *Journal of Nervous and Mental Disease, 197*(1), 35–40. https://doi.org/10.1097/NMD.0b013e31819292a6

Williams, J. F., & Kokotailo, P. K. (2006). Abuse of proprietary (over-the-counter) drugs. *Adolescent Medicine Clinics, 17*(3), 733–750. https://doi.org/10.1016/j.admecli.2006.06.006

Wilson, B., Tavakoli, H., DeCecchis, D., & Mahadev, V. (2013). Synthetic cannabinoids, synthetic cathinones, and other emerging drugs of abuse. *Psychiatric Annals, 43*(12), 558–564. https://doi.org/10.3928/00485713-20131206-08

Index